Spa Style Europe

THERAPIES • CUISINES • SPAS

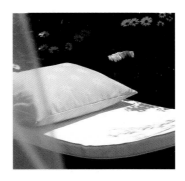

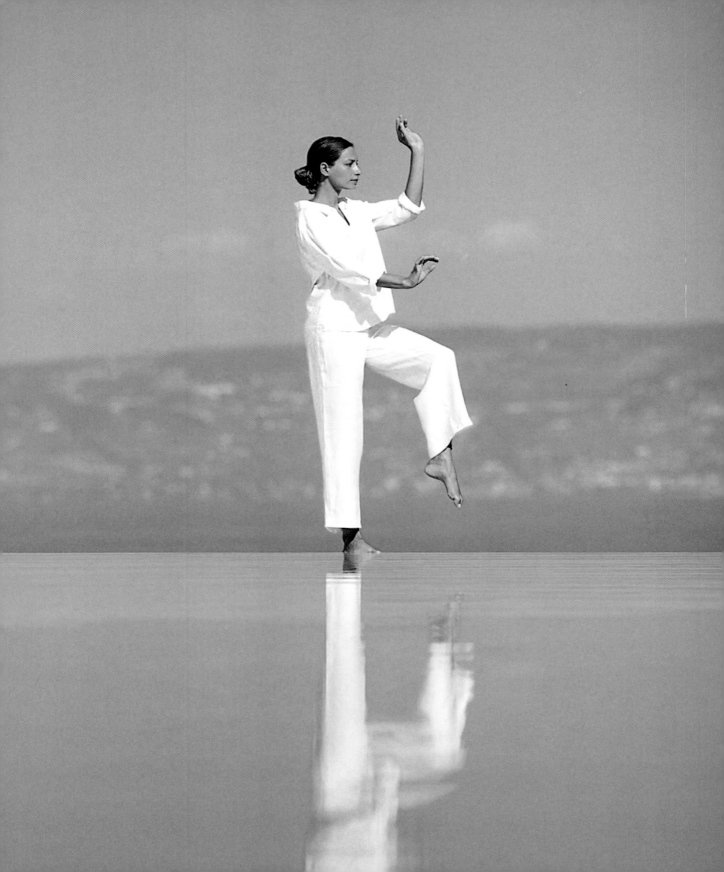

Spa Style Europe

THERAPIES · CUISINES · SPAS

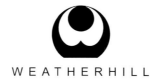

WEATHERHILL

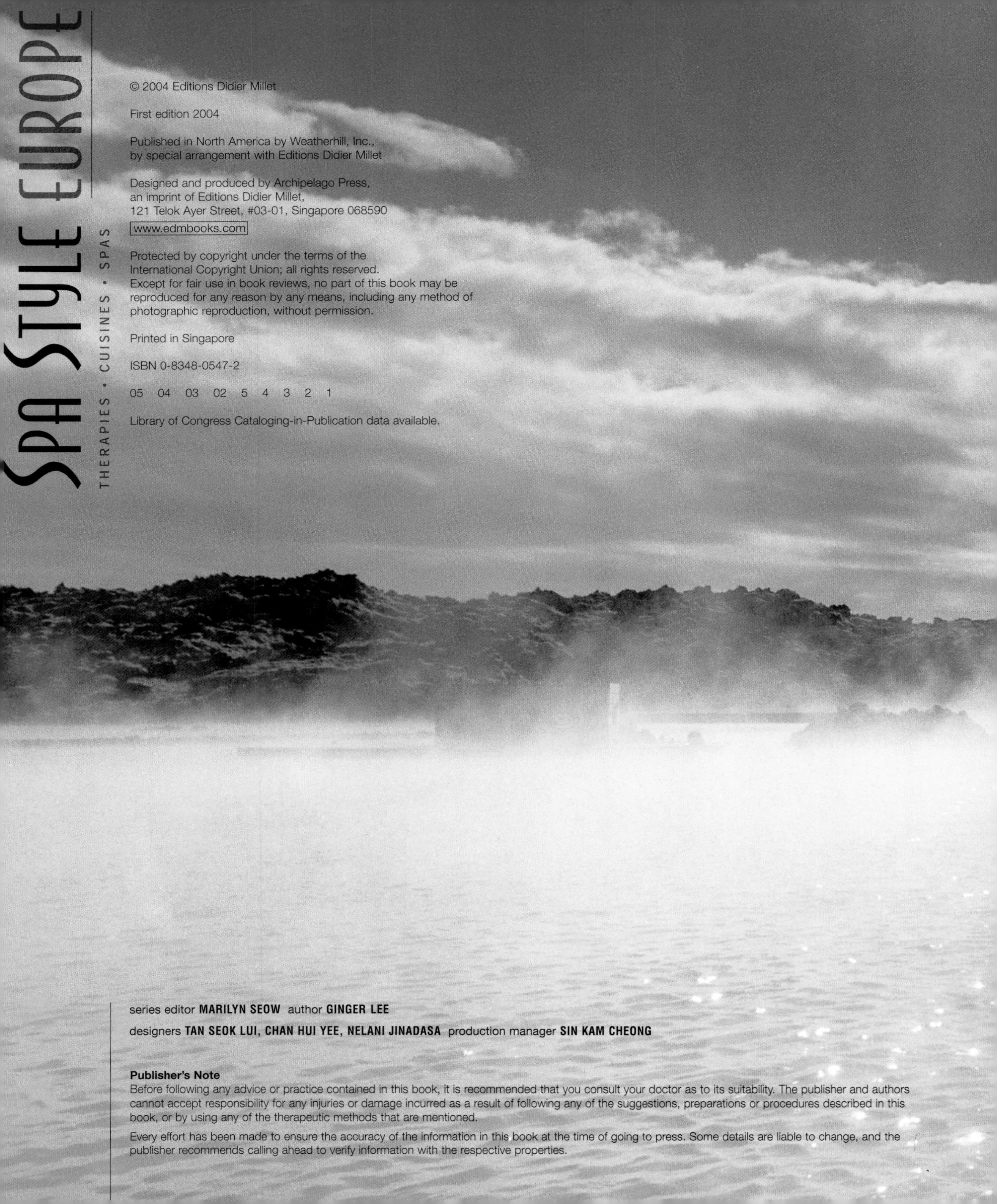

SPA STYLE EUROPE

THERAPIES · CUISINES · SPAS

© 2004 Editions Didier Millet

First edition 2004

Published in North America by Weatherhill, Inc.,
by special arrangement with Editions Didier Millet

Designed and produced by Archipelago Press,
an imprint of Editions Didier Millet,
121 Telok Ayer Street, #03-01, Singapore 068590
www.edmbooks.com

Printed in Singapore

ISBN 0-8348-0547-2

05   04   03   02   5   4   3   2   1

Library of Congress Cataloging-in-Publication data available.

series editor **MARILYN SEOW** author **GINGER LEE**

designers **TAN SEOK LUI, CHAN HUI YEE, NELANI JINADASA** production manager **SIN KAM CHEONG**

Publisher's Note
Before following any advice or practice contained in this book, it is recommended that you consult your doctor as to its suitability. The publisher and authors cannot accept responsibility for any injuries or damage incurred as a result of following any of the suggestions, preparations or procedures described in this book, or by using any of the therapeutic methods that are mentioned.

Every effort has been made to ensure the accuracy of the information in this book at the time of going to press. Some details are liable to change, and the publisher recommends calling ahead to verify information with the respective properties.

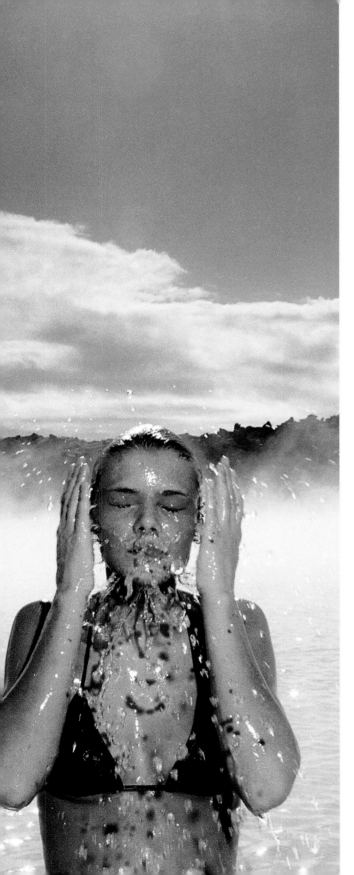

Contents

6 Introduction

8 Spa Therapies

Spa Styles • The Elements • Water • Fire • Air • Earth • Harmony

104 Spa Cuisine

La Cuisine Synergique® • Cuisine Minceur

124 Spa Digest

Austria • Finland • France • Germany • Greece
Hungary • Iceland • Italy • Monaco • Portugal • Russia
Spain • Switzerland • Turkey • United Kingdom

226 Spa Speak

229 Select Bibliography and Internet Resources

230 Spa Index

231 General Index

232 Credits and Acknowledgments and Credits

INTRODUCTION

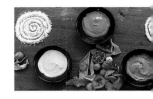

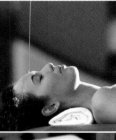

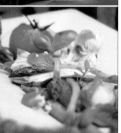

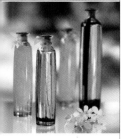

Spa Style Europe is your essential and most authoritative guide to a spa experience in Europe. It has been designed for both the spa aficionado and for those planning their first visit. This beautiful coffee-table book explains and illustrates all the major spa traditions and treatments of Europe. These range from the classic cures to cutting-edge energy-balancing therapies. Descriptions of popular treatments and spa experiences at top European spas will help you identify those retreats that are closest to your requirements so you can successfully plan your next spa visit, and realise your goals for personal wellbeing.

Spa Therapies demystifies spa treatments to help you choose those that best suit your personal objectives. Many of the featured treatments have their origins in Europe. Other treatments which have their roots elsewhere, but are now popular in European spas, are also included. You will learn about the historical and cultural backgrounds of various treatments and therapies to heighten your appreciation of the spa experience. In addition, you will find clever health- and beauty-enhancing tips and recipes for treatments that you can try at home.

Spa Cuisine gives you an appetising insight into how food is prepared in spas. It is designed to inspire you to balance your body, detoxify your system and optimise your energy in the most nutritious yet irresistibly delicious manner. Chefs Michel Lentz from Hotel Royal – Royal Parc Evian and Michel Guérard from Les Prés d'Eugénie have provided fully illustrated three-day and one-day cuisine programmes respectively that you can prepare easily in your kitchen. Recipe ingredients are measured in Metric, Imperial and American units.

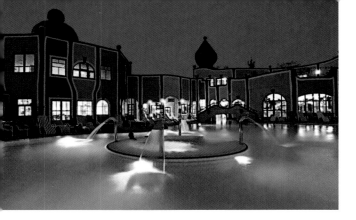

Spa Digest is a directory of 49 quality spa retreats in Europe, containing comprehensive information on treatments, facilities and services provided at each spa. Detailed descriptions of each property will help you locate the spa that best meets your own goals, interests and lifestyle. The spas are arranged in alphabetical order by country. Each spa profile includes a fact-packed 'Spa Statistics' panel so you can evaluate at a glance each spa's most important attributes and features—including its spa type, size, facilities, signature treatments, other treatments and therapies, spa cuisine, activities and programmes, services, languages spoken by the therapists and admission criteria. Full contact details are also provided.

Spa Speak explains over 200 frequently used terms related to spas and treatments.

Internet Resources lists web addresses by chapter and modality. Use these to access rich sources of information, including national organisations, and find out more about various therapies.

Spa Index helps you locate every spa featured in Spa Digest quickly and easily. Listings are organised by the spas' names in alphabetical order.

General Index gives you quick and easy reference to information about different treatments, therapeutic ingredients, interesting activities and innovative healing methods.

We hope you will enjoy this book, and your pursuit of wellness.

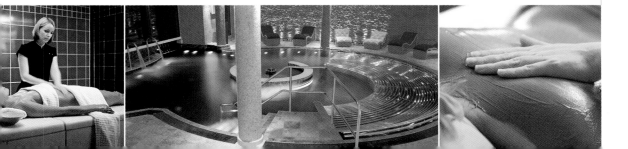

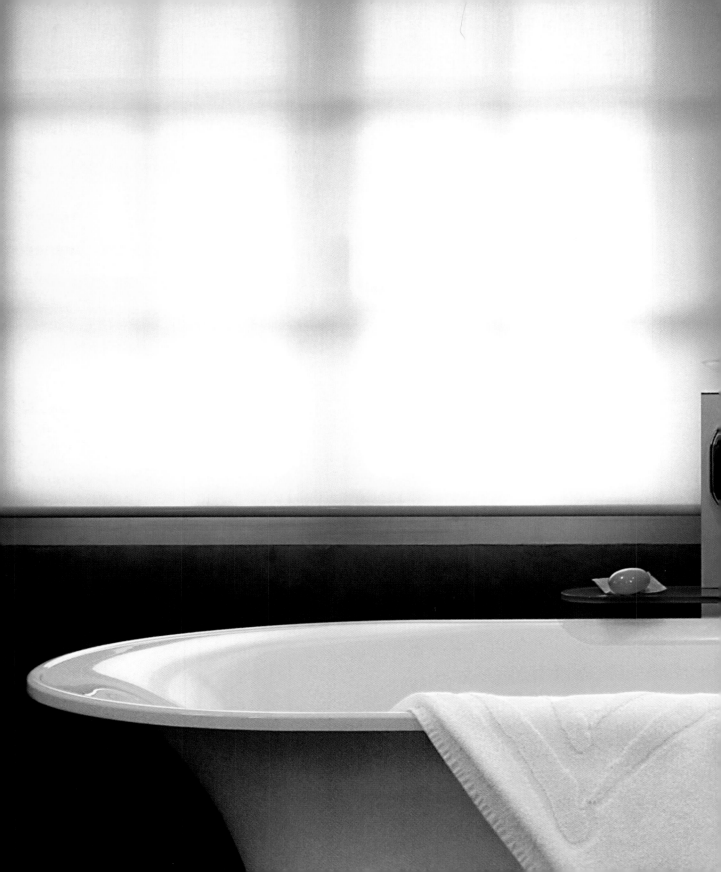

Spa Styles 10   **The Elements** 14

Water 16   **Fire** 38   **Air** 52   **Earth** 66   **Harmony** 82

SPA THERAPIES

SPA STYLES

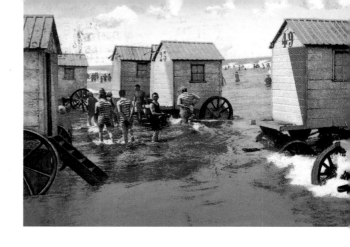

THE WORD 'SPA'

Water's ability to heal is the central theme that runs through explanations of how the word 'spa' originated—reflecting water's importance not only in ancient centres of healing but also in early European spa culture. It has been variously suggested that the word 'spa' was an acronym for a number of Latin phrases such as '*sanitas per aqua*', '*solus per aqua*' or '*sanus per aqua*', all referring to 'health through water'. Another explanation traces it to graffiti found in Roman baths, with a similar meaning: '*salut per aqua*'.

'Spa' may also be traced to an old Walloon word '*espa*' for 'fountain', or to the Latin verb '*spagere*', meaning 'to sprinkle or moisten'. Other authorities point to the town of Spa in Belgium, one of the first places to be recognised for its healing mineral springs. The term 'spa' was subsequently used to describe natural springs and health resorts offering water therapy. 'Taking the waters', or drinking or bathing in sources of water for therapeutic or medical purposes, was a fashionable social pastime in the 18th and 19th centuries.

In mainstream English today, the word 'spa' has taken on varied meanings for different people. It is unfortunate that the term 'spa' has also been diluted to refer to everything from a bath with water jets to an establishment that only offers grooming services.

In many parts of Europe, the term 'spa' still retains its strong historical associations, and many restrict the definition to establishments that focus on hydrotherapy: that is, the therapeutic use of water. In the English-speaking parts of Europe and other parts of the world, however, the term is understood to encompass a wider approach to health and wellness, rest and relaxation that aims to treat the body, mind and spirit. It is in the wider, holistic context that the word 'spa' is used in this book, to reflect the modern spa experience that aims to treat the whole person rather than an amalgamation of parts.

The modern spa is typically perceived as an establishment that integrates a range of professionally administered health, wellness and beauty treatments and services, with various fitness components, an emphasis on awareness of the self, and a focus on nutrition. This is an approach promoted by the International Spa Association (ISPA), the voice of the spa industry with members in over 53 countries.

ISPA also acknowledges the use of water as a pivotal element in the spa experience together with other facets such as natural healing methods, movement and fitness, diet and nutrition, aesthetic therapies and maintaining the harmony between the body, mind and spirit.

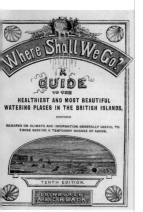

ABOVE: As with spa-goers in olden days, perhaps the hardest thing in the spa experience is deciding which beautiful spa to visit.

OPPOSITE, BOTTOM: This 1569 watercolour on paper depicts the famous baths at Vichy, France.

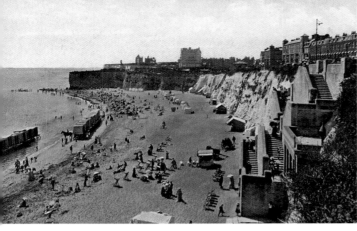

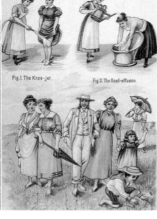

Fig. 1. The Knee-jet.   Fig. 2. The Head-affusion.

THE EUROPEAN SPA EXPERIENCE

Historically, the European spa experience focused on 'taking the waters', and 'taking the cure', which involved spending a few weeks in establishments which had therapeutic sources of water to treat certain diseases or prevent illness.

Medical centres in Europe have conventionally offered the water cure. These include balneotherapeutic centres which use mineral water and muds; thermal spas that use thermal water; German Kneipp centres that administer water and other natural therapies based on pioneering hydrotherapist Sebastian Kneipp's theories; thalassotherapy centres that focus on the use of substances derived from the sea; and climate therapy centres that take advantage of the purer air at higher altitudes for healing or relaxation.

Now, however, the European spa experience has broadened, adapting to changing times and increasing global influences. Even many of those centres built originally around healing sources of water have recently developed into resorts which offer other facilities to cater to a broader range of interests.

While many people perceive the European spa experience as clinical—a notion fuelled by 'fat farms' and 'health farms' of the 1940s and 1950s which prescribed strict exercises and meagre diets—these days the emphasis is usually on rest, relaxation, rejuvenation, revitalisation, reflection and rejoicing.

The modern spa experience is usually pampering and fun, often in beautiful surroundings, with healthy yet delicious meals. Treatments offered in European spas also reflect an increasingly global flavour. You may find complementary therapies such as acupuncture from China, an Ayurvedic head massage with oil from India, and aquatic bodywork which combines the therapeutic use of water with Eastern healing influences.

The influence of Europe's rich healing heritage, however, may still be seen in treatments for the spa-goer that have been recreated with the assistance of doctors and historians to enhance their safety, efficacy and pleasure. And the apex of the European spa revival may be seen in some spa towns in the United Kingdom, or in Greece and Spain—once left to languish, these have now redeveloped into modern healing sites, while still recreating the spirit of the past.

OPPOSITE TOP: This picture of the seaside at Ostend, Belgium, depicts a typical image at the beach in the early 1900s—the stripy bathing suits that were the fashion of the day, and the bathing machines dragged into the sea.

TOP LEFT: This image from c. 1905 shows the sweep of the beach at Broadstairs in Kent, UK. Notice the bathing machines in the water, and others waiting on the beach.

TOP RIGHT: This illustration from F E Bilz's The Natural Methods of Healing depicts Sebastian Kneipp's cures which included affusions applied to various parts of the body, and walking barefoot in the dewy grass.

Early European Spas

The development of European spas was inextricably linked with water, and also with social interaction, as shown by significant milestones along this historical time line.

2000 B.C.: Ancient Egyptians use baths for therapeutic purposes.

500 B.C.: Intellectuals gather at public baths over hot springs and mineral springs in Greece to 'exchange philosophical views'. In addition to hot water tubs, the Greeks also enjoy hot-air baths known as *laconica*.

27 B.C.–A.D. 14: There are over 170 baths in Rome during the reign of Caesar Augustus. These are at first used mainly by soldiers recuperating from war injuries, but by A.D. 43, they have become popular with the public.

C. 4 B.C.: A mineral spring, baths, sporting facilities, a hospital, and a theatre are features of the Sanctuary of Asclepius at Epidaurus, Greece, where patients rest and are given dietary recommendations and herbal cures.

A.D. 25: The first supersized bathhouse, the thermae, is built in Rome by Emperor Agrippa. As the Roman empire spreads throughout Europe, so does the Roman affinity for bathing.

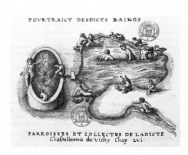

POVRTRAICT DESDICTS BAINGS

PARROISSES ET COLLECTES DE LADICTE
Chastellenie de Vichy Chap LVI.

PILLARS OF A MODERN SPA

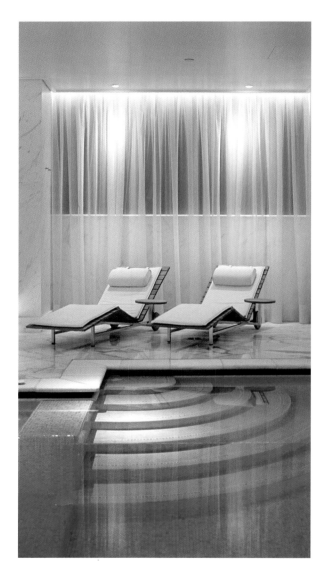

ABOVE: Beautiful and peaceful surroundings condusive to balancing the body, mind and spirit are the hallmark of the Starwood Spa Collection.

OPPOSITE, BOTTOM: While the spa experience focuses on healing traditions, it also embraces technology as seen in the Oyster Experience at GB Spa at Hotel Grande Bretagne in Greece and the Serenity Spa at Sheraton Voyager Antalya Hotel, Resort & Spa in Turkey, which combines a multi-jet massage with colour and sound therapy.

STARWOOD'S SEVEN PILLARS OF WELL-BEING

Water is still an important component of today's spa experience, though the modern spa establishment is likely to take a well-integrated and holistic approach to your health, providing comprehensive treatments, facilities and cuisine to balance your body, mind and spirit. For example, spas that belong to the Starwood Spa Collection—which has ten spas in Europe, Africa and the Middle East, eight in the Asia Pacific, eight in North America and four in Latin America, and which can be found in top luxury resorts including the Sheraton, Westin, The Luxury Collection, St. Regis and W Hotels—offer the Seven Pillars of Well-Being (below) which make each spa experience not just an isolated one, but part of a true holistic approach to fitness and well-being.

Beauty

Treatments such as facials, wraps and exfoliations help cleanse, purify and pamper your body and your skin. Such treatments go beyond being skin deep. For when you look good, you begin to feel good; it is a cycle that benefits you physically and mentally.

Harmony

Therapies such as massages harness the healing power of touch, aid relaxation and bring unity back into your entire being. Treatments on the spa menus, inspired by cultures from around the world, harmoniously embrace old philosophies as well as modern research and technology.

Life Balance

Like the ancients, who were ahead of their time in believing that physical health cannot be divorced from mental well-being, the modern spa provides an ideal environment to achieve this balance. State-of-the-art gymnasiums cater to exercise enthusiasts, while activities such as yoga and meditation help you attain fitness as well as an inner peace that is so lacking in today's fast-paced world, and treatments such as *reiki*, yoga and *tui na* help balance both body and mind.

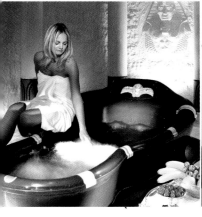
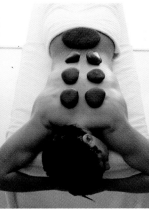
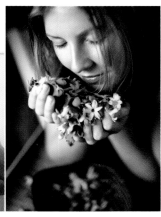

A.D. 43: In what is now Bath in England, UK, the Romans start construction of Aqua Sulis, a temple and complex of baths.

1326: A town in Belgium's Ardennes mountains near Leige is founded, adopting the name 'Spa', an acronym for the Latin phrase 'sanitas per aquas'.

Mid 1500s onwards: Physicians in the 16th and 17th centuries, such as Dr William Turner, author of *A Booke of the Nature and Properties of the Bathes of England* (1562), extol the virtues of 'taking to the waters'. Springs prescribed for treating various ailments through drinking or bathing are identified, and towns are built around mineral and thermal springs.

1600–1800: Spas flourish in Europe.

1800–1900: Aristocrats typically visit the most fashionable spas of their time at the height of the season to see and be seen in fine company. Germany's Baden-Baden is a key summer European capital.

TOP LEFT: The legendary beauty would certainly approve of the modern-day Cleopatra Bath, infused with a choice of essential oils. This exotic bath is available in spas such as Spa Trianon at Trianon Palace, A Westin Hotel, Versailles in France and Thermalife Center at Sheraton Cesme Hotel, Resort & Spa in Turkey.

TOP CENTRE: The smooth basalt stones used in the Hot Stone Massage offered by One Spa at Sheraton Grand Hotel & Spa and The Spa at The Westin Turnberry Resort, both in Scotland, UK, were picked from dry river beds in the American southwest.

TOP RIGHT: Re-connecting with nature is a pleasurable experience that awakens the senses. At Altira Spa at Mardavall Hotel & Spa in Spain for instance, the beauty of the Mediterranean is reflected through the use of indigenous building materials, and the use of colours and textures in its treatments and décor.

Vitality

The vital energy that courses through your body provides an impetus for strength, stamina and health. This vitality can be enhanced through exercises such as swimming, aqua gym and aerobics—aided by experienced tutors and teachers. Fresh air and beautiful surroundings enhance this 'feel-good factor'. A sound mind is not possible without a healthy body.

Aqua

A gamut of heat and steam facilities, thalassotherapy, bathing rituals, and hydrotherapy treatments such as invigorating jet shower massages help you connect with the cleansing, refreshing and regenerating properties of water.

Nature

A spa's connection to the environment is enhanced through its use of natural ingredients and materials in its treatments and décor. The surrounding natural elements are the inspiration and foundation for healing treatments and lingering sensory pleasures. From the remote deserts are plants, sand and stones which help heal and relax you, while the depths of the oceans provide minerals and algae that can be harvested for cleansing and nourishing.

Nutrition

A balanced meal in a spa goes beyond providing nourishment for the body. The taste, texture, fragrance and freshness of the ingredients also contribute to the pleasure of the experience felt by your entire being.

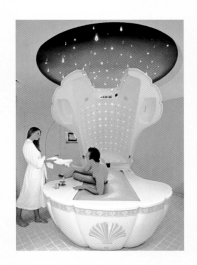

THE ELEMENTS

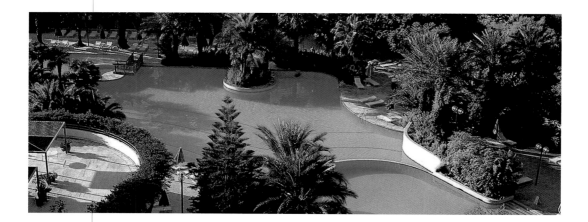

HOW THE THERAPIES ARE ORGANISED

Using the concept of the elements to categorise the spa treatments available in Europe is particularly apt, given that many therapies draw on, and are a combination of, the natural resources of water, fire, air and earth. It is also particularly fitting when we realise that the Greeks, Indians and Chinese—whose approaches to health and medicine continue to influence many treatments and therapies available in spas today—had their own versions of these concepts. A balance between the elements also reflects the balance within the body (and among the body, mind and spirit) that is central to many treatment philosophies today.

Early Greek philosophers such as Empedocles (?490–?430 B.C.), Aristotle (384–322 B.C.) and Plato (?427–?347 B.C.) attempted to order the world by theorising that all matter was formed by the basic elements of water, fire, air and earth. Empedocles dubbed these as 'roots' and proposed that they were joined or separated by the forces of harmony and disharmony. Plato named these roots 'elements', and thought they were geometric but composed of basic undefined matter. Aristotle saw each element as something that could not be further divided, and thought each was a combination of the four basic properties of hot, cold, dry and moist (for instance, water would be cold and moist, and earth cold and dry).

Indian philosophy focuses on the elements of water, fire, air, earth and ether (space); and Ayurvedic medicine associates each element with a different sensory quality and function. The elements are believed to combine to form the three *doshas* or humours (see Harmony chapter), and their balance is believed to reflect your constitution and physical and psychological health.

Chinese philosophy focuses on the theory of five elements—metal, wood, water, fire and earth—to explain relationships between humans and their surroundings. Each element is related to specific bodily features (such as the emotions, tissues and sensory organs), and specific environmental properties (such as the seasons, climatic factors, colours and directions). The

TOP: Even today, water remains a key element in the spa experience.

OPPOSITE, BOTTOM: What was a necessity in cold climates has given the world deeply relaxing and soothing heat treatments.

dynamic interplay of all these features and properties is important in the diagnosis of illness in Traditional Chinese Medicine (TCM).

While far reaching, the basic elements—water, fire, air and earth—do not have quite enough scope to include therapies such as acupuncture, reflexology, *reiki* and massages that aim to stimulate your body's vital energy to balance the body, mind and spirit. To be able to include these energy-balancing treatments, many of which have their origins in the East, Spa Therapies has been organised with an additional chapter—Harmony—a category based upon the Greek philosopher Empedocles' approach.

While a number of treatments and therapies are arranged solely according to their key essences, many of them also incorporate a balanced combination of other elements and/or the force of harmony.

Water

Therapies featured include the baths, jets and footbaths that are used in spas, as well as hydrotherapy centres, thermal and mineral spas and thalassotherapy centres. Also included are recent aquatic bodywork modalities, which are more than massages that take place in water.

Fire

Fire is manifested in heat treatments that warm the body: in particular, those that induce the body to sweat. Besides being cleansing and therapeutic, many of them have traditionally been enjoyed in a social setting.

Earth

Treatments featured use the healing ingredients of flowers, herbs, plants, muds and fruit—all nurtured by and derived from Mother Earth.

Air

Besides looking at the effects of fresh air, this chapter features oxygen and ozone treatments and other therapies that emphasise proper breathing habits, all geared towards increasing oxygen within your body.

Harmony

Treatments and therapies in this chapter, many with origins in the East, bring the body, mind and spirit into balance. They may also restore a harmonious flow of vital energy within the body.

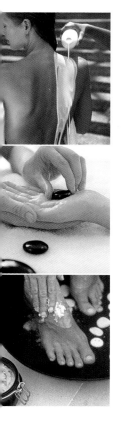

TOP: *Ingredients nourished by the earth come from various corners of the world—from alpine regions to the Amazon forests—reflecting the increasing global influence of spas.*

CENTRE: *Both therapist and spa-goer receive a helping hand from Mother Earth in a hot stone therapy.*

ABOVE: *In many urban spas, the water element is introduced early in the spa experience via a welcoming footbath, a perfect metaphor for washing away your city stresses.*

1840: The advent of the railway in the UK starts to make spas more accessible to the masses, contributing to their eventual decline as social centres for the upper classes. The railway also provides access to the seaside, contributing to its popularity.

1840 onwards: Water treatments such as mummifying clients in wet sheets, spraying them with high-pressure jets from above and below, and dunking them into cold water are administered by pioneering hydrotherapist Vincent Priessnitz at Grafenberg in the Jeseniky Mountains (now in the Czech Republic). Other spas such as Malvern in the UK subsequently offer similar treatments.

1867: The term 'thalassotherapy' is coined by Dr de la Bonnardière at a resort in Arcachon, France, that introduces the medical use of seawater. Later in 1899, Dr Louis Bagot creates France's first thalassotherapy centre in Roscoff.

1890s: Bavarian priest Sebastian Kneipp administers his water cures and herbal therapies in Bad Worishofen, Germany.

Early 20th century: With advances in medicine, many spas are converted into hospitals.

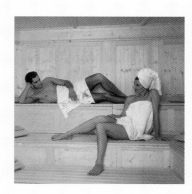

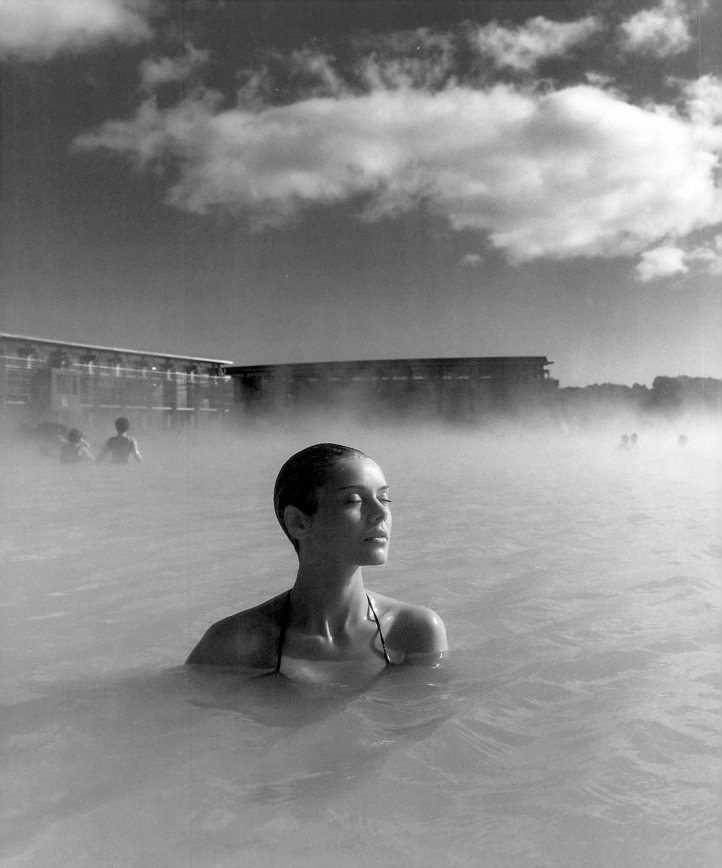

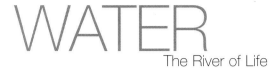

WATER
The River of Life

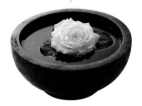

Water is thought to be the element of our origins: footprints which have been found in the East African Rift Valleys suggest that our ancestors emerged from the waters to live on land when the waters there receded 10 million years ago. Early settlers gravitated towards bodies of fresh water to feed themselves, their crops and their cattle; early towns and cities grew up around the banks and mouths of rivers.

Our affinity for water is said to be reflected in our bodies, which, like the planet, is composed of about three-quarters of liquid. Floating in water recalls the comfort and safety of being back in our mother's womb. Even being next to a mineral spring or the sea is refreshing and relaxing.

Water's therapeutic use, hydrotherapy (from the Greek word '*hydro*', which means 'water'), is based on centuries of observation that have more recently been backed by science. Water's temperature, pressure and state—solid, liquid or steam (see pp48–49)—are manipulated through a repertoire of hydrotherapeutic methods from baths (see pp20–22) to jets (see pp23–25), to elicit various responses from your body to enhance its functions. A treatment which is subsidised by the government in certain European countries, hydrotherapy has few side effects, and is prescribed by practitioners ranging from naturopaths to physiotherapists. Water is an ideal vehicle for transporting mineral salts and other additives from oils to muds to help remineralise your body. Moreover, its buoyant properties—it gives support, and aids flexibility and movement—make it particularly useful in rehabilitation work in aquatic exercise and bodywork (see pp29–32).

In a spa setting, drinking mineral water and seawater may be prescribed as part of the regime of 'taking the waters'. Water may also be administered internally in the form of enemas or colonic irrigation. Water's ready availability means we can enjoy many methods employed in spas in our own homes—from having a quick cold stimulating shower in the morning, or unwinding with a soothing warm bath after work, to relieving swollen and congested areas with an ice pack.

A RELIGIOUS PERSPECTIVE

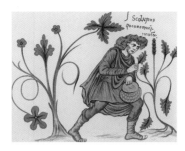

Cleanliness is next to godliness.

– Charles Wesley, founder of the Methodist Church

PURIFYING SPRINGS

Bathing in water to cleanse, heal and purify is not just a physical activity, but also one that for many millennia has been closely linked to myth, religion and ritual.

The ancients venerated the healing springs that gushed from the earth, believing them to be a gift from the gods, and built temples for various deities near them. The Romans dedicated their baths to Minerva (goddess of healing and wisdom) and Fortuna (goddess of fate), while the Greeks dedicated theirs to Hera (goddess of women, marriage and childbirth) and, later, Asclepius (god of medicine) and his daughter, Hygeia (goddess of health). Ancient bathers were also said to invoke these powerful deities for protection

Asclepius, a Greek physician who, in first century B.C. identified water—along with diets, exercise and massage—as central to combating disease, made such an impact with his holistic approach that he was elevated to a godly status. The Roman zeal for building luxurious baths extended to building temples to Asclepius next to healing springs. Records place him as the father of Hygeia and Pancea (goddess of remedies),

PAGE 16: Europe's spa traditions are deeply rooted in taking the waters for health and pleasure.

PAGE 17: A simple decorative water feature adds tranquility to any space.

TOP: Asclepius not only advocated the use of water for healing, but also herbs, as pictured in this 9th-century French manuscript reproduced in Les Arts Somptuaires *(vol. 1) where he discovers the plant betony.*

RIGHT: Since 1858 when the Virgin Mary appeared to 14-year-old Bernadette Soubirous, revealing the source of healing springs, the grotto at Lourdes has become a place of devotion for millions of pilgrims who come to drink of its waters, kiss the rock, and leave a candle or prayer petition. A medical board verifies claims of cures as miracles ranging from blindness to cancer.

OPPOSITE: The grandeur of Roman architecture and baths inspired artists such as Hubert Robert. Pictured is his oil on canvas, Ruins of a Roman Bath, *which dates back to the 1700s.*

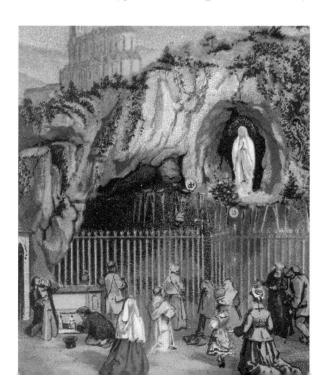

from whose names are derived the words 'hygiene', and 'panacea', a universal remedy, respectively.

Healing sources of water continue to be revered today. The most visited source in the Western world, the shrine and spring in Lourdes, France, attracts 6 million pilgrims annually who believe in its miraculous powers. Researchers studying the water at Lourdes and other healing sources in Europe surmised that these springs were not only rich in minerals, but that their powers could be attributed to the ability of water to absorb and transmit energy—in this case, the devotion projected into the water at Lourdes by pilgrims seeking its cure. Still others attribute their healing effects to pure faith or a placebo effect.

The most familiar aspect of the symbolic use of water in the Western world is that of baptism, from the Greek word '*baptein*', which means 'to bathe or dip'. This Christian ritual of sprinkling or fully immersing a baby or adult in holy water, which symbolises acceptance into the church, is a metaphor for protection, purification and rebirth. The roots of baptism are ancient, with ancient druids said to have initiated devotees by sprinkling water on their heads. Jewish cleansing rituals are also thought to have influenced baptism. This symbolism of cleansing and purification is also shared by many other cultures. Hindu devotees, for example, make it a point to bathe in India's River Ganges at least once in their lifetime.

In agricultural societies around the world where rain is crucial to the fertility of crops and survival, submersion in water is a part of rainmaking rituals. In certain parts of Russia, for instance, this involves seizing a priest and dousing him in water or throwing a total stranger—taken to represent a deity—into the river. Other methods used to bring on the rain include females, sometimes naked, dragging ploughs through the riverbeds.

Not only is there now a renewed interest in old healing sources, with New Agers visiting druidic sites to collect water for rituals; there is also a new interest in the therapeutic use of water. In the following pages, you will see that water's uses and benefits are just as diverse as the ways in which it has been revered throughout the ages.

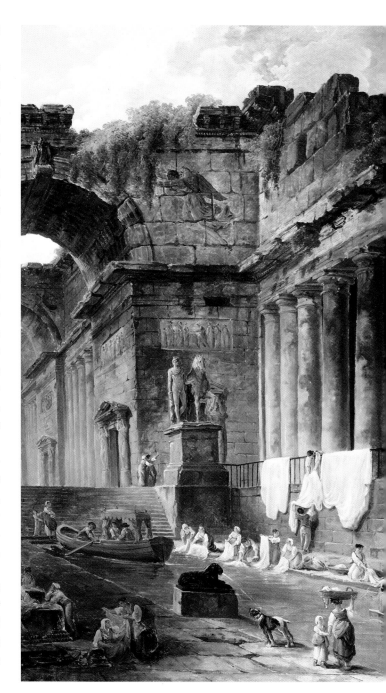

TREATMENTS AND THERAPIES

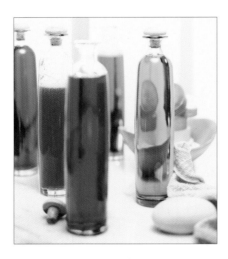

Water is best.

– Inscription over the Pump Room in Bath in England, UK, by Pindar, Greek lyric poet

TOP: *Baths of milk, mud, oatmeal, Epsom salts, coloured oils and essential oils are among those that may be found on spa menus.*

OPPOSITE: *A bathroom is a private sanctuary where you can retreat to at the end of a day. Try decorating in soothing colours such as blues or greens.*

BATHS

The ancient Greeks and Romans had their own forms of water therapy. Homer often referred to the Greek passion for bathing—from hot water tubs to hot-air baths—in the Iliad. Hippocrates, regarded as the father of medicine, suggested that joint swelling and pain could be lessened with cold water. The use of water of varying temperatures—neutral, cold, or hot—continues to be pivotal to many modern spa treatments.

Early 19th-century hydrotherapist Vincent Priessnitz, who treated the royal and not so royal at his Jeseniky Mountain spa at Grafenberg in what is now the Czech Republic, often decided what treatments to administer after seeing his patients' reaction to cold. If a patient's skin reddened—rather than stayed pale—after a cold bath, he predicted a quicker recovery. Priessnitz went on to teach his theories and methods to doctors.

Another eminent pioneering hydrotherapist, Father Sebastian Kneipp, a 19th-century Bavarian priest, prescribed hot and cold baths (see p22), compresses, footbaths (see pp26–27), sitz baths (see p21), steam baths (see pp48–49), showers (see pp23–24) and wraps—along with other natural cures such as exercise, herbal therapy (see pp73–76), nutrition, fresh air (see pp56–57), sunlight and rest—to treat a range of complaints. Kneipp's healing legacy continues in the German *kur* (cure) system. The national health programme pays for stays at a Kneipp Kurhause—a Kneipp health clinic—if prescribed by a doctor.

Neutral applications in the form of baths of water around body temperature—that feel neither warm nor cold—are so soothing that mental asylums used this method to calm distressed and violent patients before the advent of tranquillisers.

Hot treatments relax the muscles and ease stiffness. They expand the blood vessels, reduce blood pressure, and increase blood supply to the muscles and skin. They also boost the immune system, sending more nutrients and oxygen to the tissues and detoxifying the body of waste matter. However, hot treatments of more than five minutes may be exhausting and can depress circulation and metabolism. For this reason, a hot bath or steam treatment is usually followed by a brief application of cold in the form of a compress to the forehead, a cold shower, or a dip in a cold plunge pool.

Cold applications on their own are invigorating and stimulating. They constrict the blood vessels, inhibit inflammation and preserve body heat. Modern research supports Kneipp's theory that regular cold showers strengthen immunity and prevent colds. Cold baths, showers or plunge pools are usually applied for less than a minute, or circulation and metabolism may be depressed.

Contrast hydrotherapy—alternating hot and cold applications several times in succession—stimulates blood and lymph circulation, and the nervous and immune systems. It also balances the blood pressure by narrowing and dilating the blood vessels. Showering alternately in hot and cold water is a good method of hardening and conditioning the body.

Treatments with extreme and alternating temperatures should be comfortable, never reaching the point where you feel faint or dizzy, or develop chills. They may not be suitable for the elderly or very young. Always consult your doctor if you have a medical condition before undergoing such treatments.

Sitz Bath

A treatment favoured by ancient Greeks, sitz ('seat' in German) baths involve the use of two hip baths, and benefit those with conditions that affect the lower portion of the body. You sit in one—the area from your bottom to your navel soaked in water of one temperature—and immerse your feet in the other that has water of a contrasting temperature. You sit in them alternately: hips in the hot, feet in the cold, then vice versa. This treatment brings blood and nourishment to the pelvic area and flushes away any waste. Alternate sitz baths benefit those with haemorrhoids and varicose veins.

Sitz baths can also be taken entirely hot, cold or tepid. Hot sitz baths are used to treat haemorrhoids, anal fissures, atonic constipation, menstrual pain, pelvic inflammatory disease and bladder and prostate inflammation; they should not be used for diabetes. Cold sitz baths stimulate the kidneys and reproductive organs, while neutral sitz baths are used to treat cystitis.

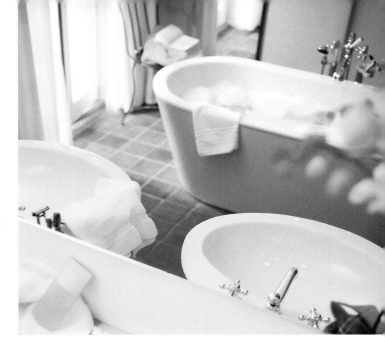

RECIPE FOR A RELAXING BATH

Light a few candles, dim the lights, put on some soothing music and enjoy this pre-bedtime bathing ritual from The Spa at Mandarin Oriental, Mandarin Oriental Hyde Park in the UK.

Ingredients
Camomile, lavender and rose essential oils
(up to 10 drops, together or separately)

- Switch off the phone, and make sure you won't be interrupted. Prepare a fresh towel and robe to put on afterwards, warmed on a heated towel rail or radiator if possible.
- Run the bath to just above body temperature (38 °C/100 °F). After filling the bath, add up to 10 drops of the essential oils together or separately. For real luxury, add rose petals. Recline in the bath for at least 20 minutes. Relax your neck against a rolled-up towel.
- Step carefully out and pat skin dry. The oils will continue working for up to 8 hours so do not wipe them away.
- Wrap yourself in your robe and drink some water or juice to re-hydrate. Alternatively, a herbal tea enhances your sense of calm and aids sleep.

Other oil blends to try are ginger, sage and rosemary (to detoxify); lemon, mandarin, peppermint (to stimulate the mind); and ylang-ylang, geranium, sandalwood (for romance).

Do not use essential oils if you are pregnant, nursing or on major medication. If in doubt, seek your doctor's advice.

Neutral Bath

The neutral bath is calming if you suffer from insomnia, anxiety, depression or nervous exhaustion. The water temperature is maintained at 33 to 36 degrees Celsius (91 to 97 degrees Fahrenheit), though it may be cooled slightly before the end of the treatment. The bath may last from 15 minutes to an hour. On getting out, dry yourself quickly but gently and rest for 30 minutes. Do not take a neutral bath if you have diabetes, fever, hypertension, chronic pain, problems with your arteries, or skin problems that could be exacerbated by water. Seek medical advice if you have heart problems or if you are pregnant.

Hot Bath

A tub of hot water draws on water's ability to transmit heat to your body without losing it too quickly. Initially stimulating, hot water has a sedating effect, easing tension and insomnia, which is why it is nice to have a hot bath before retiring to bed at the end of the day. While immersed, your body cannot regulate its temperature via sweating (except through your head), so its temperature rises, and detoxification begins. Hot water also aids muscle and joint aches and poor circulation. It is more effective than cold water in cleansing your skin.

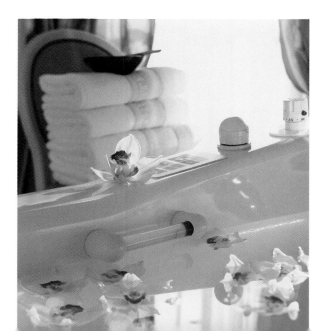

A hot bath in a spa may involve a soak in a tub of water of 40 degrees Celsius (104 degrees Fahrenheit). The temperature and timing of the bath will be monitored, a cold compress may be placed on your head, and you will be continually supervised during the session. The session may be followed with a cool sponge bath. Afterwards dry yourself well and rest for an hour. Hot water should always be comfortable—never scalding. Never take a hot bath to the point where you feel dizzy or faint.

Hyperthermia or artificial fever therapy, an extreme form of the hot bath, is used by some clinics to treat serious illnesses such as cancer or Acquired Immune Deficiency Syndrome (AIDS). Hyperthermia is exhausting, with some baths taking up to eight hours—never try it at home.

Cold Bath

A very brief application of cold water—which helps to tone the skin, increase circulation and reduce the body's temperature for a few seconds at a time—is exhilarating and invigorating. In a spa, the therapist will help you into a tub of water of about 24 degrees Celsius (75 degrees Fahrenheit) and rub you briskly with a bath mitten. The process only takes about five seconds, after which you should dry yourself vigorously. When taking a cold bath, you should be in very good health, and not menstruating or suffering from chills, diabetes, sensitivity to cold, or having problems with your heart or blood pressure.

Alternate Bath

Bathing or showering in water of alternating temperatures is an effective way to harden and condition the body. Such baths have a tonic effect, improving your circulation. They are also said to stimulate your immune system. In a warm bathroom, take a hot bath or shower for two to three minutes, followed by a cold shower of 20 seconds. Repeat this cycle three times, beginning with hot and ending with cold. You will find your energy boosted, and your complexion clearer after such a bath. It is not recommended if you suffer from bladder or kidney infections, colic, spasms, haemorrhages or heart problems.

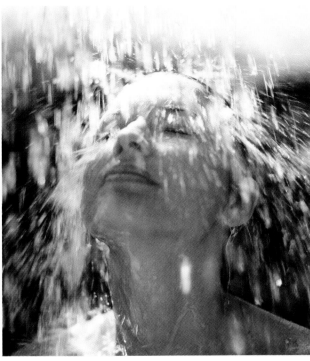

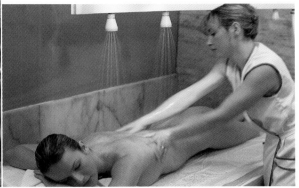

OPPOSITE: A soak is comforting, and eases tiredness, anxiety, headaches and stiffness. In modern spas, taking a full-length bath may be part of a treatment or a treatment in itself. Some baths may be a broth enhanced with additives—as diverse as sulphur (once used to disinfest people from lice!) and fragrant flower blossoms—so do inform your therapist beforehand of any allergies you may have.

LEFT: The water element is a prominent part of the spa experience, whether cooling down with a shower after time spent in a hot room such as a sauna, or washing off ingredients after a wrap.

BELOW: The affusion shower massage combines the benefits of the therapeutic application of water, and the therapeutic touch of the therapist. Some spas may employ the use of two therapists massaging you simultaneously.

SHOWERS AND HYDRO-MASSAGES

Spas and hydrotherapy centres harness the mechanical benefits of water through sophisticated showers and jets. Water is directed at various areas of the body, with its pressure varied to suit its purpose. The more powerful the jets, and the narrower the spray, the more stimulating it is to the skin, the circulation and the internal organs. Jets are useful for treating a variety of conditions ranging from arthritis to asthma.

Vichy Shower

The Vichy shower is also known as the affusion shower or rain shower. You lie on a table while water showers down on your body from five or more shower nozzles. The water temperature may be consistently warm, or it may be alternated with cool water. A light drizzle of water raining down on your body is deeply relaxing and sedative, while a heavier pressure is toning and stimulating, and ideal after sports. Your body may be brushed with a soft bristle brush to help increase circulation. The Vichy shower, initially created for paraplegic patients, is used to treat fatigue, lymphatic congestion and mild hypertension. Do not use it if you suffer from lymph oedema, open skin problems, vascular instability, or if you are pregnant.

Affusion Shower Massage

The affusion shower massage combines the hydrotherapeutic benefits of a gentle affusion shower with the healing touch of a therapist. As you lie under the light spray of rain that moistens your skin, you will be given a manual massage consisting of effleurage (stroking movements). During the treatment, oil may also be applied to your back, legs and feet. This relaxing and soothing treatment helps improve circulation and muscle tone, and combats stress and insomnia.

Scotch Hose

The Scotch hose is also known as the jet blitz. During a Scotch hose treatment, the therapist—standing about 4 metres (13 feet) away from you—directs a high-pressure hose of hot or cold water, or water of alternating temperatures at your body as you stand in a stall. The jets stimulate blood and lymph circulation and the internal organs. This shower massage is popular in slimming, anti-cellulite and anti-stress treatments, though it is often used to wash off ingredients such as mud after a body treatment. A treatment with cold water is popular as a post-exercise massage, especially with the heat built up in warm weather, and it is also used during breaks in sporting competitions and endurance events.

A treatment with hot water, which increases metabolic rate and improves the immune system, is used to treat arthritis, chronic lumbago, irregular menstruation, muscular tension, and mild blood circulation problems. Never take a hot Scotch hose shower if you have blood or heart circulation problems, inflammation, inelastic skin or varicose veins.

Swiss Shower

The Swiss shower has nine or more jet valves that spray the body with water from above the head and the sides. A shower of alternating temperatures may be a treatment in itself, though the shower may be used prior to and/or following a body scrub, body wrap or massage. It is used to ease insomnia, stress and tension, and to treat chronic back pain and vascular instability. It should not be used if you suffer from thromboses, cardiovascular problems, or venous disorders.

RIGHT: Multi-jet baths are often enhanced with ingredients such as essential oils, salts or seaweed.

OPPOSITE: Jacuzzis are becoming more ubiquitous in spas, health clubs, homes and hotels. Particularly desirable are jacuzzis perched on a rooftop terrace which offer a view of the surrounds.

Underwater Pressure Massage

In an underwater pressure massage, the therapist directs a pressured stream of water to various parts of your body as you lie in a tub of water of about 36 degrees Celsius (97 degrees Fahrenheit), avoiding sensitive areas such as your breasts and genitals. The relaxing benefits are derived from the warm water applied at variable force to your skin, subcutaneous tissues, deep-lying muscle layers, and abdominal organs. The water from the hose can be warmer or cooler than that of the bath. The water pressure is adjusted to your comfort level, and applied in circular or diagonal motions. After the 20- to 30-minute treatment, you may want to take a cold treatment to stimulate circulation, and rest for half an hour. Athletes use underwater massage as a post-exercise or post-competition treatment. It should not be used if you have had a very recent fracture, injury or wound, or if you have thromboses, cardiovascular problems, or venous disorders. Underwater pressure massage is used to treat conditions including scoliosis, dislocations, fractures, sprains, spastic paralyses, degenerative spinal disorders, and joint and muscular rheumatism.

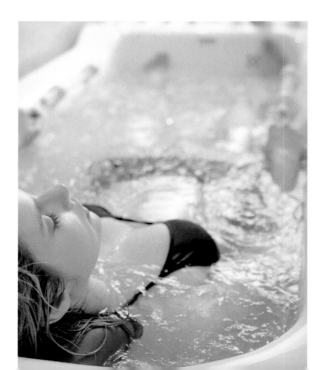

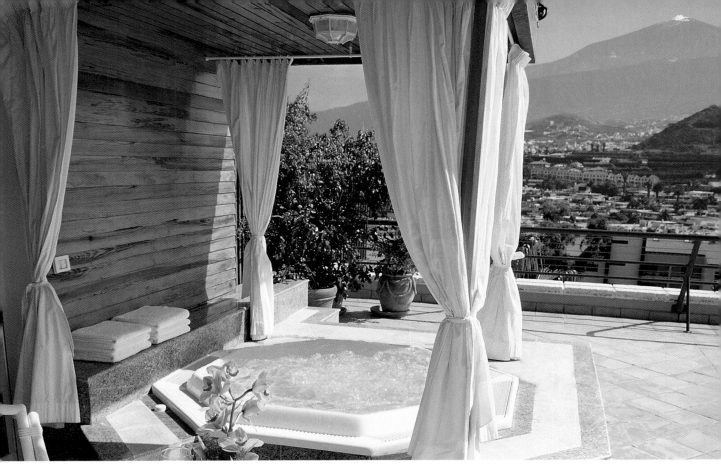

Jacuzzi

The jacuzzi, named after the American brothers who first improvised on the French-developed aerated bath with an outboard motor in a tank of water to treat an invalid boy, is also known as a whirlpool. A jacuzzi may have two types of massaging effects that can be used individually or together. The soothing effect of compressed air coming from small holes at the pool's base is ideal for preparing your body for a massage, while the pressure from jets of water from the side of the pool—with nozzles you may be able to angle—pummels and stimulates your skin. When combined, the resulting fast-moving bubbling water produces an all-over muscle-relaxing massage.

Jacuzzis may come in the form of bathtubs for an individual in treatment rooms. Sophisticated computerised multi-jet bathtubs provide massages to different parts of the body in a precisely timed and rhythmic manner.

Larger pools which can accommodate a few or several people are usually located by a swimming pool or hot or cold plunge pools. Often, the centrepiece of a thalasso centre or thermal spa is a heated exercise pool equipped with jets of water (and railings for support), which you will be instructed to use to massage various parts of your body.

Portable jacuzzi units are popular with athletes and dancers who use them in their baths to ease sore muscles and fatigue. The water temperature in a whirlpool is usually 30 to 40 degrees Celsius (86 to 104 degrees Fahrenheit).

A short session in a jacuzzi can relax your muscles, improve circulation, and produce a sense of wellbeing. Immerse yourself in the jacuzzi for about 15 minutes, then towel off, lie down and rest if you crave a relaxing experience. Otherwise, take a short cold treatment to stimulate circulation.

Medical spas and rehabilitative centres use jacuzzis to treat pain, swelling, wounds, skin sores, and joint problems. Jacuzzi baths are not recommended for people suffering from medical conditions such as diabetes or varicose veins, or for those who experience sensitivity to hot water.

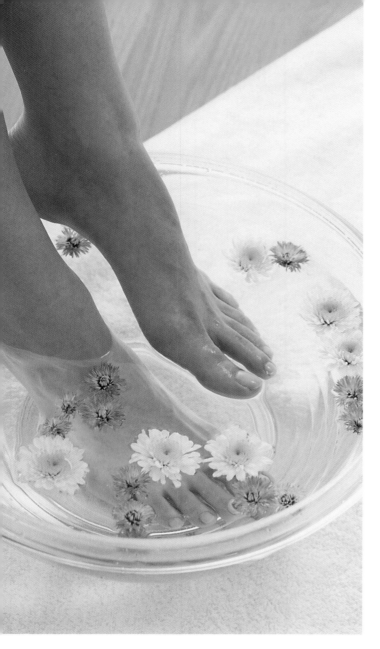

FOOTBATHS

Bathing the feet using waters of different temperatures was among the many methods of hydrotherapy expounded by the pioneering hydrotherapist Sebastian Kneipp.

Like reflexology (see pp98–99)—which works on the principle that manipulating different points of the feet, hands and ears affects organs in different parts of your body—hydrotherapy is also believed to have a reflexive effect. The skin of your feet and your hands, two of your body's main reflex connections, is said to be reflexively connected with circulation to your chest, head and pelvic regions. So a headache could be treated by a cold towel to your forehead and a hot footbath.

Warm Footbath

A soothing and relaxing footbath helps bring on sleep and increase blood circulation. After soaking your feet in water of 36 to 38 degrees Celsius (97 to 100 degrees Fahrenheit) for 10 to 15 minutes, towel dry your feet and rest in bed for at least half an hour. A warm footbath may benefit those with constipation, cold feet, circulation problems, weak immune systems, ankle or foot contusions, or infections of the nose and throat. Footbaths—often with added herbs (such as camomile, lavender, mint or rosemary), essential oils or flower petals—may also be enjoyed as a prelude to a pedicure. Do not take a warm footbath if you suffer from hypertension or have varicose veins.

Cold Footbath

A cold footbath will stimulate metabolism, increase blood circulation and influence venous blood flow return. Sitting down or standing up, dip both feet into a footbath of water of about 12 degrees Celsius (54 degrees Fahrenheit) for 15 seconds to a minute. After the footbath, wipe the water off your feet with your hands, exercise your legs till they are warm, and rest in bed. A cold footbath benefits those with circulation problems and tired feet. However, you should not take a cold footbath if you have a bladder or kidney infection, coronary deficiency, are sensitive to cold, or if you suffer from a female pelvic disorder.

ABOVE: In many spas, your treatment begins with your feet being bathed in water enhanced with essential oils and colourful blooms to relax you and ease you into the spa experience.

OPPOSITE: Kneipp water walks take place in shallow troughs filled to calf-height with water, with a handrail for support.

Alternate Footbath

An alternate footbath—which enhances your body's heat regulatory system, improves blood circulation and stabilises your nervous system—is commonly prescribed if you have cold feet, weary legs, low blood pressure, or difficulty sleeping.

Soak your feet in a receptacle filled to calf-height with warm water of 32 to 38 degrees Celsius (90 to 100 degrees Fahrenheit) for five minutes before immersing them in a receptacle of cold water of about 12 degrees Celsius (54 degrees Fahrenheit) for 10 to 15 seconds. Then repeat these two steps. After the footbath, wipe the water off your feet with your hands, exercise your legs till they are warm, and rest in bed for an hour. Taking alternate footbaths is not considered advisable for persons who have varicose veins.

Similar procedures using warm, cold or alternating temperatures may be used on the arms. In this case, two sinks placed next to each other are filled with the water.

Kneipp Water Walk

Besides admiring the forest, hikers both young and old in many German health resort towns can take off their shoes and socks, and refresh their feet in Kneipp water walks—shallow troughs fed by cold natural springs.

The technique of walking back and forth in these basins like a stork, lifting one leg after the other high out of the calf-deep water, is called water stepping or water treading. This procedure can last for between 10 and 15 seconds or 30 and 60 seconds, the duration of the exercise depending on the water temperature. However, you should never perform this treatment longer than you can bear comfortably.

Afterwards, dry off, put on dry socks, and continue your walk. The act of alternating between air and water makes the Kneipp water walk an invigorating treatment in summer.

Some spas have circuits of Kneipp footbaths in the form of dark corridors in which pebbles are placed in calf-deep water, thus combining the benefits of reflexology with hydrotherapy. A walk through one is very stimulating, even if your feet may hurt.

Water Treading at Home

You can also try water treading in your own bathtub at home, filled to calf-height with cold water. Remain clothed except for your bare feet. Use a rubber mat at the bottom of the tub and take care to ensure that you do not slip. You may also remain seated while you lift each leg out of the water.

In winter, you can try the stork-walking method in soft snow. Initially, you may only be able to do this for a few seconds (stop if you feel a cutting sensation), though you may be able to graduate up to three minutes. Avoid doing this on hard snow, and walk carefully so as not to slip and fall. Avoid frostbite by not remaining stationary or touching metal objects. After snow walking, warm your feet by rubbing them and putting on warm socks, or by going for a brisk walk. You should feel refreshed and stimulated after your walk.

Snow walking is said to benefit people who suffer from headaches and fatigue, and who are susceptible to infection. Do not attempt snow walking if you have chills, cold feet, circulation problems, urinary infections, or are menstruating or suffering from abdominal problems.

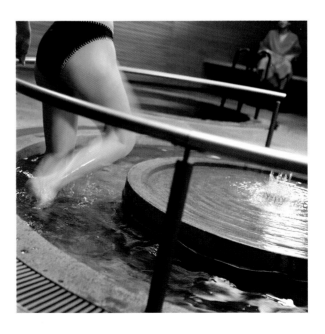

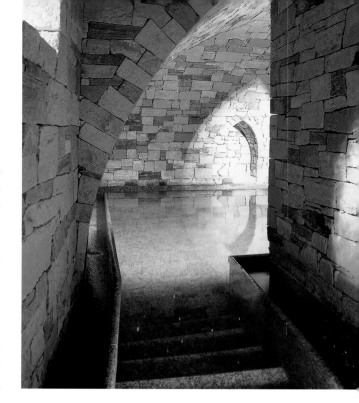

FLOTATION

Two hours of floating effortlessly in water of body temperature with your eyes and ears deprived of light and sound is said to be equivalent to eight hours of deep sleep. It is difficult to believe that confinement in a flotation tank (also known as a sensory deprivation tank) was once used as a form of torture.

The tank is traditionally a bed-sized capsule filled with 25 to 31 centimetres (10 to 12 inches) of water saturated with Epsom salts to keep your body afloat. (Many spas now have larger room-sized units.) Before treatment, remove your jewellery and apply petroleum jelly to any small cuts to prevent the saltwater from stinging. With the tank's lid closed, you will float in virtual darkness and silence except for the sound of your own breath. If you are apprehensive, you may be given a neck cushion, and soothing music may be played. Some tanks also have an intercom system. The room where the flotation tank is housed should be warm, so that you do not catch a chill when you step out of its womb-like atmosphere.

The warm buoyancy of the water encourages relaxation, eases aches and pains, and leaves you with a feeling of well-being—but the flotation tank is not recommended if you are claustrophobic or afraid of the dark, or suffer from diabetes, epilepsy, schizophrenia, or heart, kidney or skin disorders.

Dry Flotation

The dry flotation tank was developed in Austria. It resembles a rectangular waterbed with upholstered sides. You lie on a raised platform which is then lowered. Your body is suspended but protected from the heated water by a vinyl sheet, and you are left to 'float' for about 40 minutes. This method can be enjoyed on its own as a relaxing, tension-releasing treatment, often likened to being back in your mother's womb. It may also be combined with ingredients such as mud, hay (see p75), or warm oil and milk which your body has first been coated with. Do not take a dry float if you have a cold or a fever, respiratory problems, or infectious skin problems. Seek medical approval first if you have diabetes, epilepsy, or heart problems.

Floating at Home

You can enjoy the benefits of a flotation tank without the claustrophobia in your own bathroom, where afterwards you can adjourn to bed for a good night's sleep. To replicate the buoyancy and consistency of water used in a flotation tank, use the following recipe taken from Leon Chaitow's book *Hydrotherapy: Water Therapy for Health and Beauty*.

Ingredients

500 g (1 lb) Epsom salts
250 g (½ lb) sea salt
¾ tbsp iodine (clear)

- Run a neutral bath of around body temperature (37 degrees Celsius/99 degrees Fahrenheit). Add the Epsom salts, sea salt and iodine.
- Put on some soothing music, cover your eyes with a mask, and lie back for about 20 minutes. Top up the bath with warm water if the water cools.
- Towel yourself dry after the treatment—there is no need to take a shower—and get into a warm bed. Drink to replace fluids lost through heavy sweating. It may be a good idea to put a glass of water by your bed. Shower when you wake up in the morning, and moisturise your skin.

AQUATIC BODYWORK

In water, your body seems weightless. Water's buoyancy supports your weight, protects your joints from injury, allows for a greater flexibility and fluidity of movement than on land, and helps free and lengthen your spine.

Aquatic bodywork harnesses water's qualities along with the therapist's touch—in the form of cradling, massages or stretches. The sensation of lightness and being enveloped by warm water heightens this deeply nurturing experience that relaxes your body, mind and spirit, and encourages feelings of trust and security. Variations of aquatic bodywork, stemming largely from Watsu (see below), are practised in warm water, in mineral springs and therapy pools of at least 3.7 metres (12 feet) in diameter and about 1.2 metres (4 feet) deep.

Do inform your practitioner beforehand if you have a medical problem, as aquatic bodywork should be avoided in some cases—such as if you are suffering from bowel or bladder incontinence, or have open wounds or certain spinal problems.

Watsu

Watsu, derived from the words 'water' and 'shiatsu' (see p97) was developed in 1980 by Harold Dull, who married the benefits of shiatsu with that of water. He carried out these first water-based sessions of shiatsu in hot springs in California.

During a Watsu session—which is more than a massage in chest-high warm water—you will be gently floated, rocked, cradled and stretched, and your spine will be freed. Your head remains above the water as you float on your back with your eyes closed and your ears submerged.

Watsu sessions help release stress and anxiety, and in some instances, you may find pent-up emotions released as well. However, your practitioner will not interrupt the session, ask for details, or ask you to recall past traumas.

Watsu is suitable for pregnant women and for people suffering from muscular and joint problems. It has also been used to treat children with physical and mental disabilities, and people with addictions or a phobia of water.

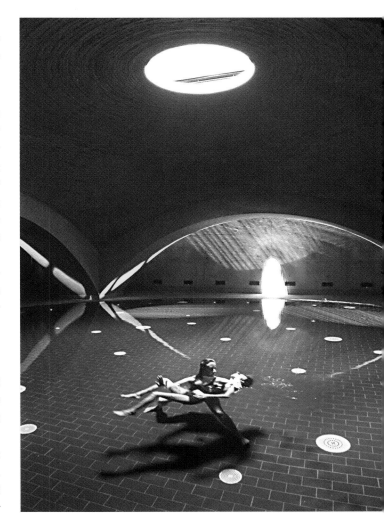

OPPOSITE: The relaxing benefits of floating on saltwater of 39 degrees Celsius (102 degrees Fahrenheit) in Sole Grotto at The Spa at the Interalpen-Hotel Tyrol is enhanced by music and light therapy.

ABOVE: Some forms of aquatic bodywork may take place in Liquid Sound pools where you can hear music underwater and see images of dolphins and whales frolicking on the ceiling, enhancing the entire experience.

WaterDance®

WaterDance®—also known as WaTa or WasserTanzen—was developed in 1987 in Switzerland by body therapist Arjana Brunschwiler and psychologist Aman Schroter. Like Watsu, WaterDance® begins with you being cradled, stretched, and relaxed above the water's surface.

Then, wearing noseclips, you will be gradually and gently taken underwater. The practitioner will cue you before each immersion. Between each underwater sequence, you will take several breaths—no more strenuous than if you were sleeping—in order to oxygenate your body.

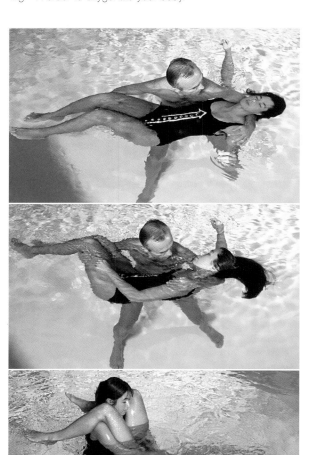

Freed from gravity, and with your head free of support, your body is manipulated in a wide variety of ways, borrowing elements from aikido, dance, inversions, massage, rolls, somersaults, and the movements of snakes and dolphins.

The lightness of being underwater induces a sense of peace, and breathing and resting between breaths is part of the healing process. The 'diving reflex' slows your heart rate, blood pressure and metabolism, enabling you to stay underwater longer almost effortlessly. The pressure of water on your body causes it to absorb higher levels of oxygen, and strengthens your heart and lungs. Tension-relieving and deeply relaxing, WaterDance® is said to bring on a blissful, even meditative and dream-like state. It also benefits those with orthopaedic and neurological problems.

Waterbalancing

This relaxing anti-stress therapy that brings harmony to the body, mind and spirit requires no effort on your part. You enter the water, lie back and close your eyes. Let the water support you, and allow a Waterbalancer to do the rest of the work.

Tension is seen as a protective posture that stems from stress or shock, but the goal of Waterbalancing is not to massage it away. Instead, you learn to let go of this resistant stance as you progress through Waterbalancing's three phases, becoming more at home in the water, and deepening your sense of confidence and relaxation.

During the first phase, flotation devices are placed under your neck and legs, and the Waterbalancer will move, massage and rock you, and use techniques from alternative therapies such as reflexology (see pp98–99), reiki (see p90), Rolfing and Tragerwork on you. The flotation aids are removed during the second phase and your body can be moved more freely. During the third phase, you will be brought underwater where directions such as up and down become blurred, opening your mind to new possibilities. Some people report feeling deeply contented, and as though they have been reborn.

Waterbalancing may be experienced one-on-one with a Waterbalancer, or as part of a group. A group session, where

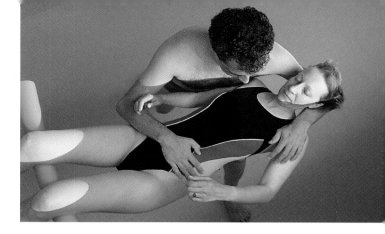

you form a circle in the pool, can also be employed as a tool of management training to foster team dynamics such as communication and cooperation. The group that forms a circle in the pool is attended by a few Waterbalancers.

Waterbalancing was developed in 1980 by the German psychologist Gunter Freude after using exercises in thermal water to treat his rheumatic fever. Besides successfully treating complaints such as rheumatism and arthritis, Waterbalancing is also used to reinforce treatment of neurological diseases, psychosomatic disorders (such as eating disorders, insomnia and migraines), and post-accident traumas.

Jahara™ Technique

Jahara™, which means 'precious stone' or 'gem filled with light', was developed by Brazilian Mario Jahara in 1995. At the beginning of the session, you will be taught playful yet educational exercises in the form of footwork patterns which, together with the support of water, help you become more aware of the way you hold and move your body. All other movements are derived from the four basic footwork patterns. Some Jahara™ principles draw on systems of body awareness such as the Alexander Technique (see p89). For instance, you are moved slowly and deliberately, with your head leading your body. Your spine receives a gentle traction against the water's resistance, expanding and releasing your musculoskeletal system and decompressing the joints. Your parasympathetic nervous system is activated, and as you approach a 'Zero Gravity Position', you soon become aware of a feeling of lightness and wellbeing as your body structure relaxes into alignment.

OPPOSITE: Waterbalancing harmonises your entire being through three progressive phases. During the first phase (OPPOSITE, TOP), you lie passively, closing your eyes, while the Waterbalancer manipulates you with gentle movements. In the second phase (OPPOSITE, CENTRE), the flotation device is removed, enabling a greater freedom of movement. In the third

(OPPOSITE, BOTTOM), you will be taken underwater.

RIGHT: In the Jahara™ Technique, a flexible flotation device dubbed the 'Third Arm™' may be used under your arms during the active exercises, or under one or both of your knees, giving support and allowing fluidity of movement during the passive exercises (pictured).

Triangular Cervical Support (TCS)™

TCS™ is a fundamental manoeuvre of Jahara™. It requires two participants—one 'Receiver' (designated A) and one 'Giver' (B)—and a Styrofoam noodle, cut to approximately 90 cm (35 in) long. The ideal pool depth is just over 1 m (3 ft).

The Exercise

- A places the noodle behind both knees, bending them until the water is above shoulder height. B stands beside and facing A, placing his forearm behind A's head. His other hand grasps the noodle next to A's hand.
- A bends her knees further, leans diagonally backwards in the water against B, lets go of the noodle and relaxes as her feet lift from the ground. B stands still, then flexes his knees, moving one foot forward so his feet are 40 to 60 cm (16 to 24 in) apart and parallel to each other. His upper pelvis tilts backwards, flattening and supporting his lower back.
- B releases the noodle, and moves his hand and forearm to rest across A's abdominal area. Shifting his weight to the front foot, B leans over A, simultaneously pressing down on three key areas: A's far shoulder using his wrist, A's near shoulder using his chest, and A's abdominal area using his other forearm and hand.
- B moves his own shoulder blades down and apart, lifting his elbows and widening his arms to apply gentle traction to A's neck. A's ears are submerged, and A's body moves slowly up and down as she breathes in and out.

To Come Out of TCS™

- B releases A's abdomen, reaches under A's legs and grasps the noodle, still giving arm support to A's head.
- B gently folds A's body, moving the noodle down until A's feet touch the ground. B uses his supporting arm to move A forward until A's weight rests on her feet.

TCS™ can be practiced daily from one to ten minutes.

Healing Dance

Developed in 1993 by former ballet dancer, teacher and choreographer Alexander Georgeokopoulos, Healing Dance was influenced by Watsu's nurturing aspects and WaterDance®'s freedom and range of motions. This therapy also draws on its developer's background in ballet, modern dance and free improvisation, as well as his experience as a practitioner of Tragerwork, a movement re-education therapy. Over the years, Healing Dance has come to include rhythmic sequences under the water, as well as a number of new ideas contributed by Georgeokopoulos' assistants and students.

As a passive receiver of the dance, your body is massaged, embraced, waved, spiralled, circled and swirled into figure eights interspersed with periods of stillness. Your practitioner's movements resemble the slow, graceful postures of *tai ji* (see p101). Practitioners may include a spiritual dimension to this therapy, working through visualisation and prayer, and invoking various divine realms for the receivers to be open to whatever they might need from the treatment.

Like a ballet in the water, the sequences of movement are unhurried and flowing, never abrupt. A Healing Dance typically lasts for about an hour. The dance awakens your enjoyment of the movements, energises you and restores a sense of balance.

THALASSOTHERAPY

In the 18th century, it became more fashionable to soak in the sea than in inland springs after the former's benefits were advocated by publications such as Dr Richard Russell's *A Dissertation on the Use of Sea Water in the Diseases of the Glands* (1750). This eventually gave rise to thalassotherapy, a complete branch of hydrotherapy. The word 'thalassotherapy' is derived from the Greek '*thalassa*', which means 'sea'.

The French have been practising thalassotherapy for over a century, but much earlier, the Egyptians used seawater and seaweed to heal burns, while the Greeks used it to cure all ills. Greek physicians Hippocrates and Galen, and Greek philosophers Aristotle and Plato recommended bathing in warm seawater. The Greeks also used mud from the sea as a remedy for stiffness and digestive problems.

The restorative power of thalassotherapy stems from the similarity between seawater's mineral composition and that of the human blood plasma that feeds and strengthens the body's cells. This similarity was recognised in the 1870s by leading French biologist René Quinton.

A true thalassotherapy centre, according to the Fédération Internationale de Thalassothérapie, is located on the sea coast, operates under medical supervision, and uses fresh (also

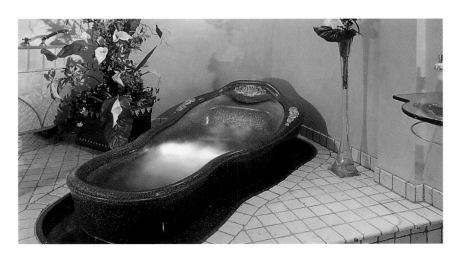

RIGHT AND OPPOSITE: A thalasso cure typically takes place over at least six consecutive days, with four treatments per day. These may include having your body bathed in warm seawater baths (RIGHT), blitzed with various types of jets, wrapped in seaweed (OPPOSITE, BOTTOM); or attending an aqua gym. At thalasso centres such as Vilalara at Thalassa Vilalara in Portugal (OPPOSITE, TOP), you will also get to soak in the beauty of often dramatic surroundings.

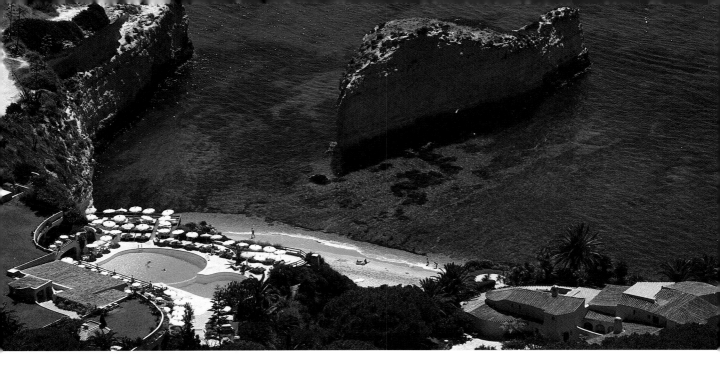

known as 'live') seawater and other substances derived from the sea. Thalassotherapy centres adhere to strict standards concerning hygiene and purity: for example, seawater is drawn from depth at a safe distance from the shore; and in France, no factories are permitted to exist within a 10-kilometre (6-mile) radius of a thalassotherapy centre.

Like hydrotherapy centres, thalassotherapy centres employ methods such as baths (see pp20–22), jet massages (see pp23–25) and large heated pools where jets massage various parts of your body and exercises are performed under the supervision of a physiotherapist. However, thalassotherapy centres focus primarily on the use of seawater and marine-derived substances including seaweed, algae, sea mud (see p79) and sand to treat a range of ailments or to enhance health. A thalassotherapy centre will often have a large pool of heated seawater where all of the prescribed exercises are performed under the supervision of a physiotherapist.

Minerals and trace elements in seawater are believed to have innate healing properties; seawater is heated to body temperature to allow these to be absorbed into our bodies. Zinc, for instance, is useful in boosting our immune defences, while iodine is thought to be useful in fat metabolism. Water with a high concentration of salt is often used to treat muscular, skeletal and skin complaints. The buoyancy one experiences

when in saltwater is also beneficial for rehabilitating the weak or people recovering from surgery, as it allows for movements that may otherwise be painful.

Seaweed is packed with minerals, vitamins, enzymes and amino acids, and contains between 5,000 and 50,000 times the concentration of seawater when micronised correctly. Its benefits include improving circulation and the immune system, regenerating and toning the skin, and reducing bloating. Seaweed applied externally in the form of body wraps, baths and poultices is often used to treat skin and rheumatic complaints, and to cleanse and tone the skin.

Seawater aerosols may also be used to help breathing problems (see p61). Even sea air (see pp56–57) is said to be beneficial, as it is richer in negative ions than air over land. These ions help reduce the levels of histamines which are produced during allergic reactions. Fresh sea air is also said to stimulate the body's immune system, and the act of inhaling it may help you combat modern-day stresses and strains.

Your visit to a thalassotherapy centre often begins with a detailed consultation with the centre's physician who will prescribe treatments tailored for your specific requirements. These thalasso treatments may focus on your personal goals such as smoking cessation, post-natal care or slimming.

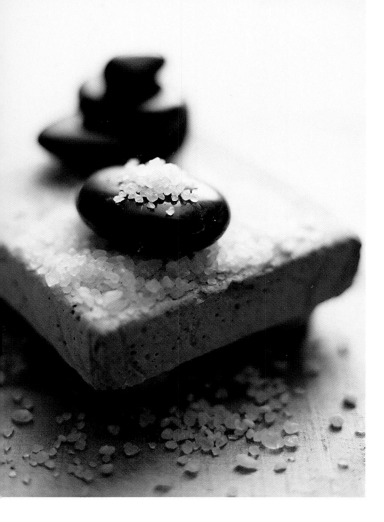

Making Your Own Salt Scrub

You can try making a home version of the salt glow for your body using the following recipe provided by Amrita Spa at Raffles Hotel Vier Jahreszeiten.

The spa recommends that you follow this procedure once a week in order to regenerate your skin and relax your mind. There is a stimulating alternative version for your feet that you can also try.

Salt Scrub for Your Back and Body
Ingredients
2 tbsp sea salt or fine- to medium-grained cooking salt
2–3 tbsp olive oil
1 drop lavender essential oil

- Mix the ingredients together in a bowl and bring it to your bathroom.
- Stand under a warm shower briefly to dampen your skin.
- Apply the salt mixture to your skin, starting from your legs up, then your arms, scrubbing in big, circular strokes towards your heart. To scrub hard-to-reach areas on your back, use a towel as if drying off.
- Rinse off under a shower, pat yourself dry, and apply moisturiser to your body.
- Keep yourself warm and rest for 20 minutes.

Salt Scrub for Your Feet
Ingredients
1 tbsp sea salt or fine- to medium-grained cooking salt
1 handful fresh basil, rosemary and mint

- Fill a shallow tub with warm water, adding the herbs to refresh your feet.
- Soak your feet in the water for 5 to 15 minutes.
- Scrub your feet with the salt, paying particular attention to your heels.
- Rinse off the salt, pat dry, and moisturise your feet with thick cream.
- Put on a pair of socks and head off to bed for a good night's rest.

Salt Glow

As its name implies, this salt scrub helps slough off dead skin cells, leaving your skin smooth and glowing. It also helps detoxify the body, and leaves you with a general feeling of wellbeing. The therapist will moisten sea salt with water and aromatherapy oil to make it sticky. Next, she will work this into your moistened skin using firm up-and-down and circular motions. Do not be afraid to ask your therapist to modify the friction to suit your level of comfort. After the treatment, rinse the salt off your body under a shower of a cool but comfortable temperature, using your hands to provide some friction.

The treatment is especially useful if you suffer from rheumatic aches and pains, poor circulation, or have difficulty perspiring. Do not get a salt glow if you have sores, wounds, rashes or sunburnt skin. Do not shave before this treatment.

Seaweed Body Wrap

Seaweed's ability to detoxify the body makes it popular as a part of detoxification or slimming programmes. Before a seaweed wrap, a warm shower followed by a short sauna session will relax you and raise your body temperature. Dry-brushing your body with a loofah sponge removes dead skin cells, and brings the blood to your skin's surface. Next the seaweed powder, mixed into a paste, is applied to your body; you are then wrapped in a plastic sheet, and then in electric and metallic blankets. A cold towel may be placed on your forehead or you may be given a head or foot massage. When you are unwrapped about 30 to 40 minutes later, take a shower—ideally a cold one—to rinse off the paste. A moisturising body massage may complete the treatment.

Drinking Seawater

Some thalassotherapy centres prescribe drinking minute doses of seawater—usually a tablespoon or two, half an hour before a meal, graduating to 4 tablespoons three times a day. The potassium content may ease fluid retention, and fluoride helps balance calcium metabolism. Seawater is often diluted with fresh water or juice for taste. It should only be drunk under qualified supervision and with strict hygiene procedures in place.

Seaweed in Your Bath

Seaweed products may be purchased from health shops and spas for use at home. Its nutrients can be absorbed through your skin in the form of face masks or baths. To make a seaweed bath, add seaweed powder or organic seaweed to a tub of warm, but not hot, water. Be prepared for the water to turn brown. You may want to put a cold towel to your forehead while you enjoy the bath for 15 to 30 minutes. You may also want to add more warm water to maintain the temperature. Showering is not required after a seaweed bath—if you want to do so, do this before your bath. Pat yourself dry, and rest for half an hour—or even better, try to schedule your bath just before your bedtime.

OPPOSITE: Salt from the sea imparts a rich mineral content and gentle exfoliation qualities to your skin.

LEFT: Seaweed's fishy scent may be reduced by adding essential oils. Although some people find its distinctive smell offensive, others view it as a relaxing component of the treatment.

BELOW: Seaweed is popularly used in bust treatments to hydrate, tone and smooth the décolletage, often regarded as an area that reveals your age.

BOTTOM: In a salt glow, the salt granules clear off dead cells which give skin its dull appearance, leaving skin with a radiant glow.

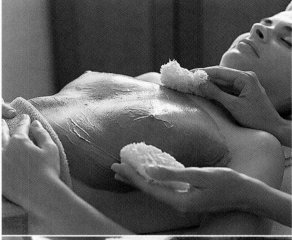

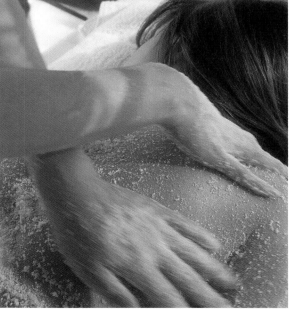

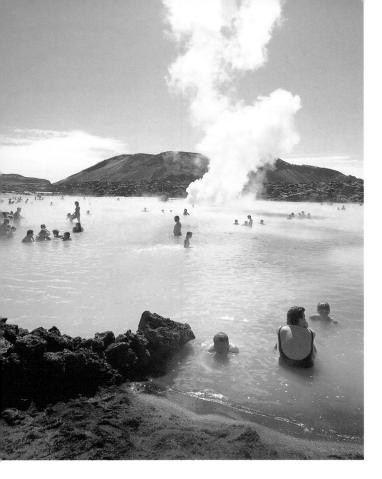

THERMAL AND MINERAL WATER

Evidence found near healing springs suggests that man has used them for over 600,000 years. The practice of using natural mineral spring water to prevent or cure disease goes back 5,000 years to the Bronze Age. In ancient times, springs were considered sacred healing sites. In recent times, scientific analysis of their chemical and medicinal properties has helped to identify how various sources of water may be used to treat specific problems. Waters rich in sulphur and sulphates, for instance, are believed to strengthen the immune system, kill bacteria and fungi, and are used to treat skin conditions.

Each spring or well is unique in temperature and mineral composition. Its content of mineral and trace elements depends on various influences such as the clays, peat, rocks and natural gases released into the water. The classification of mineral springs varies between countries. Ways in which they may be classified include temperature, mineral content, and potential of hydrogen level (pH), which varies according to the amount of calcium and magnesium salts present. The greater the amount, the lower the pH level. Waters with low pH levels, for example, are often drunk to improve digestion, and are also used to treat a variety of skin problems.

Many of Europe's spa towns built around healing springs, such as Vichy in France, trace their roots from the 14th to the 16th centuries. Visiting these sources in the past for rest and rejuvenation—known as 'taking the waters'—was a social affair, though its popularity diminished with improved domestic water supplies and advances in conventional medicine.

However, water therapies, like other natural methods of healing, are again seeing a resurgence in popularity and respectability. Centres of healing and bathing built over natural springs, once closed, have now been restored and redeveloped—such as Thermae Bath Spa in Bath, England, where five historic buildings have been restored, and the facilities now include indoor and outdoor thermal bathing, and a rooftop pool. The historical significance of such revived sites adds a new dimension to present-day bathing in these springs.

Healing springs across Europe range from natural outdoor ponds to competition-size pools in five-star resorts. Some may be naturally hot or cold, others artificially heated or cooled. They may or may not be chemically treated for purity.

In many parts of Europe, balneotherapy—bathing for therapeutic purposes—is part of mainstream medicine, paid for by national healthcare if it is prescribed by a doctor. Many spas built around healing springs have medical professionals on hand, and provide complementary treatments including homeopathy (see pp88), mud applications (see pp79–80) and fitness training. Some are geared towards pleasure and relaxation through healthy but tasty cuisine, beautiful surroundings, and cultural aspects that include museum visits, film festivals and musical concerts. Bathing (see pp20–22), therapies conducted in water (see pp29–32), hot and cold applications (see p22), inhalations (see pp58–59 and 61), jet-type showers (see pp23–25), and drinking the waters from the source (see p37) are part of their holistic approach to wellness and wellbeing.

Thermal and mineral springs are not suitable for those who are pregnant, or suffering from cancer, high blood pressure and cardiovascular disease. Medical treatment should always be supervised by a qualified health practitioner.

Drinking from the Source

Drinking mineral water from the source is not the same as consuming commercially bottled water from the same spring, whch is why it should only be prescribed by a professionally qualified healthcare professional or nutritionist.

For instance, drinking half a glass of magnesium- and calcium-rich water direct from the spring a couple of times a day may promote regularity (a sign that your body is being cleansed), whereas greater amounts of commercially bottled water may be drunk without this laxative effect.

Drinking from the source is usually done half an hour to an hour before meals. The amount prescribed will depend on the content of the water (sometimes diluted with tap water). Your age, sex and size are other factors to be considered.

Not all natural mineral waters should be drunk. Some waters such as those containing arsenic are actually dangerous when imbibed, even though they may have external uses: in treating fungal infections, for example. Waters containing sulphur and iron-rich waters are not palatable.

Drinking from the source is most frequently prescribed for gastrointestinal problems and to prevent or treat certain types of diseases, such as kidney problems.

Your Daily Dose of Water

Do not wait to visit a spa to start paying attention to how much drinking water you need every day. Our bodies' cells, tissues and organs depend on water to function, flush out waste and toxins, regulate temperature, and cool our bodies by evaporation. You lose at least 2 litres (3.5 pints) of water a day—more if you are sweating, or when you are placed in certain environments—and you should drink regularly, not just when you feel thirsty. The recommended amount is at least 8 to 10 glasses of water a day. Drink more water if you are

- Exercising.
- In a warm climate, at a higher altitude, or in an air-conditioned or heated room.
- Travelling on an aeroplane, which can be dehydrating.
- Consuming alcohol and/or caffeinated drinks (including sodas), as these can be diuretic in large amounts.
- Ill, especially if you are suffering from a fever or diarrhoea.
- Pregnant or breastfeeding.
- Elderly or very young.

Here's a popular way to calculate how much water you need a day:

$$\underset{\text{(in pounds)}}{\text{your weight}} \times \underset{\text{(pounds of water lost)}}{0.04} \times \underset{\text{(cups)}}{2}$$

To convert from kilogrammes to pounds, multiply by 2.2.

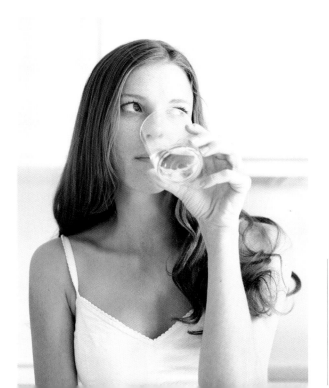

OPPOSITE: In Iceland, thermai water is also used to generate electricity (in the background), heat private facilities such as pools and greenhouses, and piped under sidewalks and parking lots to melt the snow.

LEFT: Drinking mineral water from the source should not be confused with drinking bottled water. However, it may serve to help make you aware of the amount of regular drinking water you should be consuming every day.

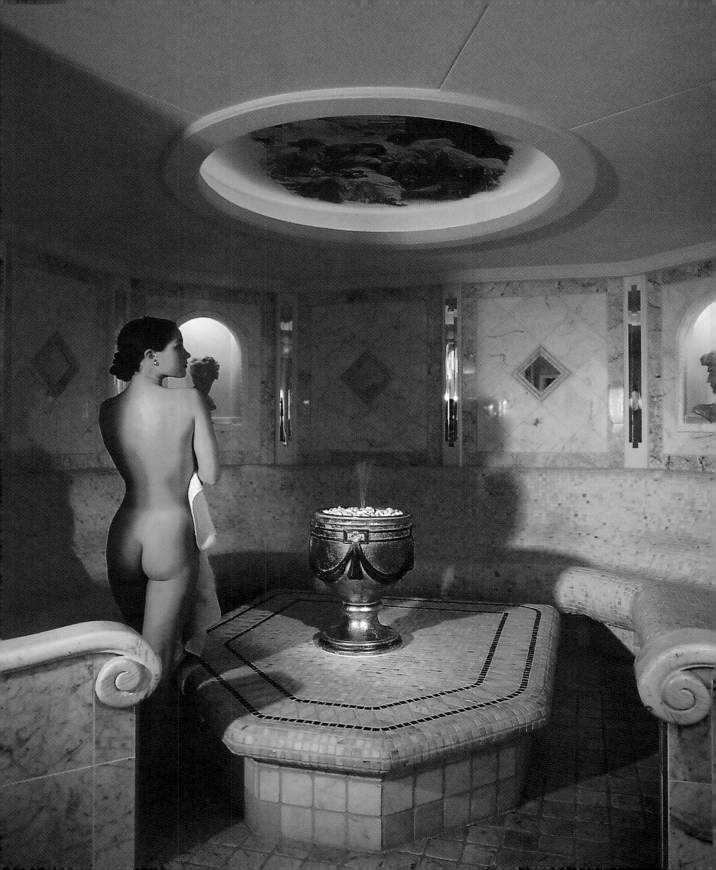

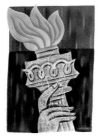

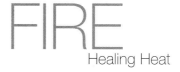

FIRE
Healing Heat

The element fire—seen as light and flame, felt as heat, and manifested through sweat—has inspired awe and respect through the ages. Before modern science explained its powers, various cultures believed that fire came from a higher force of either heaven or hell, connecting it with knowledge, creation and spiritual protection. According to a Greek myth, Prometheus stole fire from the gods and gave it to man, while in a Russian myth, a higher being created the first man through drops of sweat.

Once our ancestors learnt to harness fire's fury, a world of new possibilities was opened to them. Fire gave them light to function at night, heat to counter the cold, and fuel to cook their foods. It also afforded them protection from wild animals.

The warmth that fire gave to families in cold regions gave rise to heat treatments such as the Kraxen-Stove (see pp50–51). Man also discovered heat's ability to help rid the body of impurities, as seen in different versions of sweat baths that evolved over the years and across the cultures, from Roman baths (see pp42–43), Turkish hammams (see p44) and Russian banias (see p44) to Finnish saunas (see pp45–46).

Spas in Europe have adapted a number of heat-based treatments in novel ways to relax your muscles and prepare your body's tissues to receive treatments such as massages. Modern-day treatments such as the rasul (see p49) and Farmer's Steam Bath (see p51) were designed with the help of medical professionals to ensure their effectiveness and safety, as well as with the help of historians to reflect their historical and cultural components. Apart from using heated air and steam from heated water, spas harness the element of fire through heating substances such as water (see pp20–22), mud (see pp79–80) and herbs (see pp73–75).

A SOCIAL PERSPECTIVE

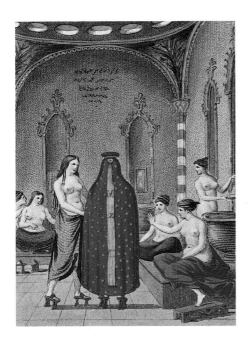

Your town is only a perfect town when there is a bath in it.

– Abu Sir, early Arab historian,
Sharing Fire's Spirit

PAGE 38: In the olden days, heat treatments had more of a function of keeping warm and cleansing. These days, heat treatments in spas—used to relax your body before other spa treatments—are enjoyed in luxurious settings such as GB Spa at Hotel Grande Bretagne in Athens, Greece.

PAGE 39: The lighting of the Olympic flame before the temple of Hera recalls the ancient Greeks' reverence for fire, which the ancients lit for their gods. As it is relayed around different corners of the globe, the modern-day Olympic flame signifies hope for peace and understanding.

TOP: Hammams gave women the occasion to inspect potential daughters-in-law for physical flaws and social shortcomings. Some would kiss their son's prospective wife to check for bad breath!

OPPOSITE: Activities within communal baths were the subjects of paintings such as Tepidarium (1853) by French artist Théodore Chasseriau.

THE SPREADER OF WARMTH

Gathering around a fire—whether a campfire, a fireplace or in a spa chamber that harnesses heat—not only warms the body and soul, but creates a convivial atmosphere. Many fire-based treatments were historically enjoyed communally, although their uses were not limited to social interaction.

Treatments based on fire arose as a function of keeping warm in the cold. The Kraxen-Stove (see pp50–51), for instance, originated from alpine regions of Europe where the head of the household enjoyed the prized seat against the fireplace as his family gathered around. Most treatments, though, revolved around the use of heat to encourage the process of perspiration which cleansed the body from the inside out, after which washing took place—giving rise to the notion of a 'sweat bath'. Experts believe that the different versions of the sweat bath practised by different cultures are likely to have evolved independently of each other.

Sweat bathing evolved in agricultural (rather than fishing or hunting) societies where there was a need to cleanse and soothe aching muscles after a hard day's toil. Resources such as firewood and water were abundant in such societies. Early sweat baths were holes dug in the slopes of hills, and were used as winter living quarters.

Sweat baths had multiple uses in cultures where they were an integral part of life. Early Finns and Russians used the hygienic confines of a sweat bath to attend to life's milestones such as giving birth, performing pre-wedding rituals, dressing dead bodies, and mourning the dead. Even private sweat baths—found in wealthy homes—had social elements to them. In Finland's past, servants would take a sauna with the family, or if the sauna was not large enough, bath times were staggered according to the hierarchy in the household.

The communal aspect of sweat baths was apparent whether the bath was humble or grand. In Ireland, sweat houses warmed by hot coals may have accommodated about eight people at a time, but someone else had to be stationed outside to shut the openings during a bath session. On the other hand,

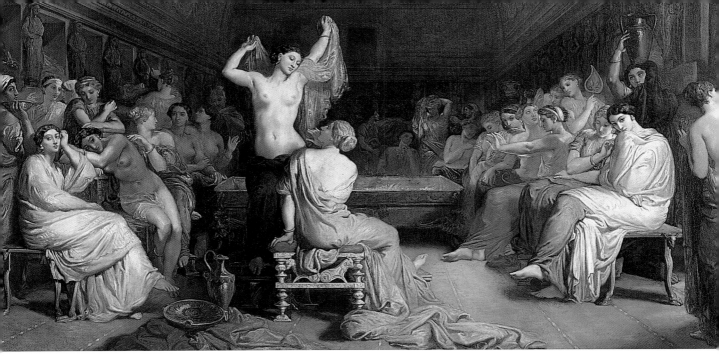

the public baths of the ancient Romans—equipped with sophisticated plumbing and heating systems—were virtual recreational cities where thousands congregated at once.

Public baths were the equivalent of a modern-day café for socialising. As urban populations burgeoned, so did Europe's number of public sweat baths. Associations with prostitution, promiscuity and venereal diseases eventually tainted the reputation of many public baths in Europe, causing many to shut their doors. However, the culture for communal sweat bathing stayed strong in countries such as Finland and Russia (and in Japan in the East) due to the fact that they were never associated with lust or sex. Finnish children, for instance, learn sauna etiquette from an early age, while the Russians would never have sex in the bania (possibly in fear of having hot rocks and scalding water tossed at them by a spirit).

Just as important as proper protocol for the sweat bather or modern-day spa-goer are the precautions to take when enjoying fire's therapeutic powers. Do not have a heat treatment immediately after a heavy meal or consuming alcohol. Remove jewellery and spectacles, as heated metal can burn. Consult your doctor first if you have any medical problems.Heat treatments may not be suitable for children, the elderly, or pregnant, and they should never be taken to the point of discomfort or dizziness: stop immediately if you feel uncomfortable.

As with hot water treatments (see pp20–22), many heat treatments are combined with rapid forms of cooling, such as a cold compress to the forehead or a dip in a cold pool. They may also be accompanied by body-brushing to remove dead skin cells and stimulate circulation.

The results of heat treatments vary depending on the type of treatment, its duration and temperature. In general, when your body is exposed to a high temperature, it works as if you were exercising even if you are relaxed. Your capillaries dilate, increasing the blood flow to the skin, and your heart and pulse rates quicken. Your nerve endings alert your sweat glands, and your body perspires, expelling water and toxins, and softening your skin. Sweating draws out the lactic acid that causes sore muscles and fatigue—which is why many athletes like to have a sauna (see pp45–46) and massage (see pp92–97) after exercising. Treatments that induce sweating are also popular in slimming programmes, though many practitioners say that such weight loss, due to loss of water, is only temporary.

While some people object to sweating, it has become even more important to sweat, given our modern sedentary lifestyles. Being constantly bombarded by pollutants and chemicals from the air, food, clothing and cosmetics causes our pores to clog, hindering our natural flow of sweat—something which could trigger a range of physical and psychological symptoms.

TREATMENTS AND THERAPIES

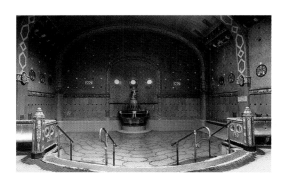

Give me the power to create a fever, and I shall cure any disease.

– Hippocrates (?460–?377 B.C.),
the father of modern medicine

TOP: *Pools such as the Saint Gellért Medicinal Bath and Pools in Hungary recall the lavish décor of olden baths.*

OPPOSITE: *The Romans built grand temples and elaborate baths in lands under their empire. Pictured here is the Great Bath, the centrepiece of the Roman baths in Bath, England in which water was piped from a sacred spring.*

COMMUNAL SWEAT BATHS

Nowhere was bathing more of a social activity than in the Roman thermae (from the Greek word '*therme*' for 'heat'). These were virtually large complexes for recreation: the baths were surrounded by sports stadiums, gymnasiums, musical theatres, halls for parties, libraries and inns for travellers. The most supersized Roman thermae were able to accommodate 6,000 people at one go.

Emperor Agrippa is credited with building the first Roman thermae in 25 B.C.. However, the Romans were already using various types of humbler baths called '*balnea*' two centuries before; these were in turn inspired by the Greek '*laconica*' or hot-air baths which were heated by coal fires or by placing heated rocks indoors. Every Roman emperor after Agrippa would try to outshine the one before by building grander and more extravagant thermae than his predecessor.

Roman baths were considered a way of life in towns within the empire. They typically comprised a series of chambers and pools of varying temperatures, depending where they were in relation to the heating furnace. The baths were heated by a hypocaust system that heated the rooms through the marble floor.

The bather would wander around the rooms, starting from the coolest and moving up to the hottest before ending in a cold plunge pool. Different Roman writers report different methods and sequences of bathing, perhaps reflecting different practices, personal preferences, or prescriptions from physicians. However, the frigidarium, tepidarium, caldarium and laconicum were typically mentioned as key rooms.

According to the Greek physician Galen, a typical bathing sequence started with the frigidarium (from the Latin word '*frigidus*', which means 'cold'). In this unheated apartment, the bather took off his clothes and proceeded to the other rooms. The bather returned here at the end of the cycle of rooms for a dip in the cold plunge pool to close his pores. It was believed that this would also help harden his body.

The next room—the tepidarium (from the Latin word '*tepidus*', which means 'lukewarm')—was a warm chamber:

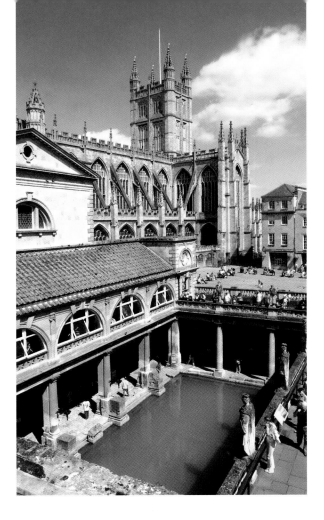

usually the biggest and most resplendent. The bather luxuriated here for an hour while oil was rubbed into his skin. This was followed by a period in the caldarium (from the Latin word '*caldaris*', which means 'warming'), a warmer room consisting of private cubicles with hot or cold water for bathing.

In the laconium, the hottest room, the bather was prepared for a vigorous massage: his body was scrubbed and dead skin removed using a strigil—a bronze or iron instrument the Romans and Greeks used to scrape off oils and perspiration after a bath.

The bath experience was usually preceded by sports or a workout. After the bath, the bather could also adjourn to the library for an intellectual workout.

Roman baths influenced other bathing cultures such as the hammams (see p44). Saunas (see pp45–47), steam rooms (see pp48–49), and hot and cold plunge pools (see p22) in modern spas echo the concept which lay behind these Roman baths.

A Modern Roman Bath Experience

In a modern take on the sequence of rooms and pools of differing temperatures that ancient Romans used to bathe in, many spas—such as Aquarias at Whatley Manor Hotel—may possess an elaborate series of thermal facilities. Recalling the Roman thermae, these are likely to be gently heated through the floor, walls and benches. It is recommended that you use the rooms in a graduating sequence of heat, though you may choose to use whichever facilities you enjoy most. However, do not at any time linger to the point of feeling dizzy or nauseous. The spa you visit will suggest that you allow time before a spa treatment to relax your body in these facilities:

- The tepidarium contains ceramic couches constantly heated to about 35 °C (95 °F). Here is where the relaxation and treatment process begins.
- The salt scrub showers are where you exfoliate and soften the skin and stimulate the microcirculation. Wet your body in the shower, then use a salt and oil sachet to gently massage your body—particularly the arms and legs—with circular movements, leaving the skin soft and supple.
- The laconium is a relaxing, dry environment of about 65 to 80 °C (149 to 176 °F), designed to recreate a Roman sauna. The temperature initiates the detoxifying process.
- The aroma grotto is typically a gentle steam experience enhanced with essential oils, which helps benefit the respiratory system, and softens the hair and skin.
- The caldarium is a more intensive steam experience. The essences used within may be changed seasonally.
- The sauna is the most intensely heated facility, and the final one used in the sequence.

You should periodically cool down during the heat experience. Hoses provided in certain thermal cabins, used to wash down benches, can be also used to cool the hands, feet or neck. Mini-basins may be provided for splashing your face. Some spas offer experience showers that feature an icy blast of water, or a tropical shower of warmer water; Experience showers with jets from above and at the sides may also combine scents and colour therapy (see pp91–92).

Apart from the mild tepidarium, thermal facilities and hydropools are not suitable for people with high blood pressure, heart conditions or epilepsy, or during pregnancy.

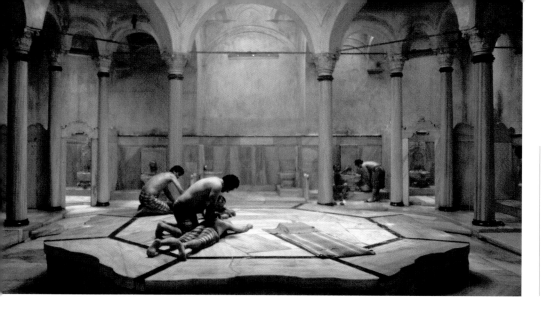

Hammam

The hammam (Arabic for 'spreader of warmth') is similar in concept to, but more modest than a Roman bath. It is usually located next to a mosque or a *souk* (marketplace), and ornately decorated with elements from Islamic art. The hammam flourished around A.D. 600 when the prophet Muhammad encouraged his followers to take such baths. Heat, he believed, enhanced fertility. It was also thought to cure small pox.

A traditional hammam has a *tellak* (attendant) who acts as usher, masseur and bouncer. He also shouts to scare off '*dijans*' (phantoms). A hammam experience starts with basting the body in heat, followed by a vigorous massage. This may be followed by being soaped down, and then exfoliated in private by the *tellak*. You then adjourn to a relaxation room.

Men and women traditionally use the hammam separately, and nudity is not accepted. Modern versions of the hammam may accommodate mixed groups, but swimsuits must be worn. Some modern hammams are limited to connecting rooms with pools of different temperatures to use while waiting your turn for a massage. Some spas have more intimate hammams to provide a luxurious ritual for just two bathers.

In the mid 1800s, author David Uquart came up with the term 'Turkish bath' in reference to hammams; his work subsequently inspired the construction of these baths in London and Europe. As a result, the term 'Turkish bath' has often been loosely applied to a variety of heat treatments that include hammams, steam baths (see p48) and steam cabinets (see p49).

Bania

If not for Russia's closed-door policy in the 1900s, the world may have become more familiar with the word 'bania' or 'banya' instead of 'sauna'. The Russian bath has been more widely chronicled than its Finnish counterpart and is widely credited for the Russians' reputation for robustness.

A Russian bania has a more boisterous atmosphere than a Finnish sauna. Bathers may whip each other with *venniks* (switches made of birch, oak, eucalyptus, linden or juniper twigs), with an aromatic scent emitting from the oils of the twigs. Ideally, a bathhouse attendant will whip you with a *vennik* to ensure that you get the most out of its massaging effect. The bania is viewed as a cure-all even today, in remote villages that still practice folk medicine.

Some banias resemble wooden Finnish saunas (see pp45–46) but the hot air within is usually wetter. Special oils such as mint or eucalyptus may be added to the water and ladled over the hot stones. Different types of banias in the former Soviet Union include Islamic- and Roman-inspired ones, and portable sweat baths akin to North American Indian sweat lodges. In Siberia, turf or clay may be used in a bania's construction. The Russian equivalent of the Finnish sauna is the black bania found in the northwest, while the white banias in cities are so popular that it is barely possible to maintain a high temperature within. Russians find the warmth of their banias especially welcome during the harsh winters, but they are also used throughout the year after exercise or sports.

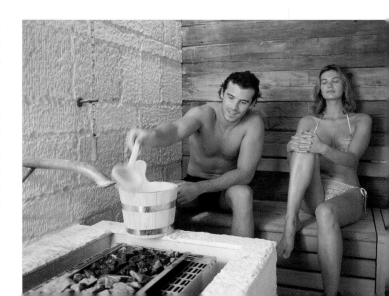

DRY HEAT TREATMENTS

While the steam room (see p48) uses the moist heat of water vapour, the air in the sauna is hot and dry. Dry heat encourages the body to perspire profusely, and thus detoxify itself. The humidity—moisture content in the air—in a dry heat room may be as low as 10 per cent, compared to that of 92 to 97 per cent in a wet heat room. Perspiration evaporates rapidly, cooling your skin and making the room appear cooler than it actually is. Your body does not feel as sweaty as it would in a steam room, but it is important to remember that you are still losing water from your body, and you should drink plenty of fluids after your treatment to rehydrate your body. It is also important to watch your time in a dry heat room to avoid running into breathing difficulties and getting your lungs parched.

Sauna

The sauna is typically a room with pine walls, floors and benches, and a stove of heated stones. Water is ladled over the stones from time to time to raise the temperature, moisten the dry air, and produce beneficial negative ions (see pp56–57) that bring about a feeling of wellbeing. Sauna connoisseurs may swear by wood-burning stoves that give off a gentler, even heat and aromatic scent, but electrical stoves are generally more feasible in many modern spas.

The heat stimulates circulation, and relaxes and refreshes your body and mind. You may even find yourself sleeping more soundly at night. Besides easing muscular and joint aches and stiffness, saunas may be used to treat certain ailments such as allergies, arthritis and poor circulation.

If you are new to the sauna experience, many sauna proponents suggest you start with a shorter session of about five to eight minutes. According to the Finnish Sauna Society, there are no rules as to how long you should stay in the sauna (though other proponents suggest 15 to 20 minutes as the average): it depends on the temperature, humidity and above all, your comfort. Do not remain in the sauna to the point of feeling faint or uncomfortable. Swimsuits are typically not encouraged in saunas for they constrict circulation and inhibit sweating. If you are bashful, wrap a towel around your waist or drape one over your shoulders.

To help your body adapt to the heat, start on the lower bench and gradually move upwards towards the ceiling where it is hotter. Sit on a towel for hygiene reasons. Follow the heat session with an invigorating and energising cold shower or a dip in a cold pool—or where available, a swim in a lake or in the sea (in winter, a hole may be cut in the ice for this purpose), or a roll in the snow. Most sauna aficionados describe this change in temperature as euphoric. With your skin temperature lowered by the cold, your body heat escapes more slowly than usual, allowing you to enjoy the cold comfortably.

You may want to have a massage before returning to the sauna and repeating the cycle. Repeated exposures are said to help your sweat flow more easily.

True Finnish saunas come with *vihtas* or *vastas* (whisks, usually composed of birch twigs) to flick water on to the stones, and to periodically beat your body with to increase circulation and encourage perspiration and detoxification.

While experts cannot say for certain if the Finns invented the sauna, taking a sauna has been an integral part of life in Finland for centuries. Saunas outnumber cars in Finland, which also has the largest number of saunas per capita. The sauna is ubiquitous, found in apartment blocks, on cargo ships, and in the parliament house in Helsinki. Finns, whose sauna tradition dates back to about two thousand years ago, use the sauna about once a week, or daily if on vacation.

Many spas and health clubs feature saunas. Within its comforting womb-like environment, users knowingly or unknowingly heed the Finnish saying, 'In the sauna, one must conduct himself as one would in church'—that is, no loud talking, no arguing, no reading of newspapers—an age-old belief so as not to disturb the spirits that reside within. Saunas in spas are often segregated, reflecting the current Finnish practise that men and women do not sauna together.

Sauna detoxification therapy uses sweating, exercise, and lifestyle changes to treat alcoholics, drug addicts, people with multiple chemical sensitivities, and people suffering from the side effects of prescription medications.

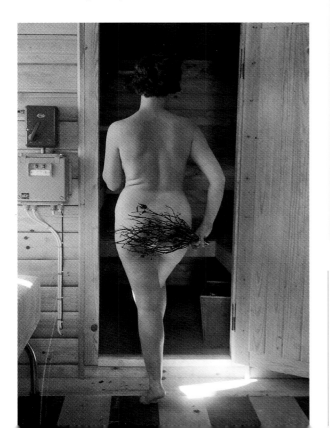

How to Take a Finnish Sauna
The Finnish Sauna Society has some suggestions for people who may not be familiar with the ritual:
- Give yourself enough time—at least half an hour.
- After changing out of your clothes, take a brief shower or dip in a pool to moisten your skin before entering the sauna. This also helps wash off any bodily odours.
- Bring a towel into the sauna to sit on.
- When you first enter the sauna, the temperature should be around 80 to 90 °C (176 to 194 °F), but no higher than 100 °C (212 °F). If the air is dry, you can increase the humidity by throwing water on the stones in the stove. Do not use your *vihta* as your skin has yet to soften sufficiently.
- Leave the sauna when you feel hot enough, and cool off by taking a shower, going for a swim or sitting outside at room temperature. Drink water—never alcohol—if you feel thirsty.
- When you re-enter the sauna, it should be more humid than before. After your body warms up, tap it with your *vihta*.
- Leave the room to cool off again.
- You can repeat the hot-cold cycle and use the *vihta* as many times as you are comfortable. Most people find two hot-cold cycles sufficient.
- Return to the sauna to warm up briefly to soften your skin before proceeding to wash up.
- After washing yourself, you may want to return to the sauna, and enjoy it at a lower temperature.
- Take a shower or go for a swim.
- Towel yourself dry or let yourself dry naturally by sitting in room temperature. You may want to lie down and rest.
- Have a refreshing drink and a salty snack.
- Give yourself sufficient time to cool down and stop sweating before changing into a clean set of clothes. Be sure to keep yourself warm after a sauna.

LEFT: Beating your heat-softened body with vihtas *creates a sensation similar to brushing your body with a loofah (which some saunas provide to enhance circulation and remove dead skin cells). The twigs also add a pleasant aroma to the experience. Before the advent of soap, the chemicals from the birch leaves cleansed the body.*

OPPOSITE, TOP LEFT: 'Avanto' in Finnish refers to a hole cut through a frozen lake or sea—often for sauna-goers to have a quick dip between or after sessions.

OPPOSITE, BOTTOM: The feel-good sensations you get in a bakery are triggered by the scent of freshly baked bread. Bread-baths work on a similar premise.

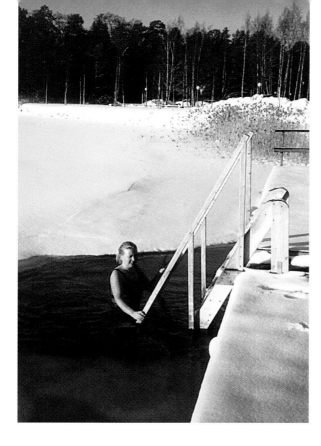

Vibratory Sauna

People with difficulty breathing in hot air or who find wooden benches uncomfortable may prefer the more personal vibratory sauna which bathes your supine body in dry heat as it is relaxed by the vibrating bed and aromatic oils, and may even be combined with coloured rays of light (see pp91–92). You can control the temperature, internal fan, and built-in stereo from within the capsule, which resembles a couch with a lid on top. It can be used in conjunction with therapies such as aromatherapy massage (see p72), body wraps and cellulite treatments, though the vibratory sauna is popularly used to help slimming, simulate exercise, and relieve sports injuries, arthritic and rheumatic pain. It is also used by jockeys and boxers, for whom weight is crucial. It is not to be used if you have certain medical conditions, a sunburn, a cold or fever.

Bread-Bath

Baking bread appears to be one of the most unlikely activities to inspire a heat treatment, yet there are several historical and cultural references to it. The Swiss were known to have shoved a patient into an oven that had just been used for baking bread, using the cooling oven's residual heat to help ease the patient's rheumatic problems. Some bakers directed the steam from sweat baths into their ovens for baking bread. This often resulted in tension between the bathhouse and the bakers. Where saunas were unavailable in parts of olden Russia and Finland, bathers—often the poor, or those with jobs such as sweeping chimneys—climbed into the household cooking oven after bread had been baked. While this did not offer the social aspect of bathing in a sauna or bania, a modern-day Bread-Bath—a warm room with a separate oven in it—does.

Many spas offer the Bread-Bath as a welcome addition to their standard repertoire of treatments, and spa-goers are discovering that the whiff of fresh bread also helps ease them into a mellow frame of mind in preparation for the spa treatments to follow. The Bread-Bath may be used as a gentle prelude to another heat treatment, or at the end of a day's treatment, to whet the appetite before dinner or before leaving the spa.

You can stay as long as you like in the Bread-Bath; most people, however, tend to linger for about 30 minutes in the room watching bread bake in the old-style oven. You will be able to sample some of the bread during the session, if not later at the spa's restaurant. The session may be shared by a group of about six to ten people. During the Bread-Bath session, you may wear a swimsuit or a bathrobe.

Modern research indicates that that the enzymes released by the scent of the baking bread trigger the release of feel-good hormones in your body. Combining the aromatic benefits of standing in front of a bakery and taking a moderate dry heat treatment, the Bread-Bath is likely to leave you with a sense of wellbeing, and feeling physically regenerated. You may want to be cautious about participating in this experience, however, if you are allergic to leavened bread.

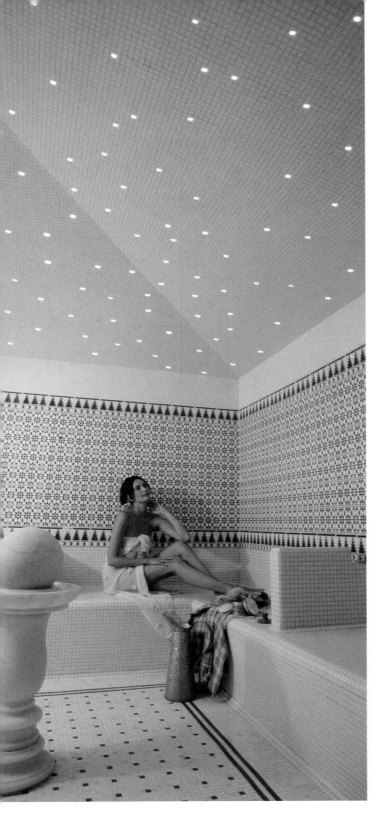

WET HEAT TREATMENTS

Unlike saunas (see pp45–46), which use the dry heat of heated air, steam baths utilise the wet heat of water vapour. Steam is produced by a boiler, but on mixing with air, it cools and condenses, leaving the air in the steam bath saturated. Your sweat cannot evaporate, so it has no cooling effect, and just runs off your skin. The steam encourages you to sweat faster and more intensely, and your skin always feels moist. European spa towns and some spas may have elaborate steam baths housed in large buildings with several rooms, like those of the Romans and the Turks; but most spas are likely to have at least a steam room or a steam cabinet.

Steam Room

Steam rooms may be designed for individuals, or for groups of up to eight people. Vents sporadically emit vapour to keep the small tiled room steam-filled. The wet heat aids detoxification and helps relax your muscles. Some steam rooms may be infused with essential oils (see pp70–72) or herbs such as eucalyptus. These give off a pleasant vapour, clear the head, and decongest the chest.

Facial Steaming with Garden Herbs

Home facial steaming using herbs is easy and fun to do, and it's a wonderful way to bring nature's freshness into your facial. Here's a recipe from The Spa at Pennyhill Park that's not only beneficial for your skin but great for your mind!

Mash and bruise your herbs so their oils disperse better into the water. Try rosemary (antiseptic; aids mental clarity); camomile (with anti-inflammatory properties); lavender (calms and heals); and rose (sweet, floral; uplifts tired skin).

Prepare your skin by cleansing and exfoliating. Then fill a large wash bowl with hot water and add your bruised herbs or flowers. Place your face just 13 cm (5 in) from the water, with a towel over your head and shoulders to block out the air.

After steaming, spritz with a facial toner, apply your mask, then follow by hydrating your skin with moisturiser.

Steam Cabinet

The forerunner of the individual steam cabinet—where a single person could sit and sweat—was a barrel heated by hot rocks and burning whisky. These Russian or Oriental Baths were popular with Europeans in the Middle Ages. Reinvented and dubbed Turkish baths in 19th-century America, such boxes were available for home use through mail order and travelling salesmen. Touted to cure without medicine, these boxes concealed one's modesty, and could be used in places that lacked plumbing. Variations included one with a boiler that fed steam under a bed cover and a four-poster canopy.

Some spas use steam cabinets with an adjustable seat adaptable to the user's height and comfort. As in a vibratory sauna, your head remains out in the fresh air, and your hair stays dry. Some people may find the steam cabinet less claustrophobic than a steam room, though others may dislike the feeling of being encased.

Rasul

A rasul is an elaborately tiled steam chamber that is crowned with a domed ceiling of starlights resembling the night sky in the northern hemisphere. After taking a short shower, you will apply different coloured therapeutic muds (see pp79–80)—the colours created from their geological composition—to different parts of your body, and bask in the steamy heat which passes through a sachet of herbs. The mud hardens, but as the humidity in the room rises, the mud gradually liquefies, and you may feel a slight prickly feeling as your body is cleansed. As you rub off the liquefying mud, you are removing dead cells and impurities from your skin. After about 20 minutes of heat, warm water rains down from the ceiling, rinsing off the mud from your body, though you may need to use the hand hoses as well. This exotic ritual is relaxing, cleansing and detoxifying. Your skin feels silky smooth and your muscles relaxed. The rasul is an excellent way to prepare your body for a massage.

OPPOSITE: Many modern steam rooms such as this one at Better Living Institute at Hotel Royal – Royal Parc Evian in France are elaborately tiled. Steam rooms in spas may incorporate the use of colour therapy (in the form of a play of coloured lights shining from above through the steam, see pp91–92) and/or crystal therapy (in the form of a large crystal, see p78).

RIGHT: This historical picture depicts a woman taking a personal steam bath, often dubbed a Turkish bath, in an attempt to curb smoking.

FAR RIGHT: A rasul provides a convivial atmosphere for couples or friends to enjoy the heat treatment together, and the playfulness of applying mud to each other's bodies. Many rasuls are designed to hold up to groups of two to four friends.

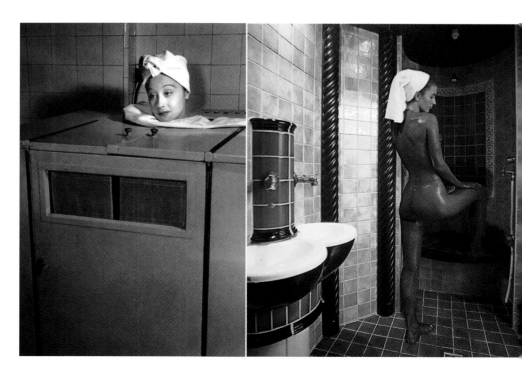

ALPINE TREATMENTS

Farmers living in cold alpine climates discovered that the powers of fire combined with plants and herbs grown at altitude produced a soothing warmth that was relaxing and regenerative, especially after a day's backbreaking work. Old documents also tell of how the ill were wrapped in herbs, flax or hemp. These centuries-old practices have since been adapted for use in a therapeutic setting with the help of historians and medical practitioners. You can enjoy these warming treatments such as the hay bath (see p75), Kraxen-Stove and Farmer's Steam Bath (see p51) at numerous modern spas around Europe that have fashioned a charming rustic setting to recreate the treatments' rural origins, as if to transport you out of a fast-paced modern lifestyle back to a time when life was simpler.

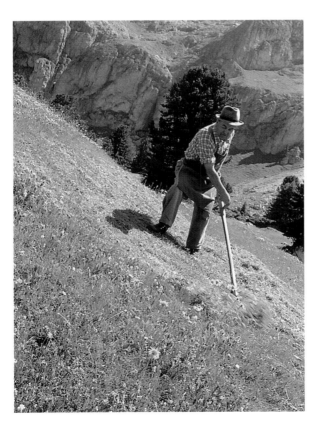

Kraxen-Stove

The Kraxen-Stove comes from 'kraxe', which in an Austrian dialect refers to the homemade baskets that Alpine farmers used to transport hay from the meadows high in the mountains to their homes in valleys. Kraxen-Stoves were inspired by stoves in the living rooms of farms in the alpine regions of Bavaria and Austria. Here, each family huddled around for warmth and companionship on dreary winter evenings. The grandfather of the household usually held the prime seat in the stove's niche, against which he placed a basket of herbs next to the stove. From this, the scent of fresh hay emanated, while the heat soothed his back, shoulders and rheumatic problems.

A Kraxen-Stove in a modern spa is designed with three or more individual niches. Each niche comes with a wooden grating which holds the alpine hay, and each spa-goer receives a pillow of hay to sit on. You will enjoy the therapeutic benefits of a gentle herbal steam on your back, shoulders, pelvis and sides of your body. The heat warms and relaxes your muscles, stimulates your metabolism, and is said to have a stronger detoxifying effect than a usual sauna session. Inhaling the herbal steam that fills the room once the stove has started also helps to relax your respiratory tract.

During this treatment, which lasts for about 30 minutes, you may wear a swimsuit or disposable underwear. Once you have made yourself comfortable on the Kraxen-Stove seat, the therapist will cover the front of your body with a fleece-lined sheet

LEFT: Besides inspiring heat treatments, the alpine region has contributed to spa treatments in terms of unique plants grown in the pure air at altitude.

OPPOSITE, LEFT: You can enjoy the social interaction that originally accompanied the Kraxen-Stove with a group of friends, or have an opportunity to make new ones among other spa-goers. You do not have to visit the Alps to enjoy the Kraxen-Stove. Spas such as Thermae Bath Spa offer this traditional yet medically based heat and hay treatment.

OPPOSITE, RIGHT: Old wooden beams and copper ceilings give the Farmer's Steam Bath the feel of an old brechelbath.

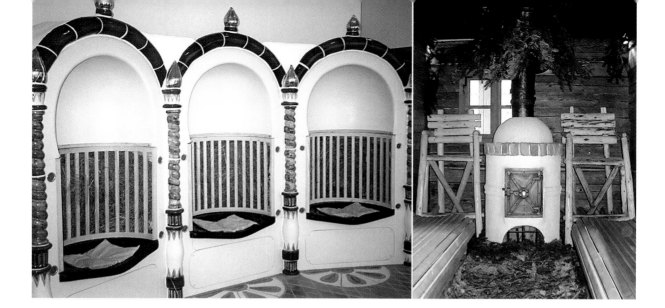

and affix it to either side of the stove to ensure that the herbal steam will stay on your body. The stove emits four minutes of steam at two-minute intervals.

A Kraxen-Stove session is best followed by a massage, as the treatment warms and relaxes your muscles. However, you should rest for at least ten minutes after this heat treatment to give your body time to relax and absorb the active ingredients of the herbal steam. The Kraxen-Stove session benefits people looking for a general relaxing and detoxifying treatment, as well as those with rheumatic diseases.

You should not take this treatment if you have any inflammations, open wounds, heart or metabolism problems, high blood pressure, or are pregnant. Avoid this treatment if you are also having a solarium session or have been suntanning.

Farmer's Steam Bath

The dry heated room where flax or hemp was prepared for weaving inspired the 18th-century *brechelbath* (from the old Bavarian word '*brecheln*', which means 'breaking'), the forerunner of the Farmer's Steam Bath. In the 18th century, flax or hemp was dried, broken (with a device known as a '*flaxbrechel*' or 'flax breaker') and steamed several times over before it could be woven into a fabric. Farmers soon noticed that herbs introduced during the process—either deliberately or by accident—gave the room a pleasant aroma and a comforting ambience. The idea for bathing in this gentle herbal steam may have stemmed from the tales of Islamic baths in the Middle East told by returning crusaders. Baths were usually taken on the eve of religious holidays, as if signifying a physical and mental renewal.

The modern-day Farmer's Steam Bath is a wooden room heated with a stove on which herbs are steamed. As you relax on the wooden seats, the herbal steam from the stove rises and penetrates the *tschurtschenkorb*—a metal basket of fir cones and conifer branches—hanging from the ceiling.

The steam, which is drawn to the ceiling and then down the walls, provides a comforting heat to your spinal area, relaxing your muscles. It also helps relax your lungs and leaves you with a feeling of wellbeing. The fir needles and branches that line the floor stimulate the reflex zones on your feet.

You may sweat profusely during a session, as the temperature is about 55 degrees Celsius (131 degrees Fahrenheit), and the atmosphere more akin to a steam room (see p48) than a sauna (see pp45–46). Natural oils released as you step on the fir needles also help fragrance the room and condition the skin on your feet. You may stay in for as long as you feel comfortable, though 30 minutes is the average. The purifying treatment will leave you with a sense of wellbeing. Depending on the culturally accepted norm in the region, guests may wear nothing or a swimsuit in this room, which is usually designed to hold six to ten people. Do not have this treatment if you feel unwell, and inform the spa beforehand if you have any medical problems, especially inflammation problems, open wounds, problems with your heart or metabolism, or high blood pressure. As always, if in any doubt, consult your doctor beforehand.

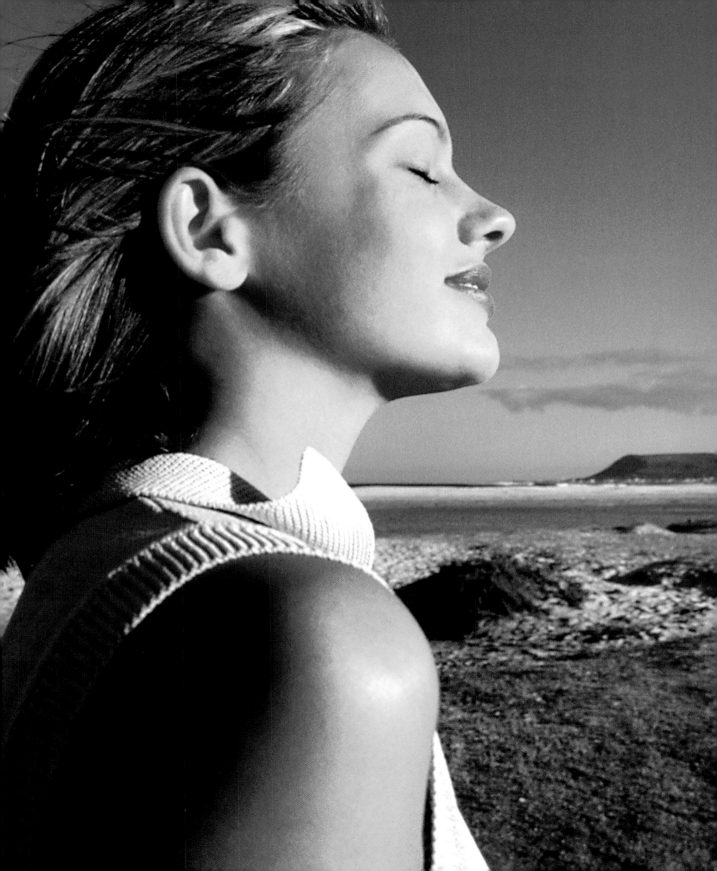

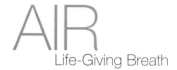

AIR
Life-Giving Breath

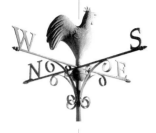

A ir is the most crucial element required for survival. You can live for weeks without food, exist for days without water, but survive only a few minutes without air. From the time you are born to the moment you die, you instinctively connect to the invisible element of air, inhaling air from your surroundings through your breath.

In the Bible, breath is life-giving and God-given. This can be seen in Genesis when the Creator breathed into Adam's nostrils when He made man. Further underscoring air's relation to breath and life, ancient Greek philosopher Anaximenes theorised that all living matter on earth was made of air, which he called *'pneuma'* (Greek for 'breath').

When you breathe, oxygen from the air creates energy that allows your body and mind to function. Paying attention to your breathing habits, and ensuring that you have adequate oxygen in your body is crucial to productive functioning and coping with stress. It is also no coincidence that many of us instinctively seek out purer air by flocking to holiday spots on the coast, by the lakes and in the mountains. Additionally, some spas promote the therapeutic benefits of pure air in what is known as climatotherapy (see pp56–57).

In a spa, you are likely to come across various breathing techniques in exercises such as yoga (see pp64–65 and 102) and *qi gong* (see pp65 and 101), and in elements of meditation (see p63) and visualisation (see p64). Your spa therapist may also guide you in your breathing to help relax your body, allowing you to optimise the benefits of the treatment, along with the use of massages (see pp92–97) and essential oils (see pp70–72), which help oxygenate your skin.

In the gym, your fitness instructor can show you how to breathe properly in order to benefit fully from exercise, which not only increases your flexibility, strength and sense of wellbeing, but also increases the amount of oxygen in your body.

The element of air may also be harnessed through inhalation, oxygen and ozone therapies (see pp48, and 58–61). Some of these have to be administered in a medical setting.

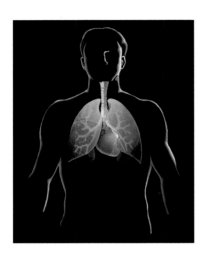

> **Oxygen is our source of life.
> The more oxygen
> we are able to enjoy,
> the more we can
> partake of life itself.**
>
> *– Nathaniel Altman,* Oxygen Healing Therapies

THE RESPIRATORY PROCESS

Air is composed of a stable composition of gases, but their proportions change as you breathe. The proportion of oxygen is lower, and of carbon dioxide higher in the air that you exhale than in the air you inhale. As you inhale, you breathe in about 21 per cent oxygen, 78 per cent nitrogen and 0.3 per cent carbon dioxide. However, when you breathe out, you are exhaling approximately 17 per cent oxygen, 78 per cent nitrogen and 4 per cent carbon dioxide.

When you inhale, air passes through your windpipe into a network of tubes known as bronchioles, and then into millions of tiny air sacs in your lungs known as alveoli. From the alveoli the oxygen passes into your bloodstream. The oxygenated blood, pumped by your heart, is then delivered to your body cells where the oxygen breaks down food to produce energy. During this process, carbon dioxide is produced as waste, and is carried back to the lungs where it is exhaled. Your blood picks up more oxygen and the cycle continues.

Our bodies need oxygen to metabolise the food we eat and turn it into energy. When we use our lungs to their full breathing potential, we optimise our energy. Besides maintaining our lungs' elasticity and strength, benefits include improved posture, reduced stress levels and increased circulation.

Carbon dioxide is often viewed as a waste gas that is excreted when you exhale. However, British doctor John Haldane debunked the widely held notion of carbon dioxide as poison, stating that the body needs a necessary balance of oxygen and carbon dioxide. The level of carbon dioxide in your body, detected by your brain, influences your breathing, and the release of oxygen to your cells. Carbon dioxide also governs your body's acid-alkali balance—or 'potential of hydrogen (pH) balance'—that helps to maintain your immune system.

The way we breathe affects the amount of oxygen in our bodies. Breathing is a natural and instinctive process controlled by our nervous system—and yet, most of us do not breathe properly. Many breathwork practitioners point out that most people breathe too rapidly and irregularly.

PAGE 52: The purity of the surrounding air and our breathing habits affect our entire psyche.

PAGE 53: The ancient Greeks, who built the first weather vanes, believed that winds had divine powers.

TOP: Be aware of the quality of the air around you, as smoke, chemicals, pollution, dust, pollens and viruses can enter your lungs with your every breath.

OPPOSITE: This c.1860 illustration on an educational plate depicts French chemist Antoine Laurent de Lavoisier (1743–1794) experimenting on the respiration of a human. Lavoisier put forward the widely held notion of oxygen as a life-giver and carbon dioxide as a poison.

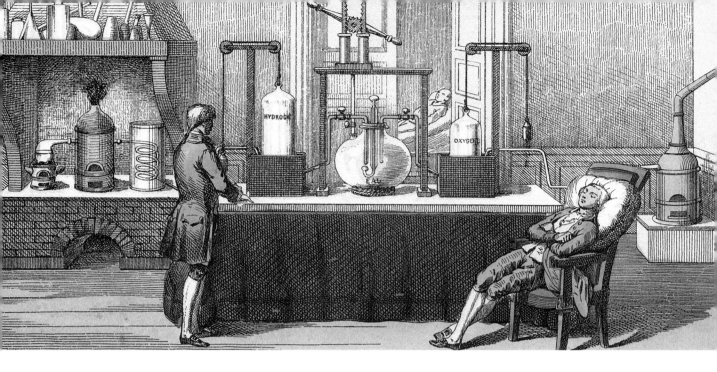

It is also true that some people, especially asthmatics, are taking in more air than their bodies can handle, say breathwork practitioners at London's Hale Clinic.

Poor breathing techniques often reflect the states of our minds and emotions. When we are stressed or tensed, we tend to hold our breaths or breathe irregularly—and over time, we forget how to breathe freely and rhythmically. In what can become a vicious cycle, our emotions influence our breathing, and our breathing can influence our emotions.

Besides our highly stressed lifestyles, by-products of modern living—pollutants in the air, and a diet high in fat—can also be to blame for oxygen deficiency. When the body is deprived of oxygen, it reacts in a negative way. Toxic residues are not completely removed, and our blood does not get enough oxygen to feed our tissues. This can lead to a host of complaints such as backaches, headaches, muscle aches, dizziness and anxiety attacks. We complain of lethargy, irritability, and difficulty concentrating and sleeping. It may also manifest itself in premature wrinkles, and unhealthy hair and nails.

More alarmingly, oxygen deficiency has also been associated with a weakened immune system, and Nobel Prize winner Dr Otto Warburg linked it to diseases such as cancer.

While Greek philosopher Anaximenes (c. 570–500 B.C.) put forward the notion that all living matter was composed of air, the concept of 'pneuma' subsequently became associated with the spirit or vital life force that is believed to pervade all living things. This connectivity between the air, your breath, and your body, mind and spirit is echoed in other cultures where the word for 'breath', too, refers to life's vital energy. In India, it is known as 'prana' and the Chinese call it 'qi'.

As the following pages show, you can help your body and mind function more efficiently through a variety of therapies that harness the element of air—and combine these therapies with a few lifestyle changes. Try to reduce your exposure to pollution, and if you are a smoker, kick the habit. You may also want to start paying more attention to getting a nutritious and balanced diet that includes food high in antioxidants.

Regular exercise not only keeps you in shape, and lifts your mood and self-esteem—it also improves your breathing by helping your body function more efficiently. It benefits your respiratory system by helping to increase the efficiency of your lungs and cardiovascular system. Your muscles require less oxygen as you make more efficient use of your respiratory system. You may find that your interest in exercise or a new activity will be piqued by a visit to a spa's gym, which offers options such as aerobics, tennis, or even more seemingly sedentary exercises such as tai ji (see p101), qi gong (see pp65 and 101) and yoga (see pp64–65 and 102).

TREATMENTS AND THERAPIES

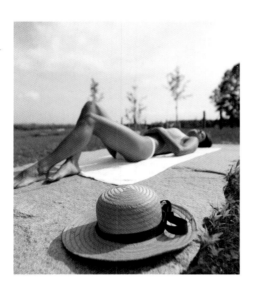

**Life is in the breath.
Therefore, he who only
half breathes, half lives.**

– *Old proverb*

TOP: *The sun's rays can also be a double-edged sword. Enjoy the outdoors, but practise safe sunning by wearing suitable sunscreen, covering up with a hat and avoiding the sun from between 10 A.M. and 3 P.M. when its rays are strongest or when the ultraviolet (UV) index is high.*

OPPOSITE: *Wide open spaces, pure air, and exposure to negative ions help increase your energy level and sense of wellbeing.*

CLIMATOTHERAPY

Climatotherapy harnesses facets of the environment—such as air, climate, atmosphere, temperature, humidity and light—to heal. It is a branch of medical climatology, which studies the environment and its influence on health and disease.

Traditionally, many people have moved from one climate to another in order to treat their health problems. Those with tuberculosis or blood problems, for example, often convalesced in the mountains, while others with bronchitis and rheumatism took to the seaside. Even earlier in history, ancient peoples such as the Incas would place their invalids on the mountaintops, exposing them to fresh air and sunlight.

These days, many people take to the mountains, seasides, lakes and rivers for a holiday to escape and recharge themselves from the stresses of modern life. Besides having the opportunity to take part in the various outdoor leisure and sporting activities that these areas offer, vacationers can get back in touch with nature, soak up some scenic beauty, and enjoy plenty of opportunities to breathe in clean, fresh air.

The air in these mountainous, wooded or seaside areas is often rich in electrically charged particles known as negative ions which are released by water in motion. Negative ions help ease tension and make us feel full of life and energy. Polluted city air, in comparison, is heavy with positive ions that hinder the brain from releasing serotonin, which contributes to our sense of wellbeing—one reason why city dwellers often suffer from high levels of lethargy and irritability.

In Europe, there are a number of holiday destinations known as climate heath resorts. Climate resorts are typically located at an altitude of over 400 metres (1,310 feet) above sea level, in sprawling grounds and heavily wooded areas.

Therapies in these resorts relate to the area and climate, and often include outdoor exercises and terrain cures—taking a walk along hiking paths within the grounds, for example. These walks not only increase your fitness—you also gain exposure to the beneficial negative ions emitted by the forest to complement other therapies you may be receiving.

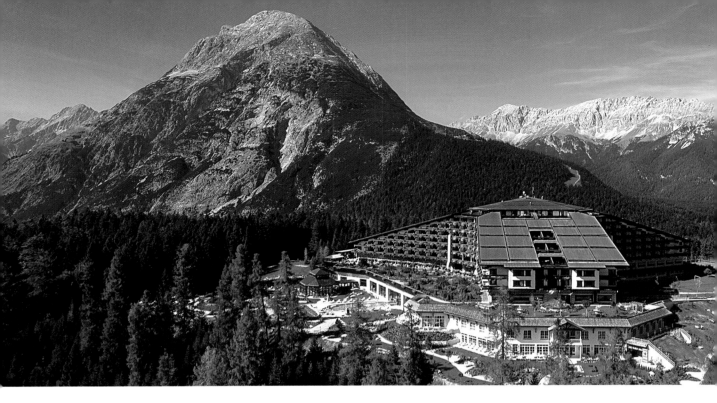

Many climate health resorts have medical staff and facilities, and also offer a range of therapies ranging from acupuncture to lymphatic drainage massage. While they are geared towards health, relaxation, and activities that emphasise a oneness with nature and the environment, many also have cultural activities related to music, regional cuisine and festivals.

Different climate conditions are recommended for various health problems. According to the Federation of Climatic Health Resorts of Germany, those destinations with a bracing climate are good for hardening the body and maintaining health, while destinations with benign climates are recommended for acute health problems and convalescence. Health problems commonly treated by climate resorts may include heart, respiratory, skin, rheumatic, gynaecological, kidney and psychosomatic problems, as well as childhood illnesses.

In a thalassotherapy centre, where the cure is administered through the focused use of seawater and marine-derived products such as seaweed, you will also be encouraged to take walks along the seashore to benefit from the maritime climate and the sea air laden with negative ions.

Climatotherapy at the lowest point on earth, Israel's Dead Sea, is recognised especially for treating psoriasis. It takes the form of a controlled exposure to the sun's long-wave ultraviolet-B (UVB) rays, and bathing in the area's exceptionally saline and mineral-rich waters. The air here is also allergen-free, and has a higher oxygen density than air at sea level.

Enhancing the Air at Home

If you are feeling sluggish in your home, it could be because there are too many positive ions present. The culprits include chemicals present in synthetic materials, chemical cleaners and pesticides, and electromagnetic radiation from electrical equipment such as computers. Stimulate and energise your living space and yourself by

- Using an ioniser that emits negative ions, especially in rooms which hold electrical equipment.
- Adding plants to help oxygenate your home and absorb toxic fumes (they also beautify your surroundings).
- Keeping your home well-ventilated.
- Opening your windows twice a day to let in fresh air.
- Ensuring that your heaters, boilers and air-conditioners are regularly serviced.
- Going outside frequently, especially to the park to take in some fresh air.

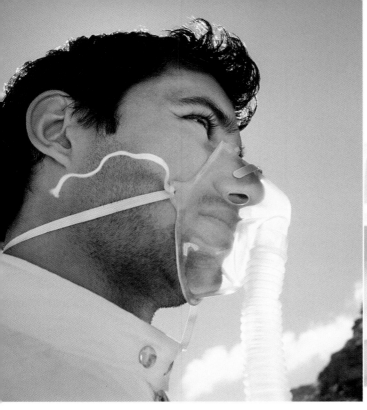

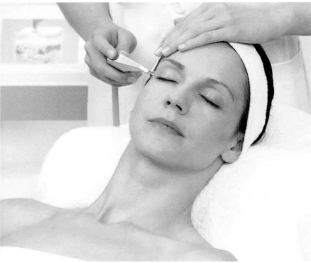

OXYGEN THERAPY

Besides making up about 21 per cent of air, oxygen also makes up about 62 per cent of the earth's crust, 90 per cent of water, and 65 per cent of our bodies, making it the most abundant element on our planet. This colourless, odourless and tasteless gas, which is essential for all life to exist, is a little denser than air and slightly soluble in water.

The term 'oxygen therapy' describes a wide range of treatments, such as medical oxygen therapy and the therapeutic use of ozone (see p60). It is also used to describe spa treatments that supplement your body and skin with oxygen, which are not to be confused with the often critical life-supporting roles that oxygen plays in hospitals.

In a spa, oxygen may be applied to your skin as part of a facial or an eye treatment, administered through inhalation (see p59), or used in anti-cellulite treatments. Oxygen may also be delivered to the body via a steam capsule or a body bag. In this procedure, your body is first exfoliated, after which oxygen will circulate around your body for about 10 to 15 minutes. A mask or wrap is then applied to your body for 20 to 30 minutes. During this therapy session, you may also breathe in oxygen to help you relax further. Oxygen may also be applied to your hair in a similar method: after the application of a hair mask, a hair bag will be placed around your hair, and oxygen and steam will be allowed to circulate.

Oxygenating products that you may encounter in a spa or that you can purchase for home use include creams and facial sprays. Suppliers of oxygenated bottled water or portable drops that you can add to your drinking water say that regular internal use increases the level of oxygen in your body, detoxifies your body, boosts your energy, reduces stress-related symptoms such as headaches and fatigue, promotes healthy hair, nails and skin, and contributes to feelings of wellbeing.

Oxygen Facial

An oxygen facial supplies your skin with more oxygen than it would otherwise receive from the surroundings, to help alleviate damage caused by free radicals, reduce the appearance of fine lines and clear your complexion.

Using a handheld nozzle, the therapist applies oxygen infused with a liquid ampoule to your face in small, deliberate motions over your muscular lines. Applied as a fine mist, the oxygen and nutrients penetrate your skin to help strengthen your collagen and elastin fibres, oxygenate your cells, and destroy bacteria that cause acne. The ampoule would have been chosen according to your skin's type and needs.

As with other facial treatments, you are likely to be kept warmly wrapped in blankets. During colder months, hot towels may be used to keep your feet warm, while in warmer months, this treatment can help bring relief to sunburn.

Alternatively, the oxygen component may be enjoyed on its own, or used in conjunction with a facial involving other products that contain substances such as botanical or marine extracts, which can also aid the oxygenation process. Oxygen may also be used before or after facial surgery or laser treatments to help enhance healing, or after microdermabrasion (see below) to help relieve the stinging sensation.

Another form of the oxygen facial uses a pulsed pressure of oxygen—likened to a needle-free, non-paralytic version of Botox. This helps deliver specially formulated serums into the deeper layers of your skin around your forehead, eyes and mouth so the active ingredients can work efficiently. The process helps relax the facial muscles responsible for the formation of wrinkles and increases the formation of collagen.

Oxygen may also be used to combat irritation during microdermabrasion: a process that resurfaces your skin by blasting its surface with a flow of fine crystals.

Oxygen Breathing Therapy

When we talk about something being 'like a breath of fresh air', we are unconsciously affirming our appreciation of the positive state of mind that results from inhaling air's most precious and life-sustaining component: oxygen.

In a spa, oxygen may be inhaled through a nasal tube or face mask as a treatment on its own, or in conjunction with a facial or body treatment to enhance your sense of wellbeing. Spas in airports in many major cities offer the use of oxygen bars and lounges to help counter the negative effects of jet lag and stale cabin air. You may also find oxygen bars in fashionable establishments in major cities, where you can also listen to music and have a drink. The popularity of such bars was fuelled by celebrity oxygen users such as actor Woody Harrelson, who opened his own oxygen bar in the United States.

During an inhalation session, you may choose to incorporate specific essential oils (see pp70–72) into the session for their various physiological benefits. These may include bergamot to combat stress and lift your mood, lemon to invigorate your mind, and lavender to balance, soothe and relax you.

Users report that oxygen inhalation helps relieve stress and awaken the mind, and helps them breathe better. Your therapist should perform a comprehensive consultation before administering oxygen inhalation. Consult a doctor first if you have heart or breathing problems, or are pregnant.

OPPOSITE, LEFT: People at very high altitudes—for example, mountain climbers—may suffer oxygen deprivation and may need to use oxygen masks to ensure an adequate supply.

OPPOSITE, RIGHT: Celebrities are among the people who swear by oxygen facials to boost their complexion, and help reduce the appearance of fine lines. The Oxyjet excretes 99 per cent pure oxygen through a refined pressure that comes out of a pen-like attachment. This refined pressure is enough to fully pump the different serums through the skin to its deepest layers.

RIGHT: Like many Japanese trends that influenced the world, Tokyo's air stations—where oxygen was dispensed through vending machines—were the inspiration behind oxygen bars. Oxygen bars are often touted as the urban alternative for people who are unable to escape to fresh air in the mountains or by the sea.

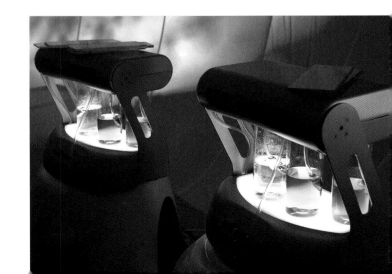

OZONE THERAPY

Ozone, from the Greek word *'ozein'* which means 'smell', was so named by German chemist Christian Frederick Schönbein in 1840 because of its particular scent.

Ozone is made up of three atoms of oxygen (O_3). It is active but unstable, and quickly breaks down into oxygen. In nature, ozone is produced when ultraviolet energy causes oxygen atoms to cluster in threes, or when there is lightning. Similarly, ozone generators work by passing an electric charge through a condenser containing oxygen.

In Europe, in particular Germany and the former Soviet Union, minuscule amounts of ozone combined with oxygen are used to treat a wide range of health problems including chronic fatigue, cancer and AIDS. Ozone can inactivate bacteria, viruses, fungi and toxins; oxidise certain poisons; and neutralise odours. It also helps increase blood circulation and strengthens the immune system. Its disinfecting properties may be used to purify drinking water or swimming pools, as it is more environmentally friendly than chlorine, which has been linked to problems such as irritated eyes and cancer.

In a medical spa, the most common method of ozone treatment, autohaemotherapy, involves mixing a small amount of your blood with oxygen and ozone and injecting this into your body. Other methods include introducing ozone through the ear, rectum or vagina. Less invasive is the ozone steam bath (see below). Ozonated water may also be applied externally to treat infections, and ozonated oil to treat skin problems.

A number of practitioners of medical ozone do not advocate breathing in ozone as inhaling it could damage the lungs. The controversy also extends to the use of air purifiers that emit ozone to purify the surrounding air and neutralise odours.

Ozone Steam Bath

An ozone steam bath may be used by both the healthy and ill. About 99 per cent oxygen and 1 per cent ozone are pumped into a specially designed cabinet and mixed with steam. You sit inside and absorb ozone through the pores of your skin. The unit should have proper seals to ensure that you do not inhale the ozone, and your neck area may be wrapped with towels.

The ozone stimulates the antioxidant system and sterilises the skin, eliminating bacteria, viruses and fungi. A session usually lasts from 10 to 15 minutes. As with conventional saunas (see p45–46) or steam baths (see p48), do not spend more time in it than is comfortable, and consult your doctor first if you suffer from any medical conditions. Alcoholics and people with platelet disorders should not have this treatment.

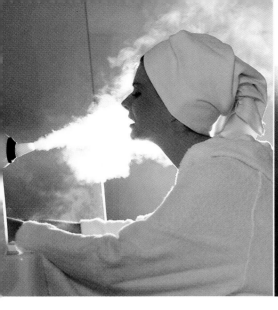

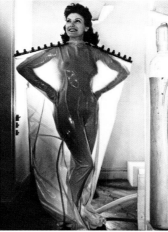

OPPOSITE: Most people associate ozone with the protective layer in the earth's atmosphere which shields us from the damaging effects of too much solar radiation.

FAR LEFT: Inhalation therapies may help you breathe easier, especially if you have a respiratory problem.

LEFT: This historical image shows a woman testing an 'ozone bath', considered in 1951 as a new beauty treatment.

INHALATION THERAPY

Inhalation therapy is not limited to oxygen (see p59). It may involve the use of steam rooms (see p48) infused with herbs and essential oils (see pp70–72) to help decongest the respiratory system; or, in thalassotherapy centres and mineral springs spas, the inhalation of a delicate spray of seawater or mineral water respectively (see below)—a procedure shown to be effective in treating lung, sinus and respiratory problems.

Marine Aerosol

In a thalassotherapy centre, the physician may prescribe inhalation of seawater vapour or use of a marine aerosol to help improve breathing problems associated with smoking or asthma, or to bring relief from a cold. It may also help clear the respiratory passages and unblock nasal mucus, and is typically used to treat respiratory infections, sinusitis and bronchitis. A fine spray of ionised seawater is inhaled through a mask. This is connected to a device in which distilled water is boiled, atop which sits a dish of seawater. A session lasts for 15 minutes.

Inhalation of Mineral Water

In a thermal spa, inhaling a fine mist of mineral water may be recommended to treat respiratory or sinus problems, allergies or asthma. The vapour may be inhaled from a device that resembles a drinking fountain, through a mask, or from an inhaler similar to the kind that asthmatics use. Some spas may also have steam rooms linked to their mineral springs.

Yoga's Nasal Douche

Jal Neti is a yogic cleansing process that douches your nasal passages with a salt solution. A Jal Neti vessel—which resembles a small teapot with a spout—can be purchased from some yoga centres. Jal Neti helps remove inhaled particles and dislodges mucus. Besides clearing your airways, nasal and eye passages, it also improves blood circulation.

Ingredients
2 tsp salt
4 glasses warm water

- Fill the pot with 2 glasses of water and 1 tsp of salt.
- Tilt your head, and place the spout in your right nostril. The water should flow through your right nostril, and out through your left. Breathe through your mouth during the whole process and not through your nose, or water will get into your nasal passages, which can be highly uncomfortable.
- Refill the pot and repeat with your left nostril.

Use Bellows Breath, also known as Bhastrika, to remove any remaining water from your nostrils:

- While standing, put your hands on your hips. Bend foward till your torso is parallel to the floor, bending the knees slightly. Keep your eyes open, and your mouth closed.
- Take a deep breath through your nostrils, relaxing your stomach. Breathe out forcefully and pull in your diaphragm.
- Breathe in and out continuously and quickly through your nose 25 times, turning your head right, left, up and down for one breath in each direction.
- Lie down on your back and relax.

BREATH AWARENESS EXERCISES

Common sayings recognise the relationship between air and our emotions. 'Heavy breathing' is associated with fear, 'second wind' refers to being re-energised, and 'aspire' (from the Latin word '*spirare*', which means 'to breathe') is linked with hope. Many breathing modalities also teach you breathing techniques to use when you feel scared, anxious or angry.

If you are a woman, you may reconnect with your breath during pregnancy when you are taught breathing exercises to help make contractions more bearable and to facilitate delivery. For others, a referral to a psychotherapist or physiotherapist may be your introduction to proper breathing techniques. Singers, actors and orators seek out methods of breathwork to help improve their voices by controlling their breath.

You will often become aware of how you breathe in a spa, as the therapist guides your breathing to help improve the oxygenation in your body, and to relax you. This helps both your body and mind to receive the optimal benefits of the treatment.

Many breathwork practices place an emphasis on your movements and your posture, as both affect your breathing habits. Some popular spa activities involving breathwork are yoga (see pp64–65 and 102) and *qi gong* (see pp65 and 101). Based on Eastern healing philosophies, they are designed to improve the flow of oxygen in the body to help it function more efficiently, and also to allow you to cultivate the flow of the vital energy (see Harmony chapter) in the body. Regular practice helps strengthen your lungs and increase their capacity.

Some experienced practitioners can take five or six breaths per minute, compared to the regular person's average of 15 to 16 breaths. This is one reason why free divers—who dive to great depths and then surface on a single breath of air—often incorporate breath control into their training regime.

These exercises also help improve balance, coordination and posture—easing associated problems such as back problems and fatigue. They are also thought to reduce the effects of ageing and increase the body's defences against illness.

Having better control over your breathing also seems to bring a sense of better control over your life, resulting in an overall sense of wellbeing, increased stamina and energy, and improved alertness and concentration.

Different breathwork practitioners offer differing views as to what constitutes proper breathing. However, they typically agree that it comprises breathing in a relaxed and rhythmic manner to ensure that your body is adequately supplied with oxygen. They also advocate inhaling through your nostrils and not your mouth, although in some instances, exhaling through the mouth is acceptable. Nasal breathing helps filter out germs and unwanted particles, keeps your nasal tract moist, and warms the air before it enters your lungs.

It is important to be guided by a qualified practitioner before trying any breathing exercises on your own. This will ensure that you gain the optimal benefits, do not harm yourself, and have some support in the event that new breathing techniques trigger the release of pent-up emotions. If you feel faint at any

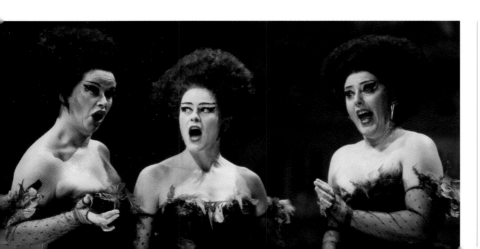

LEFT: Proper posture and breathing techniques are crucial for opera singers. They not only help with performance, but also with their nerves. Singers also train their abdominal muscles to control the amount of air needed for various singing roles. Many singers begin their day with singing exercises which energise them and help clear their nasal passages.

OPPOSITE: Taking 20 minutes out of your busy schedule to meditate can refresh your mind; people who meditate compare it to getting several hours of sleep.

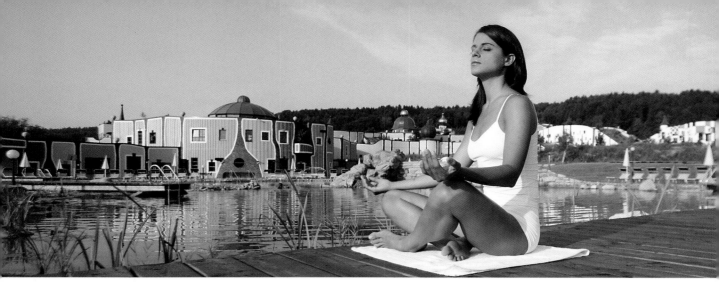

time during a breathing exercise, stop immediately and breathe normally. Certain breathing exercises may also not be suitable for people who are menstruating, pregnant, or suffering from respiratory problems, epilepsy, eye or ear problems, heart problems or high blood pressure. Inform your breathwork practitioner if you have any of these conditions.

It is also suggested that you consult your doctor before starting any new exercise, especially if you have a medical condition or have been sedentary for too long. You may need to undergo a fitness assessment programme.

Meditation

Concentrating on the flow of your breath is a basic focusing tool used in meditation to calm and quiet your mind. During meditation, your breathing, and heart and pulse rates slow down and your brain relaxes. Studies show that people who meditate suffer from fewer illnesses, cope better with daily problems, bounce back quicker from stressful situations, require less sleep, and are more in tune with themselves and their environment. Meditative elements found in religions such as Buddhism, and in the ancient Eastern techniques of yoga and *qi gong*, produce similar benefits.

The best way to learn how to meditate is to join a class, and later meditate on your own. Wear loose clothes during a session, which should take place somewhere warm and quiet. Do not force yourself to meditate longer than comfortable, and do not meditate immediately after a meal or when tired. In the rare instance that disturbing memories surface, stop immediately and seek help from a qualified counsellor. Meditation is not recommended for people with a history of mental illness.

Breathe in the Good, Breathe out the Bad

The next time you feel yourself becoming anxious or angry, try to visualise your body breathing in positive qualities such as courage or patience—and then sending out the negative emotions as you exhale (see p64).

You may also try picturing soothing warm water or healing light as you inhale, and washing away negative aspects as you exhale. Similar visualisation techniques are used in yoga.

Breath Awareness Meditation

- Find a quiet spot where you are unlikely to be interrupted.
- Sit on a chair with both feet on the floor, or alternatively in a cross-legged position on the floor. Make sure you are comfortable.
- Observe the flow of your breath without trying to change it.
- If your mind wanders, gently return it to focus on your breath.
- Do this for about 20 minutes, but never to the point where you have to force yourself.

You can also focus on your breath by
- Concentrating on the sound of your breath.
- Counting each breath either as you inhale or exhale. Count from one to ten, focusing on your breath and the numbers.
- Focusing on the sensation of your breath flowing in and out of your nostrils.

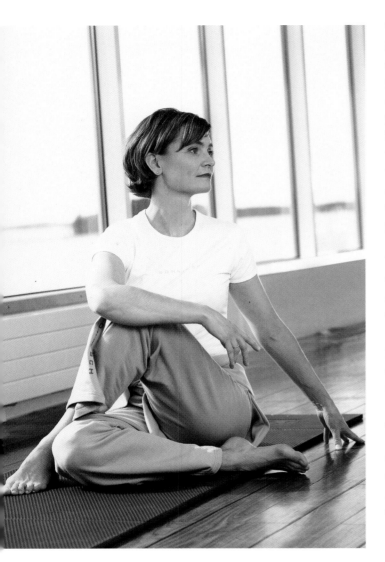

ABOVE: In yoga, you will be taught how to coordinate your breath with each movement.

OPPOSITE: Studies have shown that qi gong *can increase lung capacity from an average of 428.5 to 561.8 cubic centimetres—and up to 1,167.8 cubic centimetres during the exercises.*

Visualisation

Breathing exercises may accompany visualisation: a conscious effort to picture in your mind positive images, or changes that you want to take place in your body or your life. During a guided visualisation session (not to be confused with hypnosis), your therapist will first try to relax you—then direct you to imagine a scene related to your problem, and ask you to describe the physical and emotional sensations related to it. He may then help you to imagine positive images and outcomes to overcome these problems. Visualisation is used to boost motivation and self-image, ease stress-related conditions, eliminate phobias and change negative attitudes.

Yoga

Controlled breathing exercises in yoga are known as *'pranayama'* from *'prana'* (see p87), which means 'life force', and *'yama'*, which means 'regulation of'. *Pranayama* is one of the eight limbs of yoga (see p102), and is most commonly used in *hatha* yoga (see p102). Different schools of yoga have varying approaches, but in the traditional approach, *pranayama* techniques are only taught to advanced students. You first need to learn how to harness *asanas* (postures) to strengthen your body and mind, and how to relax and use your lungs without strain.

Breathwork in yoga includes synchronising your breath with your movements as you perform the *asanas*, and observing your breath flow to aid relaxation. *Pranayama* techniques may also be performed on their own (see p65). Not only do they foster a greater awareness of breathing, increase your lung capacity, and massage your internal organs; they also help your mind look inward to cultivate a calm and an inner strength.

As you become more proficient, you will be taught to extend and vary the ratio of inhalation, retention (holding of the breath after inhalation) and exhalation. Through breathing and concentrating, you will learn how to exercise particular muscles that you normally do not have control over. Most yoga practitioners recommend that you learn breathing techniques from an experienced teacher before trying them on your own.

Cleansing Breath (Kapalabhati)

'*Kapalabhati*' means 'skull shining', though this exercise is also known as the breath of fire. It helps revitalise the mind, clear the respiratory system and massage the organs.

- Stand or sit comfortably, but with your back straight. Close your mouth and look straight ahead.
- Inhale fully and gently through your nose, expanding your abdomen and lungs.
- Exhale quickly, pulling your abdomen towards your spine and pushing the air out of your lungs. Pause for about a second, then breathe in again, taking your time.
- Repeat 25 times.

Do not perform this exercise if you have eye or ear problems, a hernia, high blood pressure, prolapsed organs in your lower abdomen, or an ulcer.

Alternate Nostril Breathing (Anuloma Viloma)

Yogis believe that the right and left nostrils help regulate your body's thermostat and energy. To energise yourself, breathe slowly and deeply through the right nostril. To cool or soothe yourself, close your right nostril and breathe through the left.

- Sit crossed-legged on the floor, or on a chair with a straight back. Close your right nostril using your right thumb, and inhale fully through your left nostril.
- Close the left nostril with your right ring finger. Release your right thumb. Exhale through your right nostril. Now inhale.
- Close your right nostril. Exhale through your left nostril. Then inhale. Release your right nostril and exhale completely.
- This exercise is usually practised for three to five minutes.

Cooling Breath (Sitali Pranayama)

This breath cools you by soothing anger, lowering a fever, and regulating sexual and digestive energy. Initially, a bitter taste on your tongue may indicate that your body is detoxifying. With practice, the exercise may leave a sweet taste in your mouth.

- Sit cross-legged on the floor in a meditative manner with your spine straight. Fold the sides of your tongue upwards (or as far as it will go), and stick it out of your mouth.
- Inhale deeply and smoothly through your tongue. Close your mouth and exhale through your nose.
- This is practised for about five minutes at a time.

Qi Gong

Interestingly, the Chinese character for *qi* (or 'life force', see p86) also translates as 'air' or 'breath'—so in this sense, the term '*qi gong*' may be translated not only as 'energy skill', but also as 'breathing exercise'.

Besides concentrating on the breath and focusing the mind, *qi gong* exercises also involve a set series of postures and movements, all of which interact with one another, producing a continuous self-propagating cycle. Your mind affects your breathing, which in turn benefits your mind; your posture can improve your body's flow of energy, which in turn enhances your breathing and your state of mind.

As with many healing systems that originated in the East, you will typically be taught to focus on your *dan tian*—a point 5 to 8 centimetres (2 to 3 inches) below your navel that is believed to be a major storage place for *qi*—which aids your breathing, boosts your blood circulation and centres your mind.

Breathwork in *qi gong* may centre on breathing naturally and observing the flow of your breath. More advanced breathing techniques include Reverse Breathing—a *qi*-boosting exercise during which the diaphragm sinks on inhalation, and expands on exhalation. This technique may be used during specific exercises, or as a prelude to other breathing exercises. Other advanced techniques may combine alternate nostril breathing as you visualise breathing in *qi*.

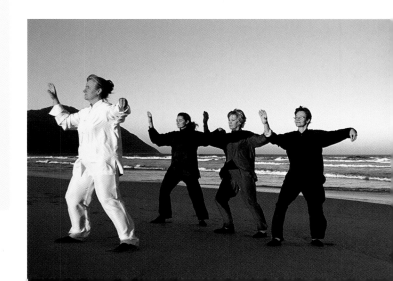

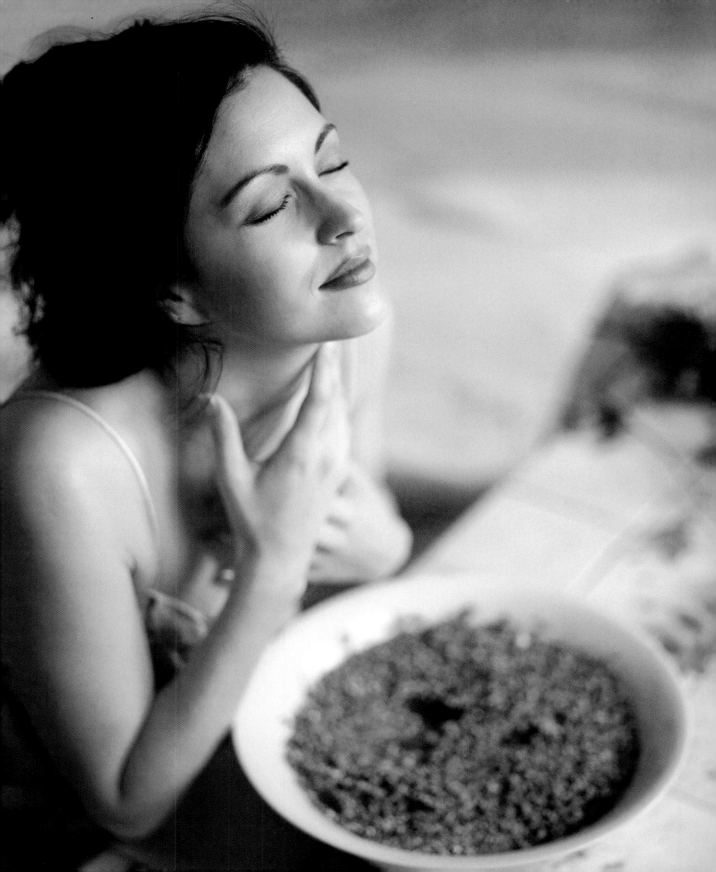

EARTH
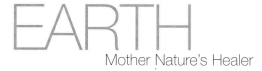
Mother Nature's Healer

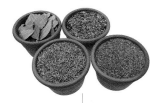

Expressions such as 'down to earth', 'grounded' and 'rock solid' are indicative of earth's status as the most stable of, and foundation of, the four elements. Its soil is where life begins and ends. Earth is often referred to as mother, protector, nurturer and giver of life, for it is from its abundant fertility that we receive materials for our shelter and clothing, food for our sustenance, and beauty to feed the soul.

As children, we romped in the mud or rolled through carpets of fallen leaves, unconsciously bonding with Mother Earth. These days, we are likely to seek this bond in a spa and absorb the earth's nutrients by having our bodies coated in mud (see pp79–80), soaked in a bath of blooms, or coddled with herbs. We may have a stone massage (see p81) in which basalt stones substitute for human hands and provide an energetic connection to earth. Many spa treatments using herbs to heal, fruit to feed the skin, and minerals and muds to nourish have been practised since antiquity. You may enjoy all these along with aromatherapy (see pp70–72)—literally, 'therapy through scent'—as you inhale the fragrance of essential oils extracted from plants.

The natural gifts of earth's own pharmacy provide our bodies with essential vitamins, minerals and trace elements, and these work not just on a biochemical level. Many people believe that these substances have energies that work on a vibrational level as well, sending out subtle signals to your body's natural energy field to aid healing. Crystals (see p78), for instance, are believed to vibrate with a particular energy that helps rebalance your body, mind and spirit. Other products of the earth which work on a vibrational level include homeopathic remedies (see p88), which are so diluted that they only contain a vibration of the original substance.

A HISTORICAL PERSPECTIVE

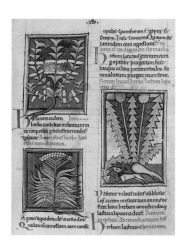

I believe in God, only I spell it Nature.

– Frank Lloyd Wright, architect (1869–1959)

PAGE 66: *Natural yet potent ingredients—such as flowers, plants, herbs and mud—feature prominently in spa menus.*

PAGE 67: *Herbs, spices and leaves, once more associated with kitchens, are now found in exotic spa treatments drawn from around the world.*

TOP: *Before the advent of the printing press in the 15th century, information on herbs took the form of illustrated representations of medicinal plants, such as this Greek manuscript which dates back to around 1200.*

OPPOSITE: *This medieval manuscript depicts the gathering of plants, which are then crushed with a pestle and mortar to prepare them for medicinal use as prescribed by the apothecary.*

NATURE'S HEALING HELPERS

Modern man is now returning to his roots with the resurgent awareness of the healing wonders derived from the fruits of the earth—even if they are plucked from health shops and supermarkets, or enjoyed in the form of spa treatments.

Just as our early ancestors were likely to have learnt of the medicinal value of plants by observing animals in the wild, zoopharmacognosy—a discipline studying self-medication by animals—has developed in the last few decades in response to burgeoning interest in natural medicines. While our ancestors may have learnt from trial and error, advances in science and technology have enabled today's scientists to improve the safety and efficacy of such treatments, backing certain practices that were once considered superstitions—the benefits of harvesting particular plants at specific times, for instance.

Herbs are still at the core of many healing cultures around the world, and are used by 80 per cent of the world's population. Archaeologists have found pollen in an excavation of a Neanderthal grave in what is now Iraq, indicating that the corpse was surrounded by flowers from medicinal plants. Findings such as these have led scientists to conclude that herbal medicine was certainly the earliest form of medicine, used many centuries before the advent of written records.

In Europe, herbs were the medicine of the people, part of oral lore. In Greece, dispensing them to the sick was the prerogative of monks who cultivated medicinal plants in their monastery grounds. Only after the invention of the printing press in the 15th century did herbal knowledge become more widely available. One notable herbalist was Nicholas Culpepper, the English apothecary who translated the *London Pharmacopoeia* from Latin into English for other apothecaries to understand. His writings in 1660 contained herbal formulae for health and beauty, many of which are still used today.

However, history also has its share of instances where herbal medicine fell into disrepute, with rogue apothecaries charging exorbitant fees, and the church levelling strong criticism against it. Practitioners of herbal medicine, who often held

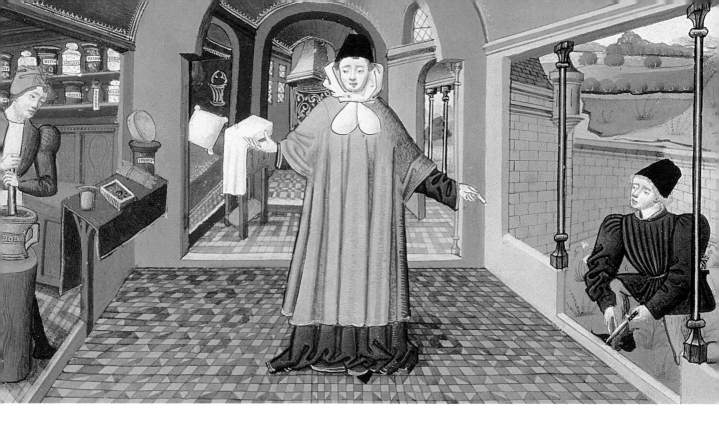

knowledge regarding fertility control, were frequently demonised and burnt as witches.

Among the cultures most prolific in their use of cures from nature's pharmacy were the Egyptians, who harnessed earthly and cosmic energies through their construction of pyramids, and imbibed medicinal potions of crushed gems mixed in liquid. The Egyptians were also thought to be the earliest users of aromatherapy, with priests making incense and perfumes, and physicians incorporating essential oils into their medicinal preparations. The Egyptians had diverse uses for oils—from embalming their dead to using oils in massages and baths as advocated by Imhotep, the Egyptian god of medicine. In fact, Egyptian papyri dating back to 1500 B.C. also refer to many ancient remedies that are still used today.

Legendary Egyptian beauty Cleopatra was famous for bathing in milk, but was also rumoured to have used body wraps as part of her beauty regime. She was said to have instigated Mark Antony's conquest of the Dead Sea region because she coveted its mud. Like Cleopatra, Biblical figures such as King David and King Solomon were also said to have had bathing palaces on the Dead Sea. Other key users of mud

were the Romans, who utilised it in the form of mud packs and firming masks to cure illnesses and to enhance beauty. Other notable figures throughout the centuries who have been drawn to sources of therapeutic mud include King Louis XV, and Napoleon and Josephine, who visited the still-famous Neydharting Moor near Salzburg, Austria. Composer Ludwig von Beethoven, European royalty, and maharajas were among the illustrious visitors who soaked up the benefits of therapeutic mud and water at the Karlovy Vary in Czechoslovakia.

More recently, spas have identified and harnessed the mineral-rich properties of different muds from a widespread variety of sources, including volcanoes, peat bogs, springs and moors. Pelotherapy, or fangotherapy (see p79–80), uses baths for medicinal purposes, while mud wraps and face masks are used to soften, firm and beautify the skin.

In this age where conventional medicine, while indispensable, does not seem to be providing all the answers in terms of safety and efficacy, modern man, it would seem, has come full circle in his re-appreciation of nature's healing wonders. With its vast diversity of flora and its wealth of beneficial minerals, the earth has much to offer us, as we are now rediscovering.

TREATMENTS AND THERAPIES

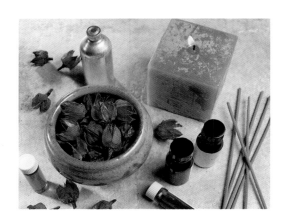

Nature does nothing uselessly.

*– Aristotle, Greek philosopher
(384 B.C.– 322 B.C.), Politics*

AROMATHERAPY

Aromatherapy, literally meaning 'therapy through aroma or scent', uses essential oils—extracted from herbs, flowers, leaves, fruit, bark, grasses and seeds—to promote physical and psychological wellbeing. The best quality essential oils come from organically grown plants, harvested at the right time.

Various methods used to extract oils from the plant parts include distillation, expression and the solvent method. As essential oils are volatile and evaporate quickly, they are kept in tightly stoppered dark glass bottles to preserve their quality.

Essential oils have mainly antiseptic properties, though they may also be antiviral, anti-inflammatory, pain-relieving, and act as antidepressants and expectorants. Their scent acts on that part of the brain associated with motivation, emotions, moods, memory and creativity—triggering the release of neurotransmitters such as serotonin (which calms and relaxes), endorphins and enkephalin (which reduce pain, and bring about a feeling of wellbeing), and noradrenaline (which stimulates and helps keep you awake). The oils are absorbed by your skin and carried to your organs via your connective and lymphatic tissues and your circulatory system, when applied in a diluted form in treatments such as baths and massages.

While aromatherapy is now commonly used to ease stress, much of aromatherapy as we know it today stemmed from treating injuries. In 1910, when a laboratory explosion burnt his hand, French chemist René-Maurice Gattefossé dipped it in lavender oil. His hand healed quickly, without scarring or infection, inspiring him to study the healing properties of plant oils. His compatriot, Dr Jean Valnet, treated wounded soldiers with essential oils in World War II. These days, aromatherapy is also widely used to treat colds, cystitis, menstrual problems, digestive problems and skin problems.

Common ailments may be treated easily using lavender oil, tea tree oil, camomile oil or peppermint oil, but it takes a skilled aromatherapist to truly understand essential oils' properties and blend a few for your use. A synergistic blend of oils used together can work more effectively than one oil used on its own.

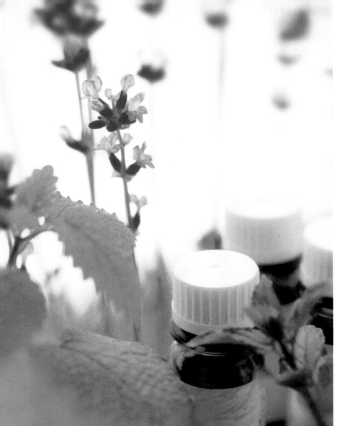

Essential oils may be also taken internally when mixed with substances such as honey or alcohol, but it is crucial only to do so under the supervision of a qualified therapist or a physician. In France, essential oils are sometimes prescribed as alternatives to conventional medicine. In UK hospitals, essential oils such as lavender oil, peppermint oil and clary sage oil may be used in the maternity ward, administered in the form of baths (see pp20–22), footbaths (see pp26–27), inhalations (see pp48, 58–59 and 61) and massages (see pp92–97).

Aromatherapy works well with Bach Flower Essences but not with homeopathic remedies (see p88). If you are epileptic, pregnant or have an allergy, high blood pressure or any medical condition, it is imperative that you seek the advice of a qualified practitioner before treatment. Young children should only be treated by experienced practitioners.

In the beauty industry, essential oils may be used in creating perfumes and cosmetics. You can enjoy aromatherapy in a spa through massages, baths, facials, herbal wraps, footbaths, inhalation, steam rooms and teas.

Some Common Essential Oils and Their Uses

Essential Oil	Main Uses	Essential Oil	Main Uses
Bergamot oil	A versatile citrus oil used in Italy to treat appetite loss, bladder infections, skin problems and sore throat. Also alleviates stress.	Peppermint oil	A cooling yet warming oil used to treat nausea, dizziness, colds and flu. Also commonly used to stimulate mental concentration.
Eucalyptus oil	A useful antiseptic oil for treating fever, skin blemishes, muscular aches, sinus and throat problems. Said to aid concentration.	Rosemary oil	An uplifting oil that enhances mental clarity and helps boost poor memory. Its antiseptic qualities benefit blemished and oily skins.
Lavender oil	A most versatile oil used for allergies, bronchitis, muscular pain, wounds and insect bites. Eases stress, insomnia and nervousness.	Sandalwood oil	A calming and harmonising Oriental oil with a warm woody fragrance. Counteracts a hectic lifestyle. It is also considered an aphrodisiac.
Lemongrass oil	A pleasantly refreshing oil. Aids digestion, reduces flatulence, stimulates lymph drainage, reduces fluid retention. Eases sports injuries.	Ylang-ylang oil	A flowery, sweet, exotic oil with aphrodisiac qualities. Induces calm and balance when used in a bath. Also boosts confidence.

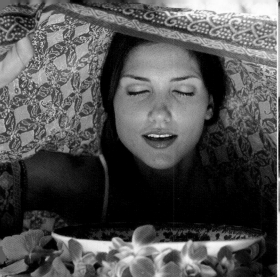
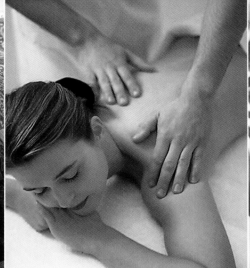
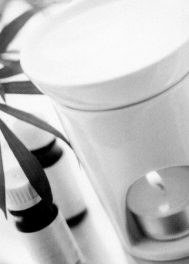

Aromatherapy Bath

A warm bath of water with added essential oils combines the benefits of aromatherapy with hydrotherapy. You can choose from a variety of essential oils and effects—citruses, which are stimulating; florals, which are soothing; and woods, which are sensual. The essential oils may be mixed with a carrier oil before being added to the bath. Or they may also be added neat under running water, or mixed vigorously with the water just before you step into the bath. The benefits of the oils are absorbed through your skin. As you relax in the tub for 15 to 20 minutes, put a cool, damp towel to your forehead.

Aromatherapy Massage

In the late 1950s, French biochemist Madame Marguerite Maury, who was unable to dispense essential oils as medicines because she was not a doctor, introduced them in massages. Aromatherapy massage combines Swedish massage (see p93) and shiatsu (see p97) techniques, and can be relaxing or stimulating, depending on the essential oils used. Essential oils are highly concentrated, and most have to be diluted with carrier oils such as grapeseed oil or sweet almond oil before being applied to your skin. Before the massage, you may want to enjoy a steam treatment (see pp48–49) to clean your skin and open your pores so that the oils can be easily absorbed and carried to your muscle tissues, joints and organs. The massage increases blood flow to the area concerned, which may encourage the oils to be better absorbed. The inhaled scent also works therapeutically on you.

Inhalation Methods

Essential oils can be inhaled in a number of ways:

- One way is to add a few drops to your handkerchief, hold it under your nose and inhale. Try bergamot, lavender, lemon, lime or mint oil.
- Another way is to put a few drops on your pillow if you have trouble falling asleep. Try lavender oil.
- You can also add a few drops of essential oils to a bowl of steaming hot water, place a towel over your head, close your eyes, and breathe deeply for about 10 minutes. End the session by splashing cold water on your face. This method can be used to open your facial pores as part of your skincare regime. It is also effective for treating respiratory problems, but not recommended if you are asthmatic, prone to nosebleeds or have broken blood vessels. Try camomile, lavender, lemongrass or neroli oil.
- To scent your room, use a vaporiser, placing 2 to 3 drops of oil in a bowl of water that is heated by a tea light. Do not leave the flame unattended. To neutralise a smoky room, try cypress, lemongrass or tea tree oil.

Never inhale essential oils directly from the bottle.

TOP LEFT: Enhance a home inhalation session through the use of beautiful props. Drape a towel or blanket over yourself and the bowl to keep the steam in.

TOP CENTRE: In an aromatherapy massage, the essential oils are fixed by mixing with a carrier oil that also helps the spreadability and absorption of the oils into the skin.

TOP RIGHT: Using an aromatherapy burner is the easiest way to bring the calming atmosphere of a spa into your home.

OPPOSITE, TOP: In Traditional Chinese Medicine, ginseng is popularly prescribed to enhance stamina, vitality and virility.

OPPOSITE, BOTTOM: Herbal remedies may be administered in forms that include teas, infusions, tinctures, baths and inhalation.

PHYTOTHERAPY

Phytotherapy refers to the use of plants for healing or therapeutic uses. Often folk wisdom from ancient texts is combined with advances in science and technology.

Parts of plants such as leaves, flowers, fruit, roots and bark may contain hundreds, even thousands of plant compounds. It is believed that the synergy or mix of ingredients in a plant—rather than an isolated active ingredient, as in a synthetically made drug—makes plant use safe and effective.

Spas offer a number of therapeutic and pampering treatments which harness active ingredients from a repertoire of plants—from the depths of the sea (algae) to deep in the Amazonian rainforest. These range from familiar favourites such as aloe vera (soothing and refreshing) and lavender (calming and healing) to more esoteric varieties such as Brazilian mimosa (healing and regenerative) and cocoa (anti-ageing). Many spas use products that blend essential oils and plant extracts.

Plant products may benefit people with sensitive skins who cannot tolerate chemicals and preservatives, but always inform your therapist of any specific allergies you have beforehand.

Western Herbalism

Once dismissed as folklore, herbal medicine gained respectability in recent times when in 1985, the World Health Organization (WHO) reported on its potential importance in modern healthcare. In the past, finding the most effective plants to heal was a matter of trial and error. These days, scientific advancements and chemical analyses have provided a better understanding of the safety and efficacy of herbs. Medical herbalism is well established in Europe, where it is studied at some universities. Herbalism's scope has also increased, and plant species from Australasia, North America and Africa are now used by modern herbalists.

Herbal medicines can be classified according to the body systems over which they have the most influence. For example, oats and Saint John's wort are used to treat the nervous system, while circulatory stimulants include gingko and rosemary.

A herbalist will take a holistic approach by looking for the cause of your illness, such as an unhealthy lifestyle, that may have upset your body's balance.

Herbal medicine is said to work gently by strengthening your body's systems. Seek expert advice, however, when taking herbs, as some may not be good for certain people such as the pregnant, the elderly or very young, or sufferers from a long-term or chronic condition.

Chocolate Heaven

This scrub from The Spa at Pennyhill Park will appeal to all your senses and is good enough to eat!

Ingredients
3 tbsp drinking chocolate
2 tbsp brown sugar
1 tbsp runny honey
Rose petals, as required
4 vanilla pod seeds

- Run a bath. Add the rose petals and vanilla pods.
- Light a few candles. Have a warm fluffy towel, a glass of red wine and a big fluffy dressing gown nearby.
- Mix the drinking chocolate, sugar and honey to a paste.
- Step in the bath. Take 2 tbsp of the Chocolate Scrub paste and warm it in your hands. Smooth it over your body in circular motions, moving towards your heart. Concentrate on your ankles, elbows and knees.
- Sit down in the water, relax and unwind for 15 minutes. Do not wash off the scrub.
- Step out of the bath, wrap up in the towel, envelop yourself in the dressing gown and relax with a glass of red wine.

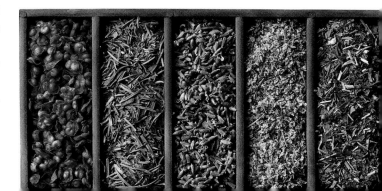

Herbal Wrap

Being cocooned with aromatic herbs next to your skin is one of the most therapeutic ways of getting closer to Mother Earth. At the same time, you detoxify your body, smoothen and soften your skin, and relieve muscle and joint aches. Wraps are used in slimming and anti-cellulite programmes. Most experts say that any weight reduction following the treatment is temporary and due to water lost via perspiration—but this reduction may motivate you to better your diet and do more exercise.

There are several methods used to wrap the body. In a herbal wrap, your body is typically wrapped in sheets steeped in a steaming herbal mixture. Your body is usually exfoliated first with a scrub before being wrapped.

Depending on the type of wrap, your body may be cocooned for 20 minutes. Additionally, you may be wrapped in blankets, or an infra-red lamp may be used to keep you warm as the ingredients start to cool. During this time, a cool compress may be placed on your head. The continuous heat encourages your body to relax and your pores to open, allowing the ingredients of the wrap to work on your skin.

Your body may begin to sweat, encouraging toxin removal. After the wrap is removed you can, if you wish, shower off the ingredients applied to your body. Drink plenty of water before and after a wrap to ensure that you stay well hydrated. Do not have a heavy meal just before a wrap, and refrain from drinking alcohol for 72 hours afterwards. As always, seek your doctor's permission if you have any medical problems. As your body temperature and heart rate will be elevated during the wrap, wraps are not recommended for some conditions, including pregnancy, heart conditions and high blood pressure.

Besides herbs, fruit, clay, mud (see pp79–80) and seaweed (see p35) are among the other beneficial natural ingredients that are popularly used in wraps. These substances are slathered on to your body which is then wrapped up.

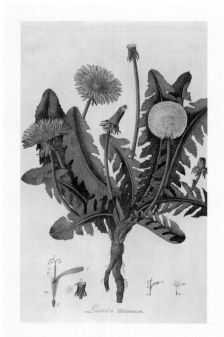

Lontodon Taraxacum.

Some Popular Herbs and Their Uses

Herb	Uses
Camomile	This gentle but powerful herb may be used in poultices to ease swollen joints and in steam inhalations to bring relief to flu symptoms. Camomile baths and teas ease tension and insomnia. Its essential oil is often used in aromatherapy.
Dandelion	This versatile herb is used to treat ailments from arthritis and constipation to kidney and menstrual problems. It is high in vitamins and trace minerals, and can be added to salads.
Sage	Mediterranean in orgin, this herb has antiseptic qualities and may be used as a gargle to treat mouth and throat infections. Sage tea is used to treat coughs and colds, cleanse the liver and kidneys, and reduce milk flow in lactating mothers.
Valerian	Popularly known for its relaxing and sedative properties, this herb is used to relieve muscle cramps, stress-related headaches, nervous conditions and insomnia. The fresh root has an earthy scent, but some people find the dried version's smell offensive.

Hay Bath

Farmers in the early 19th century who fell asleep in stacks of cut hay meant for their cows discovered that the hay helped revive them after a hard day's work. Around the same time, pioneering hydrotherapist Sebastian Kneipp advocated using hay cut from flower meadows to treat rheumatic pain and sciatica.

Hay baths have traditionally been enjoyed in alpine regions in northern Italy, Bavaria (southern Germany), Austria and Switzerland, where the grass contains aromatic and beneficial herbs and flowers. In the past, hay was harvested at dawn when it was still moist with dew and transferred to the hay baths, where it was left to ferment for three days—so hay baths could only be taken in the summer when the hay was harvested. Now, however, improved harvesting and storage methods mean that the treatment can be enjoyed throughout the year.

In a modern spa, the hay bath may take place in conjunction with a dry flotation session (see p28). Your body below the chin is surrounded by warm, moistened hay and the temperature is kept to about 42 degrees Celsius (108 degrees Fahrenheit) for around 20 minutes. The stimulation from the hay and the heat encourages perspiration and the elimination of toxins from your body. This treatment is said to be gentler on the heart and circulatory system than a sauna or steam bath.

If you prefer not to be in direct contact with the hay, a fleece sheet can be placed between you and the hay. After a hay bath, you rest in a bed for about 30 minutes, wrapped up to continue the sweating process. You should feel revived afterwards, and like the farmers who inadvertently discovered hay's therapeutic effects, find your body soothed of aches and pains.

To enhance the benefits of the treatment, follow it with a massage. You do not need to take a shower after a hay bath, as this detracts from the treatment's therapeutic effect.

Do not take a hay bath if you have just been to a solarium or have been suntanning; if you are suffering from inflammation or metabolic problems, heart disease, high blood pressure or kidney failure; or if you are undergoing treatment for cancer. This treatment is also not recommended if you are pregnant.

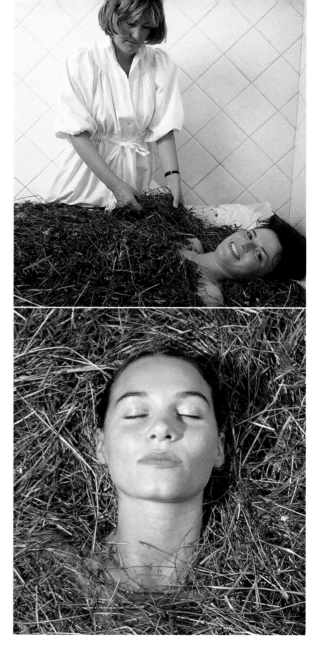

OPPOSITE, RIGHT: In the past, plants were often associated with alchemy. Camomile flowers, for example, were collected on or before Saint John's Day (24 June) to prevent witches from urinating on them. Sage in medieval times was used in magic and for prolonging life, and was even an ingredient in spells used to help young women see their future husbands.

OPPOSITE, LEFT: The Swiss have 150 names for the dandelion. The flower is also dubbed the 'shepherd's clock' because its flowers open at five in the morning and close in the evening.

TOP AND ABOVE: In the old days, hay baths were taken in groups, and the hay may have only been changed once every five days. These days, the hay bath is an individual treatment and a fresh batch of hay is used during each session.

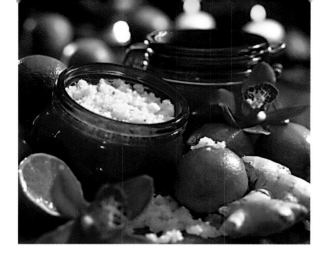

Fruit Scrub

Many face and body treatments that exfoliate the skin to improve its appearance and texture draw on the benefits of fruit. Fruit scrubs are comprised of fine exfoliating grains which are rubbed on to moist skin using circular motions. These skin-softening, complexion-brightening exfoliating treatments are very effective, but before any facial treatment, your therapist should analyse your skin, ask what skincare products you are using, and assess any possible contraindications, as some scrubs may not be suitable for very sensitive skins.

Strawberry Herbal Back Cleanse

The back is known as the 'gateway into the body' for its ability to absorb essential oils which can help cleanse and balance the skin. Treatments to cleanse and decongest the once-neglected back area have traditionally been relegated to the bottom of a spa's treatment menu. However, given the present popularity of back-revealing clothes, back cleanses (or 'back-cials') are now much sought-after. Back cleanses are also increasingly popular with men who are prone to congestion, breakouts, discoloration and excess sebum in their backs.

The Strawberry Herbal Back Cleanse developed by Elemis is like a full facial, only it is for the back. It includes cleansing, toning, the application of a hot compress, extraction (if required), a massage to ease tension, and exfoliation. A compress infused with lime essential oil stimulates circulation to help rid the skin of toxins. An aromatic herbal mask of fruit essential oils and strawberry extract is then applied. Strawberry is used for its ability to refine, purify, tone and absorb impurities from the skin—as well as for its delicious aroma.

Masks From Your Kitchen

Using fruit, herbs and other ingredients from your garden or kitchen, you can easily whip up skin-nourishing treatments in your own home. Try the following treatments by Elemis Day-Spa every three weeks as quick pick-me-ups or as a treat for your skin and scalp before a big occasion. Both masks draw their properties from ingredients which can be absorbed by the skin on contact.

Avocado and Strawberry Face Mask

This face mask will regulate oil flow, hydrate sensitive areas and restore moisture. It is recommended for dry to sensitive skins. Do not use if your skin is very sensitive.

Ingredients

½ avocado
5 large strawberries
1 sprig watercress
2 mint leaves
2 ml (⅒ fl oz) avocado or sesame seed oil

- Blend the ingredients together, if possible, using a blender.
- Apply the mixture to your face, avoiding the eye area, and leave for 8 to 10 min.
- Wipe off with a warm flannel.

Papaya and Yogurt Conditioning Mask

This mask is suited for all hair types and will restore shine, reduce oiliness and condition your hair.

Ingredients

13 ml (½ fl oz) plain natural yogurt
3 ml (⅒ fl oz) cider vinegar
2 drops rosemary essential oil
1 papaya, crushed

- Mix all the ingredients together.
- While in the bath, apply the mixture on to your scalp and hair.
- Leave on for 8 to 10 min, then rinse off with warm water.

VINOTHERAPY

While vinotherapy—the therapeutic use of wine and grapes in beauty and health treatments—is a relative newcomer on the spa scene, wine's origins as a treatment are believed to date back to before the advent of writing in Egypt in 3,200 B.C..

According to Louis Grivetti, a professor of nutrition at the University of California, the Egyptians used wine in ointments to soothe skin problems, and drank it as medicine to treat a variety of health problems from tapeworms to assisting childbirth. Women during Cleopatra's time applied red wine to their faces in the name of beauty, while in ancient Greece, Hippocrates advocated the therapeutic use of wine for maintaining health and for treating problems such as ulcers through liniments derived from wine and grapes.

Throughout the ages, wine has been condemned as a wrecker of homes for the negative societal and health consequences that excessive consumption creates. However, it has also been widely celebrated for the pleasure and health benefits it provides moderate drinkers. Research in recent times has suggested that people who regularly drink a moderate amount of wine a day are at a lower risk from heart disease, stroke and cancer than those who do not consume wine; a similar effect is not shown, however, in people who regularly consume beer and other spirits. In what is known as the French Paradox,

French scientist and alcohol researcher Dr Serge Renaud surmised that the low incidence of heart attacks in France, despite a diet high in rich foods, may be correlated with the regular consumption of wine with meals.

French pharmacology professor Joseph Vercauteren sowed the seeds of vinotherapy in Bordeaux when he noticed that the most nutritious part of the grape, the seeds, were typically discarded during the wine-making process. He scientifically proved that the polyphenols in the seeds were antioxidants, and were more effective than Vitamin E in protecting the skin-ageing free radicals that come from sources such as pollution and cigarette smoke. Before long, enterprising vineyard owners decided to capitalise on this information by harvesting the grapeseeds, and a new trend was born.

Vercauteren stabilised the polyphenols in grape seeds for use in cosmetic creams, and with his help, Mathilde Cathiard—whose parents owned a wine estate in France, and therefore enjoyed a ready supply of ingredients—developed a new line of skincare products using grape extracts.

Subsequently, Cathiard opened the world's first vinotherapy spa, Caudalie Vinotherapie Spa, in 1999 at her parent's Chateau Smith Haut Lafitte wine estate, where elements from grapes and wine combined with warm spring water are used in baths, massages, masks, scrubs and wraps.

OPPOSITE, LEFT: Lime is uplifting and helps rid the skin of toxins and waste. Ginger helps stimulate the metabolism and tone the body. Combined, they can provide an invigorating skin treatment.

OPPOSITE, RIGHT: Avocados have traditionally been used to treat skin problems. The pulp can be used to encourage healing of minor cuts, while the flesh can be used to soothe sunburnt skin.

RIGHT: At Caudalie Vinotherapie Spa, the therapeutic properties of spring water and elements from grape and wines create luxurious treatments such as the barrel bath (RIGHT), a jacuzzi in the form of a large wooden barrel, bubbling with spring water. The swimming pool at the spa (FAR RIGHT) is fed by thermal springs.

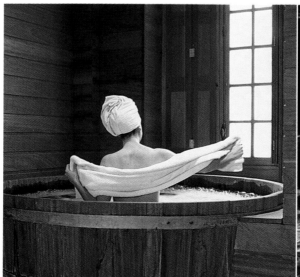
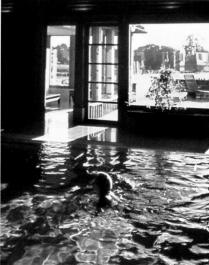

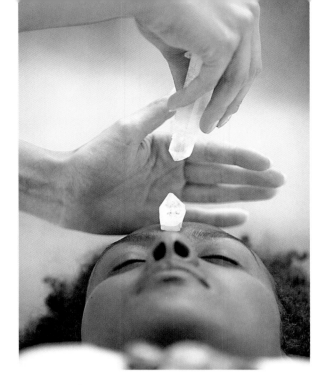

CRYSTAL THERAPY

Crystals and gems are born of the minerals from the earth, some taking hundreds of thousands of years to form. Some are pushed to the earth's surface by erupting lava, escaping gases or water. Crystals and gems have long been prized by cultures around the globe who believe they they bestow status, luck, and even health on their owners. Shamanistic cultures such as the Inuits in the Arctic and the Indians in the Amazon believe they have inherent magical and therapeutic properties.

Crystals with electromagnetic properties are believed to be able to transmit and receive energy, amplify our body's self-healing ability, respond to thoughts and emotions, and help restore balance to parts of the body experiencing disease or disharmony.

TOP: The crystal may be placed on the areas of illness or on your acupoints (see p86). Crystals may also be used to massage the body in a manner similar to stone therapy (see p81).

ABOVE: Some spas may place a large crystal such as an amethyst in the steam room to enhance your wellbeing.

OPPOSITE: The Dead Sea between Israel and Jordan is famous for both its therapeutic black mud and its concentration of mineral salts—four times more than that of regular seawater—which makes swimmers unsinkable.

Crystals are often used in conjunction with aura work (see p87) and the chakras (see p87) to increase the flow of energy in the body's energy pathways.

Practitioners of crystal therapy try to tap into the crystals' healing energy to enhance healing of an emotional or physical complaint. A practitioner may hold a crystal in one hand, rest the other on the relevant part of your body, and ask you to visualise healing energy channelling through the crystal—or he may give you a crystal to carry around, wear as jewellery, or place in your room to hold. Crystal therapy is often used with *reiki* (see p90) and colour therapy (see pp91–92).

Crystals may be used in absent healing, when a practitioner endeavours to form an intuitive link to someone not in the same physical space by projecting energies from a crystal. He may also place the crystal on top of the receiver's photograph.

Crystal Clearing

Crystals are believed to contain a healing life energy that may be charged and discharged like a battery. They are thought to be such good energy transmitters that they pick up all kinds of vibrations from the environment and from those who come in contact with them. Besides 'clearing' new crystals before use, it is essential to clear them again regularly to rid them of this jumbled energy. It is also important to clear second-hand jewellery of the former owners' energy for at least one week before wearing it. Consult your practitioner for the best methods to use on various crystals, as not all methods are suitable for certain crystals. Also use your discretion with regards to leaving particularly valuable crystals out of doors. Crystal-clearing methods include

- Leaving crystals outdoors during a full moon.
- Soaking them in a bowl of spring water with a pinch of sea salt dissolved in it.
- Exposing them to the sun for an hour.
- Burying them under the sand at a beach for a few hours.
- Standing them in a running brook.
- 'Smudging' them by wafting them with smoking herbs such as sage or sweetgrass.

PELOTHERAPY

Mud, also referred to technically as peloids (from the Greek *'pelos'* for 'mud') comprises about one-third earth and two-thirds water. Spas commonly use the term 'mud' to refer to substances that come from mineral-rich areas around natural springs, moors, peatlands, volcanoes and oceans. Some even expand the definition of mud to include algae (see p33).

Pelotherapy or fangotherapy, the use of mud for medicinal purposes, is used to treat ailments that include rheumatic, skin and digestive problems through methods such as mud packs and mud baths. Mud used for beauty and relaxation is usually administered in the form of face masks, body wraps and baths that help detoxify the body, and soften and firm the skin. Mud is water soluble, and helps the skin absorb nutrients from it. Despite mud's association with dirt, your skin will actually feel fresh and clean after a mud treatment. Mud is also used to retain heat and is commonly found in body wraps and packs. Various mud products are also sold for use at home, but as they can be messy, many people prefer to enjoy mud in spas.

Dead Sea Mud Wrap

The Dead Sea Mud Wrap, initially designed to ease joint pain, inflammation and swelling, is now a popular spa treatment used to relax the body and rejuvenate the skin. The mud's ability to help flush out toxins and excess fluid also makes it useful in treating lower back pain and pre-menstrual bloating.

A mud wrap is typically performed in a wet room with an adjoining shower. Heated mud is brushed on to your body, though some spas may apply it over a permeable fabric to facilitate removal. You are then wrapped in a plastic sheet and covered with blankets for between 15 and 40 minutes. You will next proceed to rinse off the mud and with it, surface impurities from your skin under a shower—in some spas, a Vichy shower (see p23), a Scotch hose (see p24), or a Swiss shower (see p24). The black-coloured mud from the Dead Sea's vast inland lake and hot springs contains over 20 minerals and trace elements including calcium, chloride, copper, iodine, magnesium, radium and zinc, and is also commonly used to treat skin problems such as acne, eczema and psoriasis.

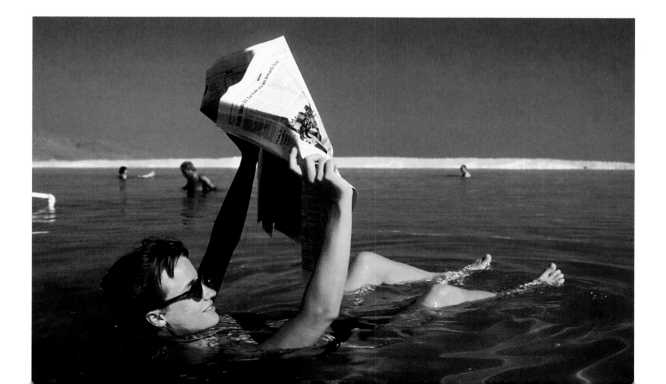

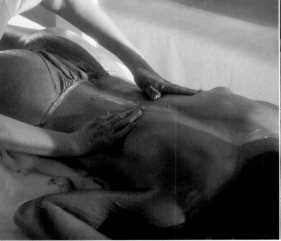
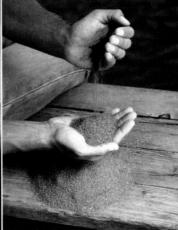
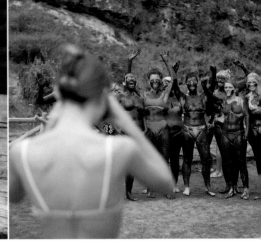

Parafango Pack

Parafango—a combination of dried fango (Italian for 'mud') and paraffin with different fusing points—was developed by German Professor Hesse as a way to improve the application and hygiene of fango. The substance also contains small amounts of talcum and magnesium oxide that prevent the fango from precipitating, and makes the substance more plastic and easier to spread and mould when melted. Parafango's ability to maintain heat longer than other peloids makes it ideal for use in packs which are applied to the joints, back, torso, abdomen, extremities or pelvis. This treatment works strictly on a thermal level without mineralisation or absorption. You may notice some sweating in the area covered by the pack and an increase in body temperature. First used in 1952, it remains a popular treatment for conditions such as rheumatism and muscle spasms. People who should avoid this treatment include those who have eczema, or heart and circulation problems.

Moor Mud Bath

Wallowing in a tub of mud—particularly the black-coloured moor mud—is a deeply relaxing spa treatment. Moor is a rich accumulation of water-logged plant deposits—some thought to have been extinct for over 500 years—including roots, flowers, fruit and seeds, many of which have medicinal characteristics. The moor bath is not a cleansing one, so you may want to shower and wash your hair beforehand. The therapist may first exfoliate your skin with a natural bristle mitt or brush. You can wear a shower cap during this treatment, but do not worry if you get the mixture on your face or hair. To create the bath, the moor is added to warm water, and mixed well to prevent it from globbing. Essential oils may also be added to the bath. You will soak in it for about 20 to 30 minutes, during which more warm water may be added if necessary. The bath may be enjoyed in a tub with jets, or you may given an underwater hose massage (see p24) to enhance results, in which case the soaking time will be shortened. After your bath, remember not to shower off. Pat yourself dry with a towel, keep warm and rest for half an hour. You may feel sleepy after this deeply relaxing treatment, so you may want to schedule it before you retire for the night. You may notice that dark-coloured towels are used in moor treatments as moor mud is known to dull light colours.

Scientific evidence shows that moor mud contains anti-inflammatory and astringent properties, ideal for detoxifying the body, and for treating skin problems such as acne and eczema. It is also used to treat rheumatism, arthritis, open wounds, and hormonal and infertility problems.

Do consult your medical practitioner before you take a mud bath. It should not be taken during pregnancy. It is also not recommended for anyone suffering from heart problems, acute rheumatic problems, kidney problems, or tumours.

Moor Drink

A moor drink does not look appetising, and may initially have a strong smell. The trick is to let it breathe overnight, after which it will have no smell or taste. Mix a teaspoonful of pasteurised moor into a glass of water or juice. This drink will detoxify you from the inside out, and can benefit people with digestive, intestinal, rheumatic and arthritic problems. Follow the supplier's instructions; the recommended dosage is usually three times a day for four to six weeks.

STONE THERAPY

Flat and smooth stones applied at various temperatures do the heavy duty work in deeply relaxing treatments known as stone massages. The stones used are generally basalt, formed from lava and shaped and smoothened by nature; these are said to be better able to retain heat and cold. Smaller stones may be used in facials, manicures and pedicures, and reflexology. Stone therapy may be used in conjunction with Swedish massage (see p93) and *lomi lomi* (a fluid Hawaiian massage). Ancient Hawaiians used lava stones in the *lomi lomi*, believing that heat from these stones warmed the body and soothed the soul.

The therapist applies these stones to your body in long, flowing strokes facilitated by oil. They are then placed on strategic energy points on your body to ease tension, on sore or tense areas of your back; between your toes or in your hands; or on different parts of your body and your face. In a Warm Stone Massage, also known as a Hot Stone Massage, only heated stones are used. Using the stones frees the therapist from straining her hands and lets her work more effectrively

Some people say the gentle, even pressure of stones gliding over your body is what makes the experience so profound, while others attribute it to the stones' magnetic and spiritual connection to Mother Earth. Some spas leave the stones outdoors during a full moon to re-energise them.

LaStone® Therapy

Modern stone therapy is attributed to Mary Nelson who got the idea of using heated stones while taking a sauna (see pp45–46) in 1993. The American massage therapist, who had injured her shoulder, was wondering how she could still work effectively on her clients when a voice prompted her to use warm stones. She subsequently used hot and chilled basalt and marble stones in a Swedish massage, and then copyrighted this technique—LaStone® Therapy—in 1994.

During a LaStone® session, heated stones are first applied to relax and relieve muscle tension, followed by cool stones to strengthen the immune system. The alternation of hot and cold applications boosts the circulation and helps the body to heal itself. You are likely to relax into a meditative state after the 90-minute session. Many receivers of LaStone® Therapy report feeling like they have just been cradled by Mother Earth herself. LaStone® Therapy may be used in conjunction with *reiki* (see p90), facials and pre-natal treatments.

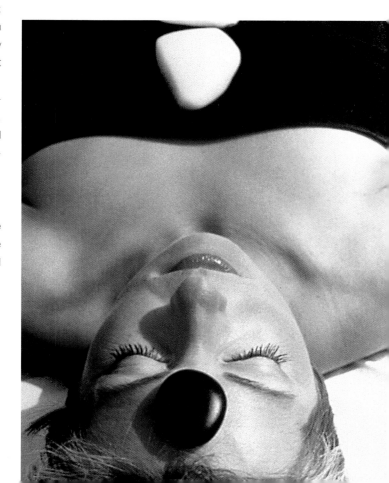

OPPOSITE, LEFT: Wraps of marine muds are popular treatments at thalassotherapy centres such as Les Thermes Marins de Monte-Carlo.

OPPOSITE, CENTRE: Contrary to popular opinion that mud is dirty, mud is popularly used in cleansing and healing.

OPPOSITE, RIGHT: Mud brings out a playful side in people as seen in this photograph of swimsuit clad women in Ilica in Daylon, Turkey.

RIGHT: Stone therapy is more than a massage; it is also grounding and balancing. Some spas offer this treatment out of doors during warmer weather, increasing your sense of connection with the earth.

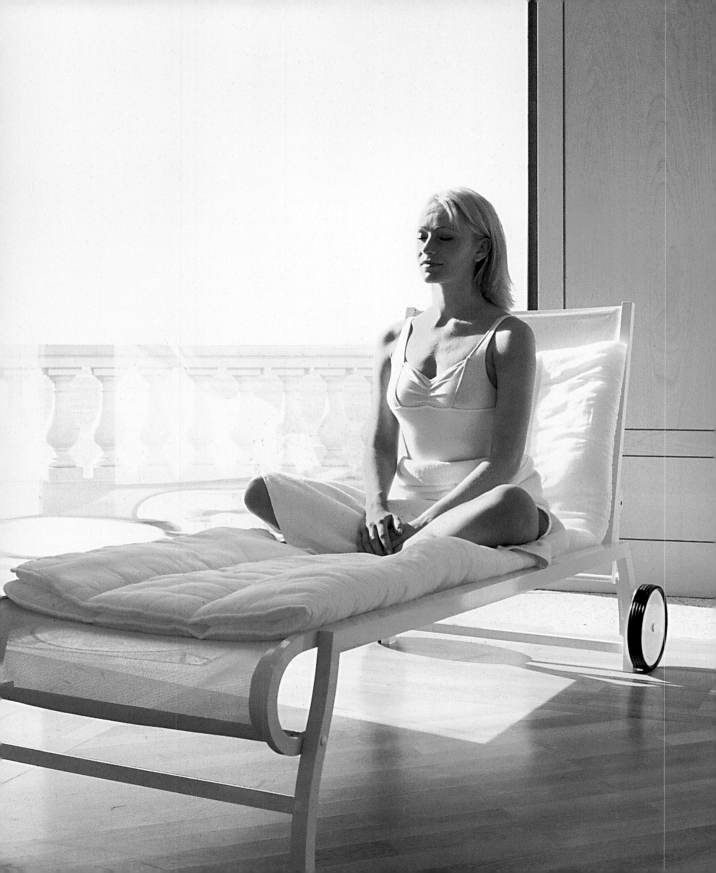

HARMONY
Balancing Body, Mind and Spirit

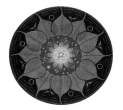

Greek philosopher Empedocles (?490–430 B.C.) held that harmony and discord are the two forces that join and separate the elements of water, fire, air and earth. This balance between harmony and disharmony is also echoed in holistic systems of healing, based on the belief that mental, physical and spiritual harmony determine the body's flow of vital energy.

Holistic health treatments and therapies aim to rebalance body, mind and spirit, bringing about overall wellbeing. Holism comes from the Greek word 'holos', meaning 'complete' or 'total'. It is based on the theory that all living things are made up of interacting wholes that are greater than a sum of their parts. Thus, a naturopath (see pp84–85), who takes a holistic approach to your health, may enquire about your medical history and symptoms like a conventional physician—but instead of treating only the symptoms, he also tries to treat the root of your problem by considering factors such as the social, psychological and environmental aspects of your life. Practitioners of Traditional Chinese Medicine (TCM, see p86) may use touch, sight and intuition to make a diagnosis, while those of Ayurveda (see pp85 and 87) may observe your gait and general appearance.

While mainstream medicine may see the body as a collection of physical systems, many other healing cultures approach it as a system through which a vital energy (see pp86–87) flows. This energy is dubbed variously as *pneuma* (by ancient Greek physician Galen), *ka* (by ancient Egyptians), vital fluid (medieval alchemists), *qi* (Chinese), *ki* (Japanese), and *prana* (Indian). Emotional disturbances or negative environmental influences can disrupt your energy flow, allowing wastes and toxins to build up that affect your body's self-regulatory powers and performance.

Body and mind naturally strive towards an equilibrium. Many treatments described in this chapter seek to restore this vital balance, which could lead to physical illness if not corrected. In addition to these health- and lifestyle-enhancing techniques, you should strive to take exercise, have sufficient rest and a balanced diet, maintain a healthy environment and positively manage the challenges that come your way, in order to achieve harmony in your health and life.

A CULTURAL PERSPECTIVE

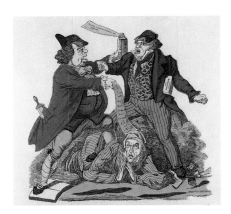

The best and safest thing is to keep a balance in your life, acknowledge the great powers around us and in us. If you can do that, and live that way, you are really a wise man.

– Euripides (?480–406 B.C.), Greek tragic dramatist

PAGE 82: Treatments that balance your energy, body-mind activities such as meditation, and the spa's serene settings are all aimed at helping you regain an inner harmony that may have been thrown off kilter by the stresses in life.

PAGE 83: This 12-petalled lotus encased within a 6-pointed star represents the middle chakra, the heart chakra, thought to be a point of balance that connects your spiritual with your physical side.

TOP: This caricature depicts the conflict between alternative methods of treatment represented by the homeopathic doctor in blue, and conventional medicine represented by the allopathic doctor in red, in the 18th and 19th centuries.

OPPOSITE, TOP LEFT: Vegetables and fruit are among the foods you should be eating more of—five to seven servings are recommended per day.

OPPOSITE, TOP RIGHT: Many healing cultures see the body as a system through which vital energy flows. In this image, an Indian doctor indicates the access points to the body's energy system.

OPPOSITE, BOTTOM: Natural healing advocates the use of good food grown in good soil. Opt for food in its natural state instead of those that are processed, or contain preservatives, artificial flavours or colouring.

HOLISM

The concept of the separateness of the body and spirit, and the conventional medical view of illnesses as a breakdown in the body's mechanisms, may be traced to the 17th century. Because of friction between the church and medicine, French philosopher René Descartes designated the attention of souls to the priests and that of the body to the physicians. However, these days, many orthodox doctors also recognise that a healthy diet and balanced lifestyle are equally crucial factors in keeping the body well tuned—principles long embraced by the naturopathy and health systems practised in the East (see TCM, p86; Ayurveda, pp85 and 87). Developments in the recent field of psychoneuroimmunology recognise that our minds, emotions and spiritual beliefs do affect our physical health, our mental well-being and our immune systems—paving the way to integrating holistic practices harmoniously into mainstream medicine.

Holistic Approaches and Diagnoses

Holistic approaches to health look at the person as a complete individual instead of isolating only the part that is ill. Treatments which are as natural as possible strive to maintain a balance, and hence health, within the body. Hippocrates, the father of modern medicine, expounded such principles around 5 B.C., emphasising treating a patient as a whole of his physical, mental and emotional states—rather than as a set of separate parts. A physician of Hippocratic times would also consider his patients' sex, race, climate, living conditions, and social and political environment in prescribing treatments geared towards helping patients help themselves. Western naturopathy and the Eastern systems of TCM and Ayurveda are now becoming popular in the West, with each having its own characteristics while sharing many holistic underlying principles with one another.

Naturopathy

The term 'naturopathy' was coined in 1895 by Dr John Scheel in New York. Rather than attack an illness, a naturopath takes a gentler approach of using natural cures that stimulate the

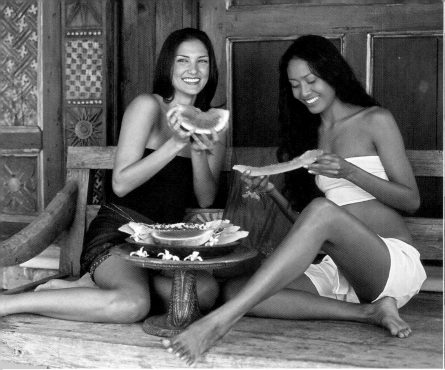

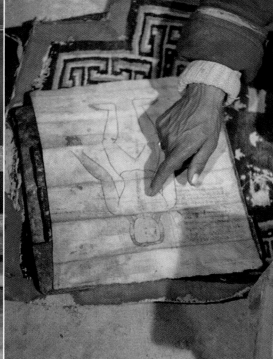

body's own vital force to fight disease and return the body to its natural state of equilibrium or homeostasis. These cures are also least likely to do your body harm. A naturopath may diagnose you by questioning you about your medical history, diet and lifestyle, observing your appearance and perhaps examining your pulse and tongue. Like Hippocrates, the modern naturopath may prescribe diet, exercise and rest. Other natural cures, such as the use of plants (see pp73–76), may derive from observations of animals self-medicating in the wild.

Naturopaths are also likely to use hydrotherapy (see Water chapter), massage (see pp92–97), fresh air (see pp56–57) and sunlight—popular in Austrian and German spa towns since the 19th century. Homeopathy (see p88) or therapies from TCM and Ayurveda may also be suggested.

Ayurveda

From India comes Ayurveda, from the Sanskrit words 'ayur' which means 'life', and 'veda', which means 'knowledge'. It is believed to be the oldest system of medicine on earth, originating about 5,000 years ago. This 'science of life' is still widely practised in India, Nepal and Sri Lanka, and Ayurvedic medicine and Ayurvedic-inspired treatments today are gaining popularity in Europe and

around the world. A traditional Ayurvedic physician—besides asking questions pertaining to your medical history and lifestyle, and observing your physical and mental characteristics—will make a diagnosis by examining factors such as your pulse, tongue, eyes, abdomen and skin, and may even ask seemingly intimate questions about your urine and stools, or your sexual lifestyle.

The physician can then determine your problem and your *dosha* type (see below), and prescribe treatments such as massages, *shirodhara* (see p95), exercises such as yoga (see pp64–65 and 102), and certain herbal preparations, while also providing dietary and lifestyle tips that he deems essential to balancing your *dosha*, and hence your body, mind and spirit.

According to the Ayurvedic 'life science', each of us is believed to possess a pattern of energy that corresponds with Ayurveda's three *dosha* types—although one *dosha* is usually thought to predominate. *Vata* types tend to be thin, creative and highly-strung. *Pitta* types tend to be medium built and driven. *Kapha* types are large-sized and stable. Each of the *doshas* is considered to be made up of a pair of the five elements—water, fire, air, earth and ether—which make up everything in the universe.

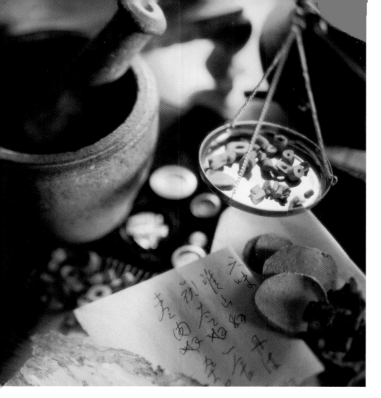

Traditional Chinese Medicine (TCM)

TCM's roots are attributed to two legendary emperors—the Red Emperor Shen Nong, and the Yellow Emperor Huang Di. The emphasis on health was so great in ancient times that wealthy households in China frequently employed their own herbalists, who were paid only when they were thought to be performing their duty of keeping the family healthy.

TCM practitioners use various diagnostic methods to assess your condition. These include taking your pulse, examining the coating on your tongue, observing your posture and the sparkle in your eyes, and questioning you extensively. Questions that may seem strange to you may pertain to your perspiration and eating habits. The practitioner is also likely to examine the area about 5 centimetres (2 inches) below your navel where your *dan tian*, or major storage area for *qi*, is believed to be located. He may then prescribe treatments such as acupuncture (see p100), the use of herbs, and exercises such as *qi gong* (see pp65 and 101), and also provide some suggestions on how to improve your diet and lifestyle.

According to the World Health Organization (WHO), TCM, especially acupuncture, is the most widespread traditional medicine practised around the world.

VITAL ENERGY

Holistic approaches to health see the body as imbued with a vital energy or life force. Ill health, it is believed, results when this energy becomes unbalanced. Treatments therefore focus on helping the body regain this balance, and hence health. Many different healing cultures focus on paradigms of energy-related balance, the key ones being the Indian chakras, the Chinese meridians, and the auras used mainly in the West.

The Meridians

According to the philosophy behind TCM, *qi*—the universal life force—courses through your body's network of 14 main meridians, 12 connected to specific organs. If a meridian is blocked, or if there is an excess flow of *qi*, illness will follow.

To regulate your flow of *qi*, a TCM practitioner manipulates those meridian points known as acupoints. The methods that he uses are quite likely to include acupressure (see p96), acupuncture (see p100) and reflexology (see pp98–99). Exercise, diet and beneficial herbal remedies are also major factors in helping to improve the flow of *qi*—not only to treat illness, but also to maintain good health.

In TCM, the human body is also viewed in terms of the complementary yet opposing forces of *yin* and *yang*. *Yin* (meaning 'the dark side of the mountain' in Chinese) is feminine, with cold, dark, quiet, static and wet properties. *Yang* ('the bright side of the mountain') is masculine with warm, bright, dynamic and dry properties. The interdependent nature of *yin* and *yang* underscores a very basic and essential principle of TCM: that it is only possible to achieve balance and harmony when these two opposing forces are in balance.

The Chinese influence can be seen in many other traditional and widely practised healing systems in Asia, including Japanese and traditional Thai medicine.

British medical researcher Sir Charles Shillington claimed in a 1930 study published in the *British Medical Journal* that he had found a network in the body which seemed to correspond with the Chinese meridians and Indian *nadis*.

Chakra Key

Each of the seven major chakras is associated with a colour in the light spectrum, an element according to Indian philosophy, and a governing principle.

Chakra	Colour	Element	Governs
Crown	Violet	-	Enlightenment and the spiritual self
Brow	Indigo	-	Insight and intuition
Throat	Blue	Ether	Communication and self-expression
Heart	Green	Air	Love and compassion
Solar plexus	Yellow	Fire	Self-worth, will, inner power
Sacral	Orange	Water	Sensuality and sexuality
Root	Red	Earth	Survival

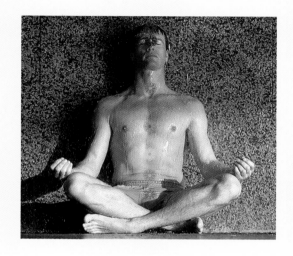

The Chakras

Ayurveda believes that good health depends on the flow and balance of *prana* (vital energy) through 72,000 channels known as *nadis*. This energy is regulated by your chakras—vortexes of energy, each thought to vibrate at a particular frequency. The seven main chakras are located from your crown to the spine along the most important Sushumna *nadi*. Each chakra is linked with different organs, Ayurvedic elements, colours and universal principles (see above table), as well as to emotions. It is believed that health is only possible when all chakras are functioning properly; imbalances may be restored through methods such as yoga (see pp64–65 and 102), breathing exercises (see pp48, 59 and 61), meditation (see p63), or by bathing the relevant area with a colour (see pp91–92) to strengthen it.

The Aura

Practitioners who work with auras believe that all living things have an electromagnetic field or body of energy that forms an oval shape around our bodies. Some energy healers or psychics claim to perceive its emanations intuitively. Others use biofeedback sensors, computers and photographic devices to record and analyse these fields. Yale University neuroanatomist Professor Harold Saxton Burr was one of the first to measure this energy field In the 1930s, calling it the L-field, for 'life field'.

Your aura's characteristics are thought to change with illness, moods or the environment, reflecting your physical, psychological and spiritual wellbeing. Auras are believed to have seven layered bands, reflecting different facets of personality, and corresponding in colour with each of the chakras.

OPPOSITE: Chinese herbalists prescribe herbs to treat and prevent not just physical illnesses, but also mental and emotional disorders.

TOP: Imbalances in chakras are often treated by using the colours associated with them.

RIGHT: The aura is often thought of as an energy field. Practitioners who work with energy or aura may use Kirlian photography as a diagnostic tool. Kirlian photography works by creating an image of your body's electromagnetic field as it comes into contact with a high-voltage, high-frequency electric charge.

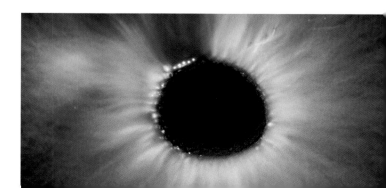

TREATMENTS AND THERAPIES

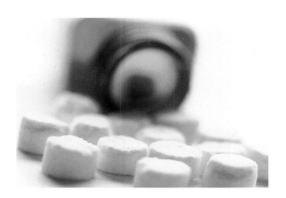

Natural forces within us are the true healers of disease.

– Hippocrates (?460–?377 B.C.), Greek physician commonly regarded as the father of medicine

HOMEOPATHY

Based on the Greek words '*pathos*' (suffering) and '*homoios*' (same), homeopathy works on a principle that 'like cures like'.

After 18th-century German physician Samuel Hahnemann experimented on himself with doses of quinine and developed malaria-like symptoms, he theorised that a cure was related to a substance's ability to cause symptoms of the same disease in an otherwise healthy person. Modern homeopaths follow the same principles, administering remedies that would otherwise cause similar symptoms in a healthy person in order to stimulate the self-healing process. Eyebright, for instance—an irritant herb—is used to soothe sensitive eyes.

Homeopathic medicines include some 2,000 remedies, generally made from minerals, vegetable and animal substances diluted many times over to make them safe to use. When the desired potency is reached, a few drops are added to lactose tablets or sucrose granules to be taken orally. The medicines may also be administered as injections, liquids, ointments, sprays and suppositories. Homeopaths believe that the more diluted the substance, the more effective it is.

A homeopathic practitioner will ask you in detail about your medical history, lifestyle and even dislikes and fears, so as to get a complete picture of you and your symptoms. A classical homeopath will prescribe a single dose of a single remedy that best matches your constitutional type; while a complex homeopath may treat your sick organs rather than your constitution using low-potency remedies, often with herbal extracts.

Some studies suggest that homeopathy works, though its action remains to be explained scientifically. Sceptics attribute its effectiveness to a placebo effect, though homeopathy continues to have a popular, high-profile following. In the United Kingdom, for example, it is accepted as part of the National Health Service.

Homeopathy is used to treat people of all ages and a wide range of illnesses, especially allergies, asthma and eczema.

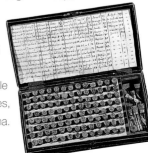

TOP: In making a homeopathic preparation, usually one part of the substance is diluted in 99 parts of alcohol, then shaken rapidly, a process known as succussion. This 1:100 dilution is known as a centesimal, or a 'c' dilution. The figure '30c', for instance, indicates that a remedy has been diluted 30 times. A 'd' (for decimal) indicates a 1:10 dilution, though some countries may use the letter 'x' in place of 'd'. When the desired potency is reached, a few drops are added to lactose tablets.

RIGHT: Early homeopathic practitioners kept phials of remedies carefully catalogued and ready to be dispensed from a box such as this one, which dates back to the late 19th century.

OPPOSITE, TOP: Your Alexander teacher will often work on you as you lie down. This semi-supine position helps restore your back to its optimal alignment, releases the muscles and joints, and eases breathing. You can also use this position at home to refresh yourself if you are feeling stressed, tired or have a backache.

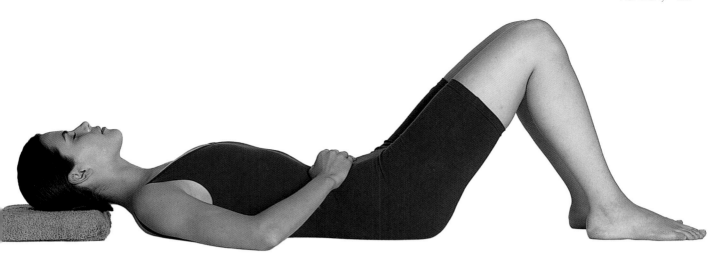

THE ALEXANDER TECHNIQUE

How you move and stand can affect your energy levels and your body, mind and spirit. Students of the Alexander Technique relearn how to stand and move correctly to help their bodies to function more efficiently.

Minor recurring complaints, such as headaches and backaches, may improve as students rebalance their posture. They also testify to profound emotional and spiritual benefits such as being calmer and more confident, having improved sleeping habits, feeling emotionally rebalanced and gaining a new perspective on their environment.

The technique was developed by Australian actor Frederick Matthias Alexander in the late 19th century. Troubled by vocal problems that could not be cured by doctors and voice coaches, Alexander used a series of mirrors to observe his movements as he spoke, and noticed that he was pulling his head backwards and downwards, tightening his throat muscles.

After extensive experimentation, Alexander devised a method to release this tension and as a result, his voice returned. His observations were ultimately to have a far more extensive application to physical and psychological problems not connected with the voice.

Alexander went on to develop and refine his eponymous technique, and eventually he moved to London where he set up his first training school in 1930. His early students included George Bernard Shaw and Aldous Huxley. In later years, Alexander took his school and his methods to the United States where they were equally well received.

Modern-day celebrity students of the Alexander Technique include musicians Sting and Paul McCartney, and actors John Cleese, William Hurt and Robin Williams. It is on the curriculum of many drama and music colleges, and is also popular with dancers and sportspeople, enabling their bodies to function at peak efficiency and avoid injury. Besides providing better coordination and greater fluidity of movement, it can also bring relief from pain or tension resulting from bad postural habits.

The Alexander Technique can be learnt at any age. A session can last from 30 to 60 minutes, and is ideally taught on a one-on-one basis. Wear loose comfortable clothing, and if you are a woman, wear trousers instead of a skirt.

Teachers vary in their approaches, but typically, the teacher first evaluates how you stand and move. Using his hands, he will make subtle adjustments to your body as you lie, sit or stand, to make you aware of your optimum posture and how it feels to move and use your muscles with minimum effort for maximum efficiency. Particular attention is paid to how you hold your head. You also learn to apply 'inhibition'—pausing and thinking before reacting—and how to project 'directions' such as 'free neck' and 'back lengthen and widen' to your body.

In subsequent sessions, the teacher can help you apply the principles to your everyday actions (such as lifting and ironing), or movements in your areas of interest or profession.

The number of sessions required varies. Practicing what you have learnt in your daily life will help you develop appropriate postural habits to help restore balance to your body, which in turn affects your wellbeing.

REIKI

Reiki, from the Japanese characters '*rei*' (universal) and '*ki*' (life force), is a calming touch therapy used to stimulate the body's own healing forces to remove physical or emotional blockages. It is used primarily to treat complaints such as arthritis, insomnia and migraine. Its numerous devotees also employ it to relieve physical pain and alleviate emotional stress.

If you are willing, *reiki* also has the potential to stimulate healing at profound emotional and spiritual levels, and can be instrumental in promoting your personal growth.

Reiki is believed to have been rediscovered in ancient Tibetan Sanskrit *sutras* in the late 1880s by a Japanese Christian theologian, Dr Mikao Usui, who was engaged in the study of the healing powers of Christ and of Buddha.

These Sanskrit symbols and mantras are believed to activate the universal life energy for healing. Dr Usui went on to practise *reiki* in Japan, and introduced it to other masters.

All practitioners of *reiki* must be attuned to the ancient symbols before they can use *ki* to heal. You may use *reiki* on yourself and others (including pets and plants) after appropriate training by a *reiki* master, who will attune you to First Degree

Reiki; once you are fully attuned, you will be able to access *reiki* any time for the rest of your life.

Second Degree Reiki is for those who wish to become practitioners, while the study of Third Degree Reiki trains one to become a true *reiki* master and a teacher.

You remain fully clothed, but have your shoes off during a session. The practitioner will place his hands over or lightly on the 12 key areas of your body, typically starting with your head. The *ki* channelled through his hands into you helps to release blocked energies, cleanse accumulated toxins and activate your body's natural ability to heal itself.

Reiki treatment sessions last for about an hour, leaving you feeling invigorated or relaxed. Shorter sessions lasting 20 to 30 minutes are suitable for babies.

Care should be taken when treating diabetics with *reiki*, as the energy released is believed to affect insulin levels. *Reiki* should also not be performed on people with pacemakers or similar devices; on someone who is anaesthetised before an operation; or on fractures before they are set in plaster. It may be successfully used in conjunction with colour therapy (see pp91–92) and crystal therapy (see p78).

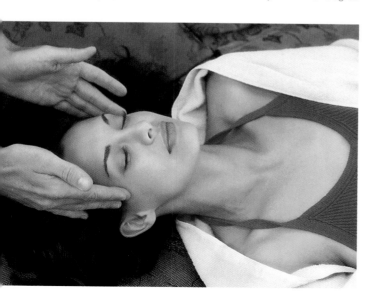

Benefitting from Reiki

A *reiki* session is a different experience for everyone, so go with an open mind, advises The Spa at The Westin Turnberry Resort.

- Drink no alcohol at least 12 hours before treatment. Limit all stimulants before, and for 12 hours after treatment.
- *Reiki* may release emotions you have not been facing up to—these may range from a few tears to insane laughter.
- You may see colours or experience a feeling of warmth or cold as energy fields help to calm, soothe and heal.
- Avoid heat treatments after a *reiki* session. Do not schedule any activities except for relaxing or swimming.
- You will feel thirsty after treatment, so drink plenty of water.
- How you feel after a session varies from person to person. You could feel very sleepy, revitalised or more in control.

COLOUR THERAPY

While studies show that colour can affect us psychologically, colour therapists go further. In the 1930s, Indian scientist Dinshah P Ghadiali devised ways of projecting coloured rays of light on afflicted parts of the body to treat ailments and injuries.

Light is made up of a spectrum of colours. When it passes through raindrops, or is refracted through a prism, we see the colours of a rainbow: red, orange, yellow, green, blue, indigo and violet. Each colour has its own wavelength and frequency, or the rate at which it vibrates. Warmer colours, such as red, are believed to have a faster vibration while cooler colours, such as blue, vibrate more slowly. Vibrational imbalances within our cells and organs are believed to be harmonised when we absorb light waves of the appropriate colours.

Much colour therapy is influenced by the theory of the chakras (see p87). It is believed that illnesses or energy imbalances can be treated by administering the correct colours. This is supported to some extent by recent psychological research.

Treatment sessions may begin with the colour practitioner enquiring about your health and preferred colours. Some practitioners employ psychological tests, or dowse a spinal chart by holding a pendulum over each illustrated vertebra—the way it swings is believed to indicate stagnation or blockages in energy. Others prescribe colours without such aids.

Two main methods used to administer colour to your body include contact healing and exposure to coloured lights. In contact healing, the therapist places her hands on or near you to sense blockages in your aura. She then visualises the colours you require and channels them to you through her hands.

For colour illumination therapy, you typically sit in front of a computerised colour therapy instrument that emits alternating coloured lights. The therapist may also shine a torch through stained glass discs into a quartz crystal point, which is then directed to various parts of your body. Exposure to your treatment colour (for example, blue) as well as its complementary colour (orange in this case) is believed to stabilise your condition. Wear white so as not to distort the colours administered.

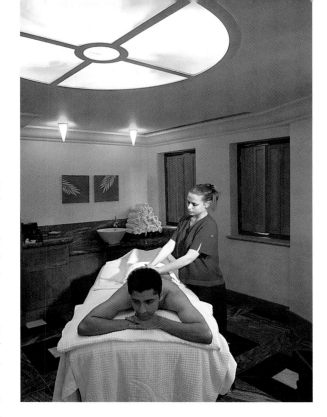

Drinking water 'solarised' by the sun's energy through a coloured filter; wrapping yourself in coloured silks; or adding non-toxic colours to your bath are other ways to absorb colour.

Some spa treatments employ colour therapy principles. Your massage therapist may perform massages in front of stained glass windows where certain colours fall on certain parts of your body. Colour therapy may also be used in saunas and steam rooms fitted with coloured lights, and colour therapy may be combined with visualisation (see p64) and breathing exercises (see pp62–65).

OPPOSITE, LEFT: During a reiki session, as the healing energy is channelled to you, you may feel a warm, cold or tingling sensation. Some people find themselves crying as their emotional blockages are cleared.

TOP: The Spa at Pennyhill Park is equipped with the most advanced computerised lighting systems in which the lighting changes through a kaleidoscope of colours as your spa treatment progresses. These sequences are believed to enhance your wellbeing, to aid relaxation and to create a sense of calm and serenity.

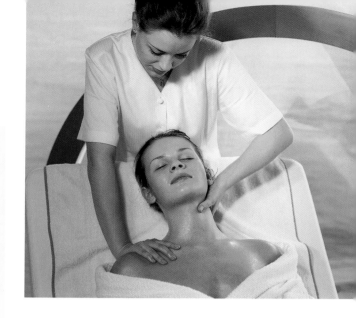

Colouring Your World

You may already be using colour to affect your mood in the clothes you wear, or the colours you use in your home. The following table shows the colours of the rainbow and traits they are commonly associated with, and includes suggestions on how to use them, and instances where you may want to avoid them.

 Red
Red is associated with strength, sexuality and stimulation. Wear red if you are feeling cold or when you need to give yourself an energy boost. Use red in an activity room or a passageway. Too much red may lead to aggressiveness.

 Orange
Orange is associated with energy and life. Wear orange to lift your spirits if you are feeling down. Use orange in your study room to boost creativity. Too much orange may lead to complacency.

 Yellow
Yellow is associated with vigour and vibrancy. Wear yellow to help enhance your self-esteem. Use yellow in your study room to enhance concentration, or in your dining area to help stimulate your digestive system. Too much yellow may make it hard to calm down.

 Green
Green is associated with nature, balance and harmony. Wear green to balance your emotions. Use green in your family room to strengthen harmony within the family. Too much green can be too calming when you need to stay alert.

 Blue
Blue is associated with relaxation, peace and inspiration. Wear blue to help you cool down on a warm day. Use blue in your bathroom or in other rooms where you need to unwind after a day's work. Too much blue can be overly sedative.

 Indigo
Indigo is associated with intellectual ability and insight. Wear indigo to help enhance your intuition. Use indigo in those rooms which you use to quiet yourself. Too much indigo may intensify feelings of mental trouble or depression.

 Violet
Violet is associated with a connection with the divine. Wear violet if you need inspiration, or if you want to step out of the past and look to the future. Use violet in rooms where you meditate. Too much violet may not be a good idea for people with mental-, alcohol- and drug-related problems.

MASSAGE

Massages originating from the East are based on the theory of energy flowing through the body, while massages from the West are typically based on the anatomy and physiology. Massage in general leaves you feeling relaxed, refreshed and restored, both physically and mentally. It is perhaps the earliest form of medical care, practised by many cultures including the Egyptians, Greek, Romans, Chinese and Indians since ancient times. A large proportion of treatments which can be classified as massage therapy have been developed since the 1970s, when people started taking a greater interest in leading a healthier lifestyle. Interest in massage is surging as more people seek ways to lower their stress levels and prevent any resulting problems such as insomnia and migraine.

During a massage, body tissues may be manipulated either manually or mechanically. The touch of a manual massage often feels nurturing, and helps bring about a sense of peace. Touch helps stimulate endorphin levels, reducing anxiety and pain, and minimising tension. Mechanical massages such as the G5 (a gyratory vibrator, the most commonly used type of mechanical massage machine) are less personal, but they do provide a greater depth and are especially useful for treating muscular male spa-goers. Machine massages may also be used to ease muscle ache and help break down fatty tissues.

Besides aiding relaxation and positively affecting the body's muscular, vascular and nervous systems, the main benefits of massage include improving blood and lymph circulation, easing

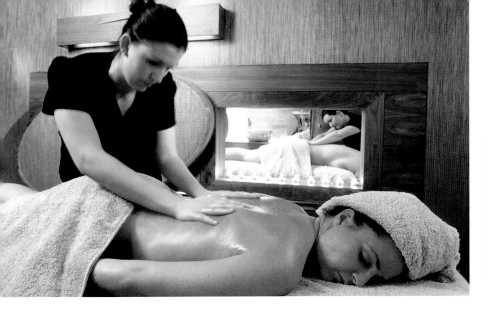

muscle and nerve pain, improving the texture of the skin, and promoting an overall sense of wellbeing.

Depending on the techniques and oils used (see pp70–72), you may feel invigorated or calmer after a massage. Do inform your therapist beforehand—or during the massage—if there are specific areas you would like her to concentrate on or to avoid.

There may be a number of instances where massages in general, or to specific areas, should be avoided. Seek medical advice on the suitability of different massages, for example, if you suffer from any medical condition or are pregnant. Conditions for which massages are contraindicated include problems with the heart, blood pressure, lungs and skin. Do not have a massage if you have haemophilia, a suspicious lump, high fever, sunburn, or are in a late stage of pregnancy.

Swedish Massage

What is possibly the most widely used massage was developed in 1813 by Swedish fencing master and gymnastics instructor Per Henrik Ling, who used it to cure himself of rheumatism. Grounded in anatomy and physiology, this massage, the first modern systemisation of massage in the West, has served as a basis for many other massage techniques developed since.

A Swedish massage involves five main strokes, all done on the more superficial layers of the muscles, and generally in the direction of the blood flow towards the heart. The massage begins with effleurage (French for 'flower-like'): long gliding strokes which the therapist uses to apply lubricant—such as a

mix of essential oils—to your skin, to help her examine your muscle tissues and relax them. The benefits of this stroke are numerous, but most importantly, it helps increase blood and lymph circulation. The massage also ends with this stroke.

Effleurage is followed by petrissage, or kneading, whereby the therapist uses movements that roll, pinch, wring, or lift up your skin. These strokes improve circulation, stimulate weak muscles, and provide heat to the body. Friction, or rubbing, is used to break down knots of muscle fibres formed after any muscular trauma or strain. It is applied in transverse movements across the fibres of your muscles and soft tissues, or in circular motions to a joint. In tapotement, or percussion, the therapist taps your muscles using beating, hacking, slapping and cupping movements to release tension and cramping.

The final stroke, vibration, is a rhythmic shaking of hands or fingers in a stationary or 'running' position. When performed for over ten seconds, it may assist in easing muscle spasms. Swedish massage is used for relaxation, rehabilitation, or for maintaining one's health.

Deep Tissue Massage

Known also as deep muscle therapy, deep tissue massage works on the muscles and connective tissues to treat pain (especially chronic, lower back and neck pains), release muscular knots, and help circulatory problems. The therapist begins by identifying your areas of pain and affected connective tissues. Your body must be relaxed before she can work on your problem area. The massage works on your fascia, the sheath that surrounds your muscles and organs. It usually begins lightly, but graduates to a level which many refer to colloquially as 'hurting so good'. At this level, physical correction is believed to occur—but it should never be agonisingly painful.

Deep tissue massages include sports massage catering mainly to athletes, dancers and exercise enthusiasts. The therapist starts with superficial strokes to identify problem areas and overstrained muscles—these are usually hard and tense compared to the surrounding tissues. Many top athletes use it as part of their daily training regimen; before events to warm up the ligaments and tendons to prevent injury; and to enhance performance and endurance. After an event, this massage is restorative and useful for muscles which have been overexerted; it also helps accelerate recovery from injuries.

Avoid a deep tissue massage if you have a low threshold for pain, are pregnant or breast-feeding, or have torn muscles, bruises or vascular problems.

Lymphatic Drainage Massage

British vacationers in Cannes around 1932 were among the first recipients of this massage. Pioneered by Danish massage therapists Dr Emil Vodder and his wife, their technique, which went against the approaches of the time, eased their patients' chronic colds and the swollen lymph nodes in their necks.

This gentle connective tissue massage technique—which involves stationary circles, pumping, scooping, rotary and thumb circle movements—helps stimulate the movement of the lymph: the milky fluid that bathes our muscles and organs and delivers nutrients, antibodies and other immune constituents to our cells. The procedure is based upon the premise that a healthy lymphatic system is necessary to keep the body's tissues and cells free from waste and excess water so the body can function efficiently and maintain its immune system.

Manual lymph massage is also used to treat conditions such as skin ailments and swelling related to surgery in otherwise healthy people. It is also a popular treatment for reducing stretch marks. You should seek the advice of your doctor before having a lymph massage, especially before or after surgery, or if you have any medical conditions such as cancer, heart problems, thrombosis, kidney problems or viral infections.

Champissage

For thousands of years, Indian women have been keeping their locks lustrous and men have fended off baldness through the use of head massage. Even today, Indian children are regularly

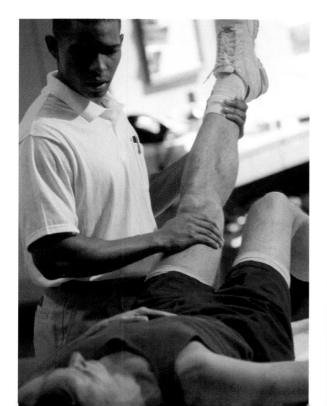

LEFT: The sports massage is a specialised form of Swedish massage designed for athletes. A sports massage may take less than an hour; and could take just 15 minutes if a particular muscle group is being worked on.

OPPOSITE, LEFT: A head massage boosts your concentration, recharges you mentally, calms your mind, and helps relieve insomnia.

OPPOSITE, RIGHT: One who applies oil on his head regularly does not suffer from headache, baldness, greying of hair, nor does his hair fall. Strength of his head and forehead is especially enhanced; his hair becomes black, long and deep-rooted; his sense organs work properly; the skin of his face becomes brightened; applying oil on the head produces sound sleep and happiness.
– Ayurvedic physician Charaka, in Charaka Samhita, the first text on Ayurveda, written over 2,000 years ago

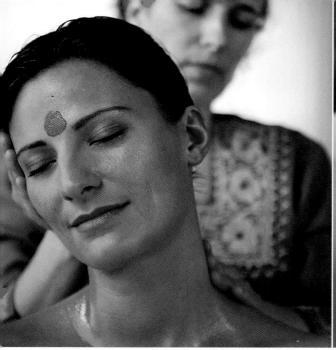
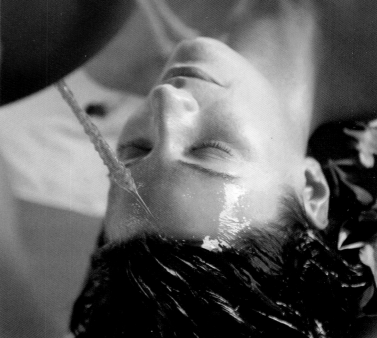

massaged from birth, inheriting at a tender age the techniques that have been passed down from their ancestors.

Champissage—from the Hindi word '*champi*', which means 'head massage'—was developed by blind Indian manipulative therapist Nehendra Mehta, who popularised his technique in London in the 1980s. Besides nourishing your hair, the massage calms your spirit, easing stress-induced tension such as eyestrain, headaches, and neck-and-shoulder aches. It is also believed to improve blood and lymph circulation.

You may remain fully clothed during the 20- to 30-minute session, which can be performed with oils chosen to suit your hair condition. However, if you have a social engagement or are returning to the office after this energy-balancing treatment, you may want to opt for an oil-free head massage. Your therapist may use techniques that include pulling and squeezing your shoulders with her thumbs and fingers, ironing down your shoulders and upper arms with her palms, grasping and pulling your neck, and ruffling your hair with her hands or combing through your strands with her fingers. As a head massage improves blood flow to your brain, you may find yourself working more productively after the session.

In Western-style versions of the Indian head massage (which has its roots in Ayurvedic medicine), it is not just your scalp and neck that are massaged, but also your face, ears, shoulders and upper arms. Anger and stress tend to manifest themselves as tension in your head, neck and shoulders, which are considered major energy centres in your body. Head massages are not recommended for those with eczema, head injuries, for those who are epileptic or psychotic, or with certain other medical conditions, so check with your therapist beforehand.

Shirodhara

Shirodhara, from the Sanskrit words '*shiro*' (head) and '*dhara*' (flow), is considered one of the most powerful Ayurvedic treatments available. It is also known as the 'massage of the third eye' as, during this treatment, you will lie on your back as a thin, steady stream of heated medicated oil is dripped between your brows. The oil, held in a brass bowl pot with a hole in its base suspended above you, trickles down into your hair, and may be massaged into your scalp to enhance the effects of this treatment. Oils are chosen to suit your *dosha* type (see p85).

This treatment may last for between 30 and 40 minutes, and is used to treat problems such as anxiety and insomnia that typically affect Ayurvedic *vata* types. A session helps relax your central nervous system and relieve mental tension. You may find the deep, meditative state you are in during the treatment leaves your mind feeling calm and balanced. *Shirodhara* is also used to treat amnesia, epilepsy and migraine.

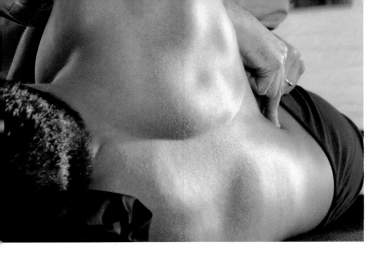

Acupressure

This ancient Chinese massage system—often described as 'acupuncture (see p100) without needles'—is believed to have been practised for over 4,000 years. The practitioner may stimulate acupoints along your meridians using not just finger and thumb pressure, but also knuckle and palm pressure, with a gentle rotating motion to boost *qi*, restore imbalances in the flow of energy, ease tension and help the body heal itself. Pinching movements may be used on the nails, fingers and toes where major meridians begin, and a wooden knobbed instrument may be used to stimulate acupoints.

Acupressure releases tense muscles, increases blood circulation and may remove toxins from the tissues. It is used to treat many complaints including headaches, sinus complaints and menstrual problems. Western theory attributes acupressure's effectiveness to the release of endorphins, which ease pain and produce a feeling of wellbeing

Several techniques, such as the Japanese shiatsu (see p97), have evolved from acupressure. The Chinese *tui na* (see right) is a variation of acupressure massage. Do not have acupressure immediately after a meal or exercise, or if you have a fever, infection, skin problem or a serious medical problem.

Press Away Nausea

A common way to relieve nausea is to apply pressure to the point 5 cm (2 in) below your wrist on the underside of your arm for 1 to 2 minutes using the thumb of your other hand. This technique is useful if you suffer from travel sickness. Acubands available from pharmacies work on a similar principle.

Tui Na

This ancient Chinese system of massage aims to remove any blockages and restore a harmonised flow of energy within the body. It may have been used as early as 500 B.C., and it has influenced major bodywork systems from Thai massage (see p97) to shiatsu (see p97). *Tui na* is now taught in traditional medical schools in China and practised in hospitals.

The massage is deep and vigorous, and not recommended for people with a low pain threshold. It may be applied to the whole body, though more gently to sensitive areas such as the face and neck. A gentler system is used to treat children.

Eight fundamental techniques are used: pushing *(tui)*, grasping *(na)*, pressing, rubbing, rolling, pulling, beating and shaking. The therapist uses hands, arms, elbows, and even feet to stimulate the acupoints and treat soft tissues. Traditionally, *tui na* is performed though clothes, and an extra cloth may be wrapped around the area being treated, but in some instances, your upper body is uncovered. Herbal preparations, oils or powders are occasionally used.

Tui na is used to treat a variety of problems including musculoskeletal ailments, and digestive and respiratory problems. A session usually lasts for 20 to 30 minutes. It is not recommended for people with cancer, fragile bones or heart problems.

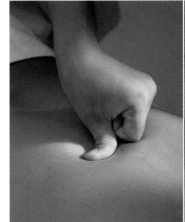
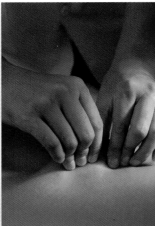

Thai Massage

This massage, known in Thai as *nuad* (massage) *bo-ram* (ancient), has been practised for over 2,500 years. It is also called Thai medical massage. Ancient medical texts etched in stone may still be seen on the walls in Bangkok's Wat Poh Temple, the most famous school where the massage is taught.

Based on TCM (see p86), Ayurveda (see pp85 and 87) and yoga (see pp64–65 and 102), it aims to create a smooth energy flow within your body. You will wear loose, comfortable clothes during this massage, given on a floor mat so the therapist can use her body's weight to provide a deeper level of pressure and allow for movements that would otherwise be impossible on a table. Using her hands, thumbs, fingers, elbows, forearms, knees and feet to apply pressure along acupressure points known as *sens*, she will also pull, twist and manipulate your body in yoga-like stretches and a gentle rocking motion. Thai massage is given meditatively and slowly, minimising the risk of injury. It typically lasts for two hours and is believed to help loosen joints, stretch muscles and tone the internal organs. You should feel deeply relaxed afterwards.

Shiatsu

Shiatsu, derived from the Japanese characters 'shi' (finger) and 'atsu' (therapy), combines principals of TCM (see p86) with a knowledge of physiology and anatomy from Western medicine.

You lie on a padded mattress or futon on the floor, clad in loose, comfortable clothes. Specific areas or your whole body may be treated in a session lasting from 60 to 90 minutes. The therapist will apply firm pressure for three to five seconds on points called *tsubos*—vital points along your energy pathways—and perform body stretches along your meridian passages. Besides fingers, she also uses the palms and heels of her hands, her knuckles, as well as forearms, elbows, knees and feet to apply a constant pressure. Designed to relax your muscles and soft tissues, boost stamina, and improve digestion, this holistic therapy also relieves stress and calms nerves. Do not exercise or take a hot bath before shiatsu or afterwards.

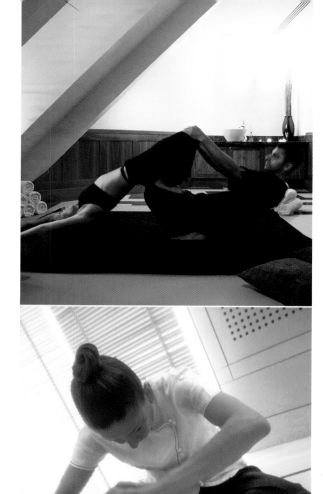

OPPOSITE, TOP LEFT: In acupressure, pressure lasting between ten seconds and three minutes is said to be sedative, while pressure lasting under ten seconds is stimulating.

OPPOSITE, BOTTOM: Literally translated, tui na means pushing (LEFT) and grasping (RIGHT), though six other key strokes are also used.

TOP: In Thai massage, you may be manipulated into elegant stretches. Your therapist's meditative state of mind contributes to your healing experience.

ABOVE: Unlike many other massage methods which may be vigorous and moving, the pressure is sustained and stationary in shiatsu.

REFLEXOLOGY

Reflexology is the art of stimulating various points on certain areas of your body to improve energy blockages and restore a smooth flow of energy. It is commonly associated with the feet—the most sensitive part with 7,200 nerve endings in each foot—though reflexology is also performed on the hands and ears. Stimulating your reflex points on these areas with thumb and finger pressure is believed to affect the organ and gland each point is associated with. The pressure helps remove any congestion in the corresponding part, improve circulation and blood supply, and enhance the body's ability to heal itself.

Proponents of reflexology recommend that you have regular sessions to maintain your health. Studies have shown that regular reflexology is useful in easing stress and pre-menstrual symptoms; it also reduces pain and increases mobility for people with back pains. A study conducted in Denmark in the 1990s on postal workers who had reflexology twice a month showed that absenteeism went down by 13.3 per cent.

Various cultures—including the ancients in China, India, Japan, Greece and Egypt, and the indigenous people in Africa and America—have their own variations of reflexology. However, much of reflexology that is practised in the West today stems from the work of American ear, nose and throat specialist Dr William Fitzgerald. In the early 20th century, Dr Fitzgerald observed that pressure on specific parts of the body had an analgesic effect on other parts. He divided the body longitudinally from the head to the toes into ten zones with five zones—one per toe—on each side of the body. Each finger is also associated with a particular zone. Pressure on any part of the zone is believed to affect parts along that longitudinal line.

American physiotherapist Eunice Ingham took Dr Fitzgerald's zone therapy further in the 1930s, developing it into what is now foot reflexology. Focusing on the feet, she noticed that tension in a certain part of the foot reflected tension in a corresponding part of the body. She designed foot maps that are still in use today and developed the technique of alternating pressure.

While many people associate reflexology with pain, more recent work by British reflexologists such as Patricia Morrell show that a gentler approach is also effective. It is important to find an experienced, qualified reflexologist, as this treatment is contraindicated in some instances. Extra care needs to be taken if you are pregnant or have a serious disease. Avoid reflexology if you suffer from vein problems or thrombosis.

Foot Reflexology

Before a foot reflexology session, lasting between 30 to 60 minutes, you remove your socks and shoes, and your feet will be washed and dried. Your reflexologist will identify areas in your body that may be congested by looking for signs such as calluses, and feeling your feet for tenderness or grainy areas.

You lie on a massage couch or sit in a chair with your feet on a footrest as the therapist works on each foot, using techniques such as thumb and finger walking, thumb hook and back up, rotating on a point, flexing on a point, pivoting on a point, and finger rolling. She should adjust her pressure to your comfort level—some areas may feel more painful than others, indicating an area that may be congested. Afterwards, many people report feeling revitalised, though others may feel tired, or notice themselves perspiring more or using the toilet more frequently—signs that toxins are being removed from the body.

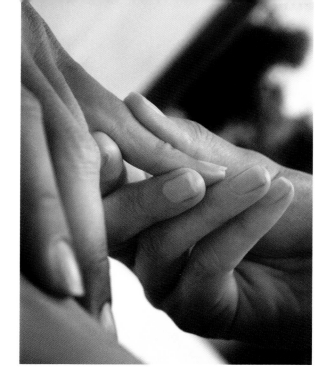

Hand Reflexology

While our hands may not be as sensitive as our feet, hand reflexology is helpful for people who may not like their feet being touched, or who are shy to reveal their feet. It may also be used to precede a foot reflexology session. As in any form of reflexology, you should tell your reflexologist in advance if you suffer from any unusual symptoms or medical problems.

Your therapist will use techniques such as deep thumb or finger pressure to feel underlying bones or muscles, or pressing and rolling, or pressing and pulling thumb movements to feel out sore areas. Accessories such as combs may also be used to create sustained pressure during a session.

Ear Reflexology

Ear reflexology using simultaneous finger pressure on both ears may be given as a session on its own, or included at the beginning or end of a foot reflexology session. You may also have your ears manipulated during treatments such as facials and head massages. As with the feet and hands, specific auricular points on the ears are believed to correspond with certain organs and body areas—thus, swelling, redness and discomfort around certain parts of the ear may indicate a problem in the correspondent part.

Relieve Stress with DIY Reflexology

The next time you feel stressed, The Spa at The Westin Turnberry Resort recommends you try stimulating the solar plexus reflexes on your feet and hands. It will bring about a feeling of relaxation.

On Your Feet:

- Put your hands around your toes and squeeze them together. This pushes in the underside of the foot, creating a soft area in the middle.
- To find your solar plexus reflex, trace down between your first and second toes to the area between the ball of your foot and your arch.
- Press this point gently, for about a minute.
- Do the same on the other foot.
- If you suffer from backache, you may also want to try rubbing along the whole inner edge of each foot, moving from the tip of the big toe to the base of the foot that represents your spinal area.
- It may be easier if you can get a friend to massage these areas for you.

On Your Hands:

- Squeeze the fingers of one hand together so that you create a soft area in the middle of the hand.
- Your solar plexus reflex is located in the middle of the hand under the middle finger.
- Press this point gently and give it a little rub for a minute. This can help to relieve stress, anxiety, nausea and give you a feeling of relaxation.
- Do the same on your other hand.

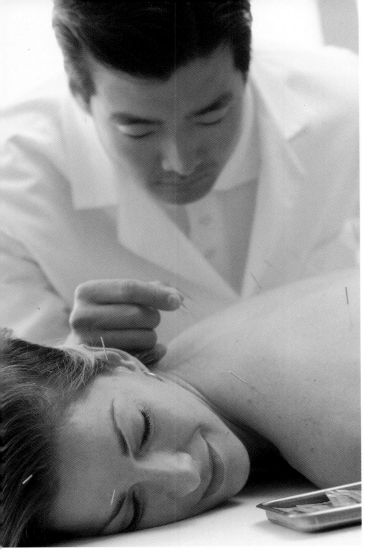

ACUPUNCTURE

A vital component of TCM, acupuncture involves inserting needles quickly and painlessly at various acupoints around your body, often synchronised with your breathing. While commonly used to manage pain, acupuncture is also typically used to treat illnesses by removing energy blockages, or stimulating the flow of *qi* among the 365 acupoints along the body's meridians.

The needles are inserted to a depth of 4 to 25 millimetres (⅛ to 1 inch) at various acupoints in the location of pain or problem, or along the acupoints that lie on the corresponding meridian pathway. Depending on the condition being treated, between 6 and 12 needles may be used during a session.

The practitioner may gently twist the needles or even electronically stimulate them to help the flow of *qi*. The needles may be removed immediately, in a few minutes, or retained up to 30 minutes or longer, depending on the area of the body and the nature of the problem that is being treated.

According to the WHO, acupuncture is effective in treating digestive, gynaecological, neurological and respiratory problems. However, it is important to seek out a qualified and experienced practitioner. In the West, acupuncture may be used in place of anaesthesia before surgery.

Auricular Acupuncture

Auricular acupuncture, or acupuncture to the ear, practised in the West, is attributed to the research of French neurologist and acupuncturist Dr Paul Nogier in the 1950s.

Dr Nogier was influenced by TCM, but his work in return sparked off new research and a resurgent interest in the ancient Chinese practice of ear acupuncture. As a result, Chinese researchers subsequently mapped out about 200 auricular acupuncture points.

Eventually, the WHO, in conjunction with the Chinese Acupuncture and Moxibustion Association, officially recognised 90 ear acupuncture points. These were standardised in 1982 as the International Standard Auricular Points.

ABOVE: *Acupuncture is applied in order to supply what is lacking and in order to drain off excessive fullness.*
– Yellow Emperor Huang Di

RIGHT: *Ancient Chinese warriors injured by arrows on certain parts of their bodies noticed that some of their health problems disappeared, and acupuncture operates on a similar principle. In the past, acupuncture needles were made of flint, bone, bamboo, gold, silver or copper. These days, they are made of disposable stainless steel and are likely to range from 2.5 centimetres (1 inch) to 30.5 centimetres (1 foot).*

OPPOSITE: *Tai ji is best performed at dawn when nature's* qi *is believed to be at its strongest.*

BODY-MIND EXERCISES

Exercises stemming from the ancient Eastern healing arts aim to bring the body, mind and spirit into balance through manipulating the body's vital energy. *Qi gong, tai ji* and yoga each have their own paradigms, but share an emphasis on breathing (see pp48, 59 and 61), posture, gentle movement, and focusing the mind. Regular practice may help improve your suppleness and energy, strengthen your body, and help your bodily systems function more efficiently. Many users also report that regular practice helps bring about an inner stillness, enhances mental clarity, and gives them a better handle on life. Some adopt these exercises as part of their fitness routine, as a form of relaxation or to help beat stress. Others may be attracted to incorporate the exercises' philosophical or spiritual aspects into their lives. It is a good idea to consult your doctor before trying a new exercise programme, especially if you have a medical condition or have been leading a sedentary lifestyle for too long, and to undergo a fitness assessment programme.

Qi Gong

Qi gong literally means working with *qi* (see p86), the life force believed to be within our bodies and the universe. Thought to have been first practised over 2,000 years ago, *qi gong* has several variations that revolve around breathing, meditation, postures and movements to help cultivate the *qi*, aid relaxation, and enhance physical and emotional wellbeing.

In TCM (see p86), *qi gong* is one component used to treat illnesses ranging from migraines to high blood pressure. Some Chinese hospitals have *qi gong* practitioners who impart these techniques to treat patients with serious illnesses such as cancer. However, some practitioners may prefer not to work with the seriously ill or people with psychotic disorders.

Qi gong exercises are considered ineffective if you do not begin and end with sequences: first to activate the *qi*, and then to return it to its storage areas in the body. A practitioner can teach you the exercises—which may be performed while sitting, standing or lying down—which you can practise at home.

Tai Ji

Gentler and more graceful than *qi gong*, the Chinese martial art of *tai ji* or *t'ai chi ch'uan* is also intended to help build an inner stamina by cultivating your *qi* through a slow, liquid sequence of movements and precise postures coordinated with controlled, calm breathing. Besides helping to relax the body, calm the emotions and focus the mind, *tai ji's* benefits include improving your breathing habits, circulation, posture, balance, flexibility and muscle strength.

Tai ji (Chinese for 'the supreme ultimate fist') was believed to have first been developed during the Song dynasty by a Taoist monk and martial arts exponent. *Tai ji* has five major styles. Originally developed as a martial art, the self-defense components were de-emphasised by the Communists who took over China in 1949 and promoted a modified version. Today, *tai ji* is popularly used as an exercise to encourage relaxation, alleviate stress-related disorders, and aid the recovery of injuries.

The Chinese believe that *tai ji* promotes health and longevity. Research shows that old people who regularly practice *tai ji* have better breathing and cardiovascular functions than their counterparts who do not. *Tai ji* is also popular with athletes, who use it to enhance their concentration.

A *tai ji* teacher will teach you the breathing and concentration techniques and the sequences of movements. These may look deceptively simple, but take a long time to master.

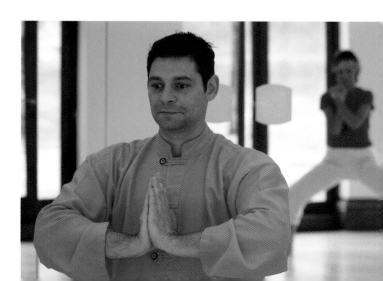

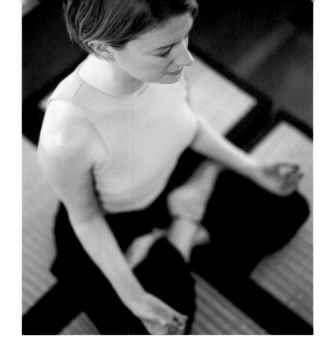

Yoga

Yoga—derived from the Sanskrit word for 'union' or 'yoke'—is popular for its fitness and meditative components that aid relaxation, ease tension, and improve balance, flexibility and posture. Some students, however, find it inspires them to try to attain a higher consciousness or enlightenment, achieved by the ancient Indian sages believed to be yoga's first practitioners.

The eight 'limbs' of yoga are *yama* (moral codes), *niyama* (daily observations), *asana* (postures—which may involve standing, sitting, kneeling and lying down), *pranayama* (controlled breathing exercises—see p65), *pratyahara* (withdrawal of the senses), *dharana* (mental focus and concentration), *dhyana* (meditation) and *samadhi* (attaining a superconsciousness). This framework was laid down in the 4th century B.C..

The third and fourth limbs of *asana* and *pranayama* are most commonly used in *hatha* yoga, the most familiar form of yoga in the West. Different forms of yoga vary in their approach to balancing your body, mind and spirit.

Directing *prana* may be achieved by restricting certain muscles which also affect various parts of your body. This use of *bandhas* or 'energy locks' was traditionally only taught to those students who had mastered *asanas*.

Some exercises are not recommended if you suffer from medical problems such as high blood pressure or heart disease, are pregnant, or menstruating, so do inform your teacher of any conditions you have beforehand. If you are on medication or have any disability, consult your doctor. There are certain yoga courses that are specifically geared for pregnancy.

Styles of Hatha Yoga

You should choose a form that best meets your interests, needs and *dosha* type (see p85). These are just four styles:

Ashtanga Vinyasa

Comprises a physically demanding sequence of exercises linked with breathing. It appeals to the very active and very fit.

Iyengar

Emphasises precise *asanas* and employs the use of props. Classes may be modified to suit the elderly or the injured.

Sivananda

Embraces postures, breath work, relaxation, nutrition, positive thinking and meditation to encourage people of all ages to pursue a healthy lifestyle. It is good for everyone.

Vinyoga

Comprises gentle movements coordinated with your breath. It is often used therapeutically and can be adapted to suit different needs and *dosha* types.

LABYRINTH

A spiritual and psychological tool for meditation and self-evaluation, the labyrinth is meant to be a metaphor for a journey to the centre of your self, and back out into the world with a clearer, deeper and better understanding of who you are.

Not to be confused with a maze that has high walls, dead-ends and several paths leading to the centre, a labyrinth is usually marked out on the ground, and is unicursal: that is, having only a single path from the mouth to the 'goal'. Labyrinths come in all shapes and sizes, but walkable ones typically range from 6 to 20 metres (20 to 66 feet). In a spa, a labyrinth may be situated in a lush, secluded area in a garden, and may include space around for people to watch or meditate.

Unlike walking a maze, which is a left brain activity that demands problem solving, walking the labyrinth calls on the right brain's intuition and creativity.

There is no one way to walk a labyrinth, which is said to provide a completely different experience for different people. You can be joyful or sombre, playful or prayerful during various parts of your labyrinth walk.

A facilitator may brief you about the history and approaches to walking a labyrinth, as well as the etiquette involved if walking in a group. One suggested method of walking a labyrinth is to quiet and centre yourself, and give a gesture such as a nod or bow before entering the labyrinth.

During your walk, pay attention to the experience and the sounds around you, and release your concerns and worries. When you reach the goal, stop and meditate quietly for a few moments to receive any illumination or insight that may come to you, before turning around and following the same path out.

During your walk out of the labyrinth, you are believed to be integrating the insight you have received. Before leaving the labyrinth, you may wish to offer some form of acknowledgment, perhaps by saying amen.

Some people walk into the labyrinth with their palms down (to symbolise release)—and at the centre and on the way out, with their palms up (to receive guidance and insight), ending the walk prayerfully with their palms together.

Labyrinths in the ancient world were typically built over power centres of the earth and were sacred to many cultures. Though the concept of the labyrinth stems from the West, and may be used in a church to aid meditation and prayer, its iconography is similar to that of a mandala, a spiritual symbol and meditation tool used by Buddhists in Asia.

Finger Labyrinth

On a wall outside Lucca Cathedral in Italy, there is a labyrinth that dates back to the 12th century. Pilgrims to this cathedral trace this labyrinth with their fingers, supposedly to still their minds before entering.

Today in this age of technology, finger labyrinths may also be found on the Internet. If you are unable to visit a physical labyrinth, try tracing a printed one with your finger or your mouse to receive similar benefits. Using your non-dominant hand, trace the path in and out of the finger labyrinth. Repeat the sequence several times.

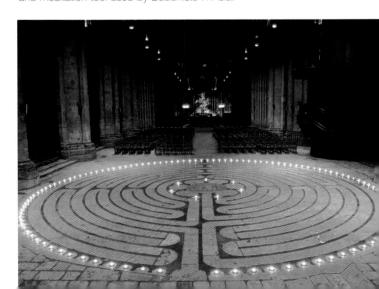

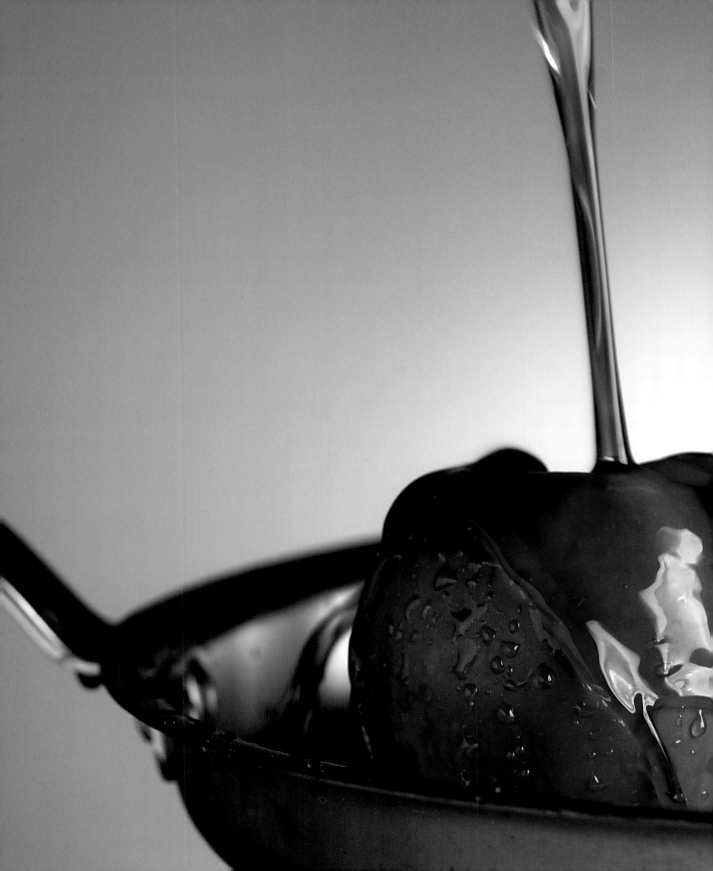

La Cuisine Synergique® 106   Cuisine Minceur 120

SPA CUISINE

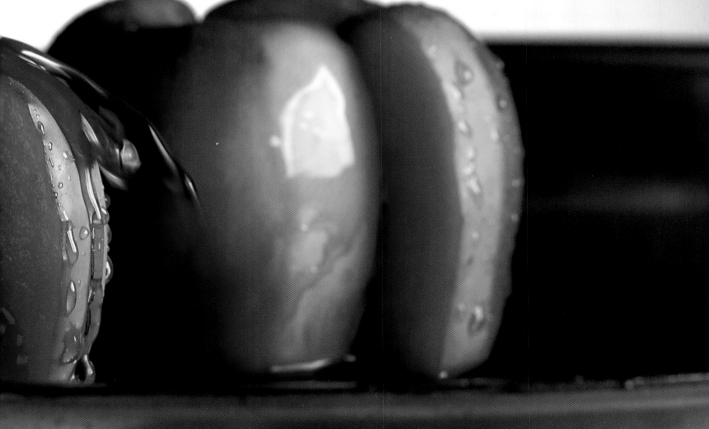

LA CUISINE SYNERGIQUE®

Royal Parc Evian

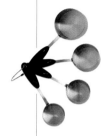

Contrary to popular belief, spa cuisine transcends meals that are merely low in fat, low in calories and low in salt. These days, meals served at spas are delicious yet inventive, and have been designed to balance your body, detoxify your system and optimise your levels of energy to benefit your overall health and wellbeing.

At the Royal Parc Evian, healthy eating takes the form of La Cuisine Synergique®: an imaginative approach to food developed over 15 years by Chef Michel Lentz to help guests lose weight. Lentz's synergetic cuisine—which is both low in calories and high in energy—draws from the philosophies of nutritherapy, phytotherapy, and Chinese medicine. It is based on linking different foods, spices and herbs with cooking methods carefully chosen to preserve the integrity of all the nutrients, while at the same time coaxing out the true flavours of the ingredients used.

Depending on the benefit sought, La Cuisine Synergique® associates the properties of each food, herb or seasoning with a specific cooking method. On the following pages, Lentz introduces you to his innovative gastronomic style and inspires you to cook your way to better health by sharing a three-day programme—comprising three main meals and two snacks per day—that you can prepare easily in your kitchen.

Each day's menu revolves around a theme or objective: purity (to rid your body of toxins and negative energy), lightness (to help shape and tone your body), and energy (to replenish energy drained by stress and poor eating habits). All La Cuisine Synergique® menus guarantee weight loss, and each one offers additional benefits such as neutralising toxins, chasing out free radicals, aiding digestion, stimulating drainage and providing high vitamin content.

Day 1 • Purity: The First Step This alternating menu of vegetables, cereals, pulses and fruit improves digestion, cleanses the system, generates weight loss and provides internal tranquillity.

Day 2 • Lightness: Rebirth Flavourful dishes of fish, shellfish and poultry combine with vegetables in season and herbs. Their aim is neutralising toxins, draining the body and weight loss.

Day 3 • Re-Energising: The Joys of Life Low-fat meat and fish, rich in proteins, join a variety of green vegetables to supply nutrients and vitamins, stimulate weight loss and make you feel on top of the world.

DAY 1 • BREAKFAST

PURITY BREAKFAST

Serves 1 • 125 Cal • 11.5 g protein • 57.6 g carbohydrate • 2.5 g fat per serving

100 ml (3⅜ fl oz/1⅜ cups) fresh papaya juice
40 g (½ oz) *sérac* goat's cheese
60 g (2 oz) breast of chicken
10 g (⅓ oz) rye bread
Unlimited tea
Unlimited Evian mineral water

PREPARATION
- Prepare and serve immediately.

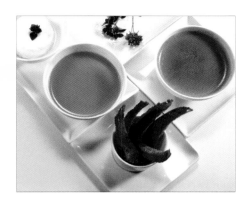

DAY 1 • 10 A.M. SNACK

PURITY SNACK

Serves 1 • 108 Cal • 4.18 g protein • 20.4 g carbohydrate • 1 g fat per serving

100 g (3½ oz) crudités
20 g (¾ oz/4 tsp) fat-free yogurt
100 ml (3⅜ fl oz/⅜ cup) fresh vegetable juice

PREPARATION
- Prepare the crudités, and serve immediately with the yogurt and juice.

DAY 1 • LUNCH

YOUNG VEGETABLE ROOTS COOKED IN A HERACLEUM STOCK

Serves 4 • 75.4 Cal • 2.25 g protein • 8 g carbohydrate • 3.7 g fat per serving

10 g (⅓ oz) root of fresh heracleum
Fromage blanc, as required
Seasonal vegetables, as required
1 large tomato
3 carrots
3 white turnips
30 g (1 oz) salsify
1 peppered artichoke
20 g (¾ oz) fresh broad beans
250 g (9 oz) new cabbage

50 g (1¾ oz) cooked beetroot, cut into strips
1 ltr (2 pt 1⅞ fl oz/4¼ cups) vegetable stock
1 tbsp colza (rapeseed) oil
1 tsp olive oil
90 ml (3 fl oz/6 tbsp) cider vinegar
Salt and pepper to taste
20 g (¾ oz) spinach shoots, for garnish
Wheat and sunflower buds and shoots,
 as required, for garnish

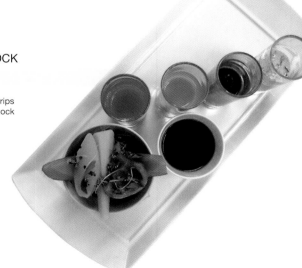

PREPARATION
- Scoop out the tomato, and season with salt and pepper.
- Wash and peel the carrots, turnips, salsify, artichoke, broad beans, cabbage and seasonal vegetables.
- Add the heracleum root and a few drops of colza oil to the vegetable stock, and bring to a boil.
- Cook the vegetables in the heracleum stock, family by family, keeping them crunchy, then remove. Reduce the stock.
- Add some stock to the scooped-out portion of the tomato. Cook again for 15 min, then blend to a purée in a liquidiser and season with salt and pepper.
- Repeat the above step with the seasonal vegetables.

PRESENTATION
- Place the beetroot then the cooked vegetables into a bowl.
- Sort and dry the spinach shoots, wheat and sunflower buds and shoots. Sprinkle with a little of the olive oil and the cider vinegar.
- Place the tomato and seasonal vegetable purées and the *fromage blanc* in matching recipients and serve on the side.

CHICKPEA FLOUR PASTA WITH PAPAYA SAUCE

Serves 4 • 122 Cal • 4.9 g protein • 17.95 g carbohydrate • 3.39 g fat per serving

Pasta
80 g (3 oz/¼ cup) chickpea flour
1 egg yolk
80 g (3 oz) basil
1½ tsp sea salt
120 ml (4 fl oz/½ cup) water
20 ml (⅝ fl oz/4 tsp) olive oil

Sauce
100 g (3½ oz) papaya, cubed
200 g (7 oz) fresh tomatoes, cubed
1½ tsp honey
10 ml (⅜ fl oz/2 tsp) white vinegar

Garnish
260 g (9 oz/4¼ cups) cooked
  chickpeas

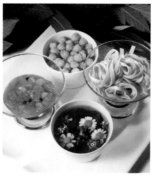

PREPARATION
Pasta
* Put the chickpea flour, egg yolk, basil and sea salt into a bowl. Add the water and knead well.
* Leave it to rest, then cut into tagliatelle shapes.
* Divide it into small quantities, cook in boiling salted water and bind with olive oil.

Sauce
* Reduce the honey and vinegar and add the papaya and tomato cubes. Leave to cook until soft, then blend very well.

PRESENTATION
* Serve the pasta in a bowl, with the chickpeas and the sauce each served separately in matching recipients.

FRESH FRUIT WITH SORBET AND LEMON CRISPS

Serves 4 • 47 Cal • 0.23 protein • 11.21 carbohydrate • 0.09 fat per serving

Fruit
1 kiwi fruit, sliced
2 Victoria pineapples, sliced
2 passion fruit, sliced

Sorbet
180 ml (6 fl oz/¾ cup)
  Evian mineral water
20 g (¾ oz/4 tsp) kara sugar
100 ml (3⅜ fl oz/⅜ cup)
  lemon juice

Lemon Crisps
1 lemon
100 g (3½ oz/½ cup) caster sugar
100 ml (3⅜ fl oz/⅜ cup) water

Garnish
Mint leaves, for garnish

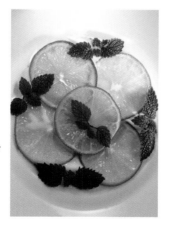

PREPARATION
Sorbet
* Heat the water to 45 °C (113 °F).
* Add the sugar and bring the heat up to 80 °C (176 °F).
* Cool by adding the lemon juice.
* Blend when the mixture is cool (a mixer can be used).
* Freeze for about 12 hours.

Lemon Crisps
* Cut the lemon into thin slices.
* Boil the sugar with the water. Pour over the lemon slices and cook at 80 °C (176 °F) for 20 min.
* Strain the lemon slices, and place on a sheet of cooking paper.
* Put into the oven at 70 °C (158 °F) for 4 hours.

PRESENTATION
* Divide the fresh fruit into 4 bowls and top each with the sorbet. Cover with the lemon crisps and garnish with mint leaves.

DRIED VEGETABLE TEA

Serves 4 • 6 Cal • 0 g protein • 1.22 g carbohydrate • 0.06 g fat per serving

100 g (3½ oz) carrots
100 g (3½ oz) leek
100 g (3½ oz) celery
100 g (3½ oz) onions
1 ltr (2 pt 1⅞ fl oz/4¼ cups) water
5 g (¼ oz) salt
A pinch wild thyme
A pinch star anise
2 leaves fresh lemon grass
  (citronella)
6 tsp fresh green tea leaves,
  for garnish

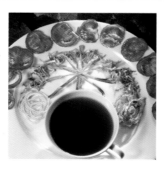

PREPARATION
* Wash and peel all the vegetables. Cut into fine strips.
* Steam-dry them at 30 °C (86 °F) the day before, and leave them for 2 days.
* Bring the water to a boil. Add the herbs and seasonings.
* Remove stock from the heat and add all the vegetables. Leave to brew overnight.
* Serve iced in large glasses, garnished with the fresh green tea leaves.

DAY 1 • 4 P.M. SNACK

VEGETABLE 'SANDWICH' WITH CHICKEN

Serves 1 • 108 Cal • 9.7 g protein • 15.88 g carbohydrate • 0.62 g fat per serving

50 g (1¾ oz) breast of chicken, sliced into batons
2 leaves iceberg lettuce
20 g (¾ oz) tomatoes, sliced
5 g (¼ oz) carrots, grated
5 g (¼ oz) flat-leaved parsley, chopped

10 ml (⅜ fl oz/2 tsp) rice vinegar
Salt and pepper to taste

125 g (4½ oz) *fromage blanc*
50 g (1¾ oz) grape juice
Unlimited tea
Unlimited Evian mineral water

PREPARATION
- Lay the lettuce leaves flat.
- Arrange the chicken batons, tomatoes, carrots and parsley on each lettuce leaf, and season with rice vinegar, salt and pepper.
- Roll up each lettuce leaf like a sushi, folding in the ends as you go along to prevent the stuffing from falling out.
- Follow with the *fromage blanc*, tea and mineral water.

DAY 1 • DINNER

RED PURSLANE SALAD

Serves 4 • 310 Cal • 15.05 g protein • 35.5 g carbohydrate • 11.81 g fat per serving

Salad
120 g (4¼ oz) purslane

Vegetable Crisps
40 g (1½ oz) shallots
200 g (7 oz) carrots
200 g (7 oz) tomatoes
200 g (7 oz) asparagus
200 g (7 oz) white turnips

Sauce
1 tsp cider vinegar
1 tsp wine vinegar
1 tsp ginger juice
20 ml (⅝ fl oz/4 tsp) vegetable stock
20 ml (⅝ fl oz/4 tsp) colza (rapeseed) oil
A pinch espelette chilli
Salt to taste

PREPARATION
Vegetable Crisps
- At least one day in advance, wash, peel and cut the vegetables very finely with a mandolin.
- Place flat on a Teflon plate and dry in the oven at 60 °C (140 °F) for 1 night or longer.

Sauce
- Make the sauce by mixing the 2 vinegars, ginger juice and salt in a dish. Dissolve well. Add the vegetable stock, colza oil and espelette chilli, and blend.

Salad
- Cut off most of the purslane stem. Soak in cold water for 10 min. Change the water, then take each bunch by the stem and plunge it up and down in the water for 10 to 40 sec.
- Put the bunches of purslane into a receptacle of clean water. Then drain and place on a large cloth or absorbent paper.

PRESENTATION
- Season the purslane with the sauce, and sprinkle with the dried vegetables. Serve.

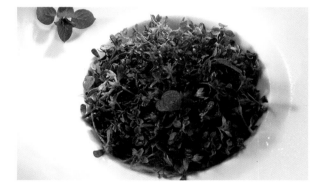

QUINOA RISOTTO WITH MUSHROOM CASSEROLE, HERACLEUM ROOT BROTH AND BEAN CURD

Serves 4 • 276 Cal • 21.56 g protein • 21.45 g carbohydrate • 11.74 g fat per serving

Quinoa Risotto
1 white onion, cut into small cubes
120 g (4¼ oz) quinoa
1 tbsp colza (rapeseed) oil
1 ltr (2 pt 1⅞ fl oz/4¼ cups) soya milk

Mushroom Casserole
400 g (14 oz) shitake mushrooms
400 g (14 oz) enoki mushrooms
60 g (2¾ oz) red onions, chopped

Bean Curd
320 g (11¼ oz) bean curd
A dash soya sauce

Heracleum Root Broth
1 ltr (2 pt 1⅞ fl oz/4¼ cups) poultry stock
1 tsp turmeric
20 g (¾ oz) heracleum root

Garnish
40 g (1½ oz) sprouted sunflower shoots
Fresh mushrooms, as required, sliced

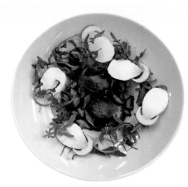

PREPARATION

Quinoa Risotto

- Heat a saucepan, add the colza oil and then the onion cubes. Leave to cook gently for a few minutes.
- Wash the quinoa by placing the grains in a fine strainer. Hold under cold running water until the water runs clear.
- Add the quinoa to the saucepan with the onion. Stir until coated with oil, then add the soya milk to cover. Bring to a boil, taste to check seasoning and add salt if necessary.
- Cover and cook in the oven at 180 °C (350 °F) for 20 min.

Bean Curd

- Strain the bean curd, cut into 1-cm (½-in) cubes and toss in a non-stick pan over a high flame for 2 to 3 min. Deglaze with a dash of soya sauce.

Mushroom Casserole

- Dry the shitake and enoki mushrooms and cut off the rough portions of the stems. Cut into slivers and cook on a bed of red onions over a high flame for 3 to 5 min.

Heracleum Root Broth

- Boil the poultry stock and the turmeric for 2 min. Add the heracleum root and leave to brew for 5 min.

PRESENTATION

- Mix the bean curd and quinoa risotto, and place in the centre of each dish. Add the heracleum root broth, then top with the mushroom casserole.
- Garnish with the sunflower shoots and fresh mushroom.

POACHED PEACHES WITH VERBENA ON STRAWBERRY COULIS

Serves 4 • 73 Cal • 0.93 g protein • 16.7 g carbohydrate • 0.23 g fat per serving

4 large white peaches
24 verbena leaves
1 ltr (2 pt 1⅞ fl oz/4¼ cups) Evian mineral water
Sugar substitute equivalent to 8 tbsp sugar
200 g (7 oz) wild strawberries
Juice from 1 lemon

PREPARATION

Verbena Syrup

- Boil the Evian mineral water with half of the sugar substitute.
- Allow the verbena leaves to brew for 10 min away from the heat.
- Remove the leaves from the syrup, retain them, and strain the syrup.

Strawberry Coulis

- Wash the wild strawberries and remove the stalks.

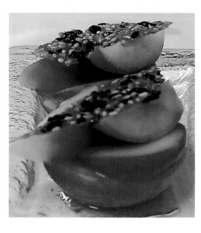

- Blend in a liquidiser with the remaining sugar substitute and the lemon juice.
- Keep this coulis on ice until just before serving.

Peaches

- Wash the peaches. Bring the verbena syrup to a boil, place the peaches in the syrup and poach for 20 min.
- Drain the peaches, peel them and cut them in two. Remove the stones and leave to cool.

PRESENTATION

- Pour a little of the strawberry coulis into 4 little dishes, place a rejoined peach on each coulis and decorate with verbena leaves.

BITTER CUCUMBER TEA

Serves 4 • 0 Cal • 0 g protein • 0 g carbohydrate • 0 g fat per serving

1 ltr (2 pt 1⅞ fl oz/4¼ cups) camomile tea
Skin from 1 bitter cucumber

PREPARATION

- Prepare camomile tea in the usual way, but using mineral water instead of tap water and adding the skin of a bitter cucumber.

DAY 1 • EVENING TEA

WILD VANILLA TEA

Serves 4 • 0 Cal • 0 g protein • 0 g carbohydrate • 0 g fat per serving

8 tsp wild vanilla tea leaves
1 ltr (2 pt 1⅞ fl oz/4¼ cups) Evian mineral water

PREPARATION

- Brew as you would normal tea and serve.

DAY 2 • BREAKFAST

LIGHTNESS BREAKFAST

Serves 1 • 321 Cal • 21.9 g protein • 14.85 g carbohydrate • 17.38 g fat per serving

100 ml (3⅜ fl oz/1⅜ cups) fresh mango juice
40 g (½ oz) white *tomme* cheese
60 g (2 oz) fillet of beef
10 g (⅓ oz) wholemeal bread
Pure Arabica coffee
Unlimited Evian mineral water

PREPARATION
• Prepare and serve immediately.

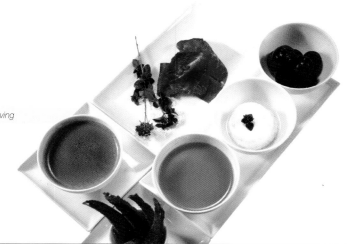

DAY 2 • 10 A.M. SNACK

LIGHTNESS SNACK

Serves 1 • 108 Cal • 4.2 g protein • 20.4 g carbohydrate • 0.1 g fat per serving

100 g (3½ oz) crudités
20 g (¾ oz/4 tsp) fat-free yogurt
120 ml (4 fl oz/½ cup) Mémises cocktail (see boxed recipe below)

PREPARATION
• Prepare the crudités, and serve immediately with the yogurt
  and cocktail.

MÉMISES COCKTAIL

Serves 1

20 g (¾ oz) watercress
2 grapefruit
5 drops green Tabasco
50 ml (1¾ fl oz/¼ cup) Evian mineral water
5 ice-cubes
Sugar substitute to taste (optional)

PREPARATION
• Wash the watercress, thin out the leaves, and put into an
  electric mixer bowl.
• Juice the grapefruit and pour the juice into the bowl.
• Add the Tasbaco, mineral water and ice-cubes, and mix
  for 30 sec.
• Filter through a strainer and pour the juice into a glass.
  Add the sugar substitute according to taste.

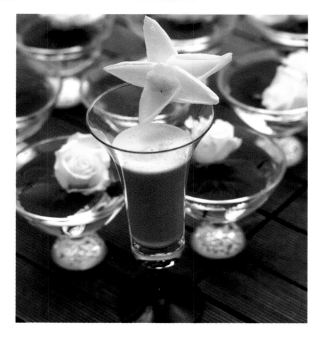

DAY 2 • LUNCH

ELDERBERRY TEA

Serves 4 • 0 Cal • 0 g protein • 0 g carbohydrate • 0 g fat per serving

40 ml (1⅜ fl oz/⅛ cup) elderberry essence
1 ltr (2 pints 1⅞ fl oz/4¼ cups) Evian mineral water

PREPARATION
• Mix the elderberry essence with the mineral water. Serve.

ROYAL DUBLIN BAY PRAWNS

Serves 4 • 160 Cal • 13.89 g protein • 16.45 g carbohydrate • 4.04 g fat per serving

Prawns
16 Dublin Bay prawns
Water as required
Salt to taste

Garnish
4 fresh sage leaves
4 sprigs thyme
1 tsp caraway seeds
1 tsp sesame seeds
2 shallots
Espelette chilli to taste

Dandelion Salad
100 g (3½ oz) dandelion leaves
4 tbsp reduced prawn stock
2 tbsp Zen sauce (see boxed recipe below)
1 tbsp carrot juice
1 drop green Tabasco
1 drop Worcestershire sauce
15 g (½ oz/1 tbsp) cooking salt
1 tsp cider vinegar
Ground pepper to taste

PREPARATION

Prawns
- Shell the uncooked prawns, remove the black gut, trim the tails and keep them cool.
- Crush the prawn shells, put them in a saucepan, cover with water and salt lightly.
- Bring to a boil and leave to cook on low heat for 20 min. Strain and discard the shells. Then boil again to reduce to half the quantity.
- Bring the reduced stock to the boil, then add salt and pepper. Plunge the prawns into the stock to cook for 5 min.
- Put the prawns aside and strain the stock. Set aside.

Dandelion Salad
- To prepare the dressing, put 4 tbsp of the reduced prawn stock into a bowl. Add the rest of the ingredients except the dandelion leaves and whip till a smooth sauce is obtained.
- Sort, wash and carefully dry the dandelion leaves. Season with the dressing.

Garnish
- Dry the sage leaves, thyme and caraway seeds overnight in an oven preheated to a maxminum of 60 °C (140 °F).
- Grill the sesame seeds very lightly in a pan.
- Peel the shallots and chop them finely.
- Mix all these ingredients with some espelette chilli.

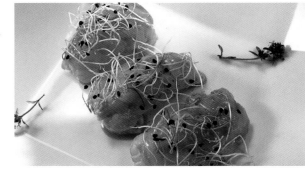

ZEN SAUCE

540 ml (1 pt 2³⁄₈ fl oz/3 cups)

A pinch sea salt
A pinch sesame, grilled and crushed
20 ml (⅝ fl oz/4 tsp) lemon juice
20 ml (⅝ fl oz/4 tsp) soya sauce
100 ml (3³⁄₈ fl oz/⅜ cup) rice vinegar
100 ml (3³⁄₈ fl oz/⅜ cup) peanut oil
150 ml (5 fl oz/⅝ cup) vegetable stock
150 ml (5 fl oz/⅝ cup) Evian mineral water

PREPARATION
- Dissolve the sea salt and sesame in the lemon juice, soya suce and rice vinegar. Mix well.
- Add the peanut oil, vegetable stock and mineral water. Mix well.

PRESENTATION
- Place 4 prawns on each dish. Top with the dandelion salad and sprinkle with the garnish of seeds and herbs.

POLLOCK ON A BED OF TURNIP

Serves 4 • 202 Cal • 33 g protein • 10 g carbohydrate • 4 g fat per serving

Fish
4 pollock fillets, each weighing 120 g (4½ oz)
4 sprigs horsetail
600 ml (10⅛ fl oz/1 ¼ cups) fish stock

Purée
200 g (7 oz) parsley
200 g (7 oz) nettles
4 sprigs horsetail
Water as required
Fish stock as required
Salt to taste

Turnip Bed
100 g (3½ oz) Swede turnips
Juice from 4 segments of lemon
500 ml (1 pt 1 fl oz/2⅛ cups) vegetable stock
100 ml (3³⁄₈ fl oz/⅜ cups) fish stock
20 g (¾ oz/2¼ tsp) salt

Garnish
4 drops olive oil
4 sprigs chervil, for garnish

PREPARATION

Fish
- Trim the fillets nicely and cut into square blocks.
- Place the horsetail into the fish stock and boil to reduce to 100 ml (3³⁄₈ fl oz/⅜ cup).
- Fry the fillets on both sides until golden brown.
- Place the fillets in a deep dish, fill halfway with fish stock, and cook in the oven for 10 min at 200 °C (390 °F).

Purée
- Wash and sort the parsley, nettles and horsetail. Cook in boiling water. Salt them, drain and then blend into a purée. Dilute this purée with a little of the fish stock.

Turnip
- Wash and peel the turnips and rinse with lemon juice. Cut the turnips into cubes and cook for 30 min in the vegetable stock. Remove the turnip cubes and put aside.
- Mix the vegetable stock with the fish stock. Boil to reduce to a quarter of its volume. Add the cooked turnip cubes, and thicken.

PRESENTATION
- Arrange the turnip cubes at the bottom of each dish. Place 1 fillet on each bed of turnip.
- Surround each fillet with the purée, and add 1 drop of olive oil and a sprig of chervil.

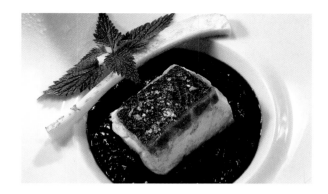

ROAST APRICOTS WITH ICE-CREAM

Serves 4 • 165 Cal • 2.78 g protein • 38.22 g carbohydrate • 0.12 g fat per serving

Apricots
100 g (3½ oz) apricots
10 g (⅓ oz) honey
8 sprigs lavender, for garnish

Ice-Cream
120 g (4¼ oz) sheep's milk yogurt
100 ml (3⅜ fl oz/⅜ cup) Evian mineral water
4 g (⅛ oz) glucose
40 g (1½ oz) fructose

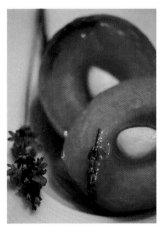

PREPARATION
Apricots
- Preheat the oven to 210 °C (410 °F). Cut the apricots in 2 and remove the stones.
- Close the apricots and arrange in an ovenproof dish. Sprinkle with honey and bake in the oven for 10 to 15 min.

Ice-Cream
- Whip the sheep's milk yogurt, incorporating the mineral water, fructose and glucose.
- Pour into an ice-cream maker and leave running until a creamy consistency is obtained.
- Leave to set for about 2 hours in the freezer.

PRESENTATION
- Divide the warm apricots among the plates with a roll of ice-cream in the middle, moulded with a spoon. Decorate with sprigs of lavender.

DAY 2 • 4 P.M. SNACK

VEGETABLE 'SANDWICH' WITH SALMON

Serves 1 • 132 Cal • 13.017 g protein • 10.95 g carbohydrate • 4.06 g fat per serving

40 g (1½ oz) cooked salmon
2 leaves iceberg lettuce
10 g (⅓ oz) celery, grated
Juice from 1 lemon
1 g (¹⁄₁₆ oz) wasabi

125 g (4½ oz/½ cup) *fromage blanc*
40 g (1½ oz) fresh strawberries
Unlimited tea
Unlimited Evian mineral water

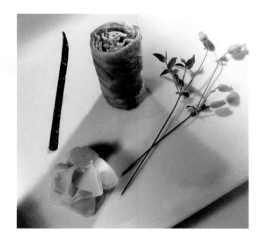

PREPARATION
- Lay the lettuce leaves flat.
- Arrange the salmon and celery on each lettuce leaf, and season with the lemon juice and wasabi.
- Roll up each lettuce leaf like a sushi, folding in the ends as you go along to prevent the stuffing from falling out.
- Follow with the *fromage blanc*, strawberries, tea and mineral water.

DAY 2 • DINNER

SALMON MARINATED IN SEA SALT

Serves 4 • 68 Cal • 8 g protein • 0 g carbohydrate • 4 g fat per serving

Salmon
160 g (5⅝ oz) salmon fillet,
   40 g (1⅜ oz) per person

Salad
2 bunches dill
80 g (3 oz) alfalfa
1 tbsp Zen sauce (see boxed
   recipe on p112)

Marinade
5 g (⅛ oz/¾ tsp) sea salt
2.5 g (¹⁄₁₆ oz/½ tsp) sugar
A pinch star anise, crushed
A pinch pepper

Garnish
20 g (¾ oz) marinated ginger,
   cut into fine strips
4 wedges lemon

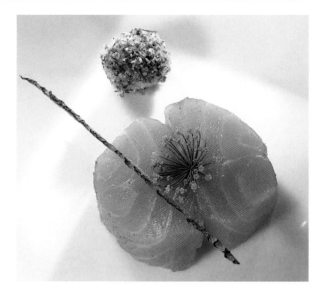

PREPARATION
Fish
- Mix the ingredients for the marinade together well.
- Rub each salmon fillet thoroughly on both sides with the marinade and leave to marinate for 48 hours.

Salad
- Wash and sort the dill segments and the alfalfa.
- Mix the dill and alfalfa together and season with the Zen sauce.

PRESENTATION
- Cut the salmon into large cubes, allocating 3 cubes per person.
- Serve the salmon with the dill and alfalfa salad, and serve the ginger and lemon wedges separately on the side.

QUAIL WITH SAGE UNDER THE SKIN

Serves 4 • 255 Cal • 9.73 g protein • 28.67 g carbohydrate • 11.2 g fat per serving

8 quails
40 g (1½ oz) celery
40 g (1½ oz) onions
400 g (14 oz) curly green
   cabbage
½ bunch sage
40 ml (1⅜ fl oz/⅛ cup)
   lemon juice
200 ml (6¾ fl oz/⅞ cup)
   chicken stock
80 g (3 oz) candied lemon
Salt and black pepper to
   taste
2 g (⅛ oz) juniper berries
Juniper berries, as required,
   for garnish
80 g (3 oz) candied lemon,
   for garnish

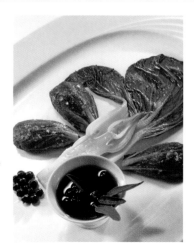

PREPARATION
Sauce (to be prepared one day in advance)
- Bone the quails and flatten them. Cut into fillets and put aside. Keep the carcasses to make the sauce.
- Boil the carcasses with a little celery and the onions for 20 min, then strain.

- Continue cooking the liquid until almost dry.
- Add the lemon juice and set aside.

Cabbage
- Wash, remove the stalk and cut into fine strips. Cook in water with a little lemon juice.
- Strain and place the cabbage in a casserole with the remaining celery and sage. Cover with chicken stock.
- Cover and cook in the oven for 1 hour at 180 °C (350 °F). Remove and strain. Sprinkle with finely crushed juniper berries.

Quail
- Spread out the quail fillets. Season with salt and black pepper.
- Slip a leaf of blanched sage under the skin of each quail. Close each quail to form a cylinder shape and wrap in in the cooked cabbage.
- Preheat the oven to 180 °C (350 °F). Cook in the oven for 15 min. Remove and leave to rest for 20 min.

PRESENTATION
- Divide the wrapped fillets into 4 portions.
- Place 1 portion on each plate and garnish with the remaining cabbage, candied lemon and juniper berries.
- Serve the sauce on the side.

GRAPEFRUIT PLATTER WITH 'LING MY' GREEN TEA JELLY

82 Cal • 6.07 g protein • 14.5 g carbohydrate • 0 g fat per serving

6 grapefruit
250 ml (8½ fl oz/1 cup) orange juice
Star anise, for garnish
50 g (1¾ oz) acacia honey
3 sheets gelatine
'Ling My' green tea, as required
A few leaves peppermint, for garnish
Unlimited Evian mineral water

PREPARATION

Green Tea Jelly

- Remove the skin from the grapefruit. Peel the segments, taking care to keep the juice.
- Soak the sheets of gelatine in cold water.
- Infuse the star anise for 5 min in the hot green tea.
- Incorporate the gelatine into the syrup and add the grapefruit juice.
- Add the gelatine, syrup and grapefruit juice to the green tea.
- Leave to cool on a bed of ice.

Orange Syrup

- Cook the orange juice on low heat with 1 star anise and the honey until a smooth syrup is obtained.

PRESENTATION

- Divide the peeled grapefruit segments into 4, and arrange each portion in a circle in a shallow dish. Pour the green tea jelly halfway up. Leave to set.
- Pour a spoonful of orange syrup on each dish and garnish with the star anise. Serve very cold.

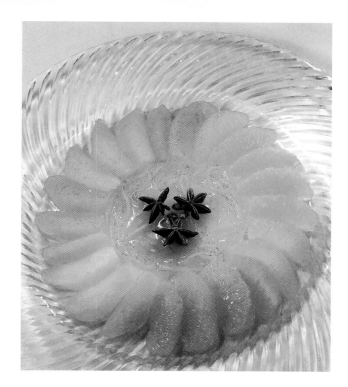

ELDERBERRY TEA

Serves 4 • 0 Cal • 0 g protein • 0 g carbohydrate • 0 g fat per serving

40 ml (1⅜ fl oz/⅛ cup) elderberry essence
1 ltr (2 pt 1⅞ fl oz/4¼ cups) Evian mineral water

PREPARATION

- Mix the elderberry essence with the mineral water. Serve.

DAY 2 • EVENING TEA

ROSEMARY TEA

Serves 4 • 0 Cal • 0 g protein • 0 g carbohydrate • 0 g fat per serving

8 tsp rosemary tea leaves
1 ltr (2 pt 1⅞ fl oz/4¼ cups) Evian mineral water

PREPARATION

- Brew as you would normal tea and serve.

DAY 3 • BREAKFAST

RE-ENERGISING BREAKFAST

Serves 1 • 214 Cal • 16.5 g protein • 17.64 g carbohydrate • 8.46 g fat per serving

100 ml (3⅜ fl oz/1⅜ cups)
  fresh pineapple juice
40 g (½ oz) soft white cheese
60 g (2 oz) cold roast veal

10 g (⅓ oz) black bread
Unlimited tea or pure Arabica coffee
Unlimited Evian mineral water

PREPARATION
• Prepare and serve immediately.

DAY 3 • 10 A.M. SNACK

RE-ENERGISING SNACK

Serves 1 • 98 Cal • 4.1 g protein • 18 g carbohydrate • 1 g fat per serving

100 g (3½ oz) crudités
20 g (¾ oz/4 tsp) fat-free yogurt
100 ml (3⅜ fl oz/⅜ cup) vitamin
cocktail (see boxed recipe)

PREPARATION
• Prepare the crudités, and
  serve immediately with the
  yogurt and juice.

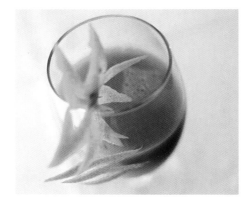

VITAMIN COCKTAIL

Serves 1

1 stick celery
15 ml (½ fl oz/3 tsp) fresh lemon juice
80 ml (2¾ fl oz/⅓ cup) pasteurised carrot
  juice

PREPARATION
• Put the celery through a juicer.
• Mix the celery juice with the lemon
  juice and carrot juice and serve
  immediately.

DAY 3 • LUNCH

STEAMED SPROUTED CEREALS WITH MINT YOGURT

Serves 4 • 107 Cal • 7.6 g protein • 14.34 g carbohydrate • 2.42 g fat per serving

Vegetables
100 g (3½ oz) alfalfa shoots
5 g (¼ oz) fenugreek leaves
80 g (3 oz) roquette sour lettuce
100 g (3½ oz) sprouted lentils
50 g (1¾ oz) wheat sprouts
50 g (1¾ oz) shallots, very finely
  chopped
2 red tomatoes, sliced into 8ths
2 green tomatoes, sliced into 8ths

Yogurt
80 g (3 oz) fat-free yogurt
½ bunch mint
10 g (⅓ oz) charroux mustard
Salt and pepper to taste

Vinaigrette
½ tsp soya sauce
½ tbsp safflower seed oil
20 g (¾ oz) lemon juice

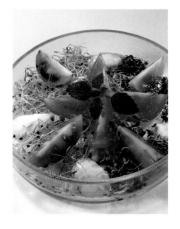

PREPARATION
• Mix the ingredients for the yogurt, and season with salt and
  pepper.
• Mix the ingredients for the vinaigrette.
• Cut the alfalfa shoots and fenugreek leaves with a scissors.
  Sort the roquette sour lettuce and wash it well. Combine the
  alfalfa shoots, the fenugreek leaves and the roquette sour
  lettuce, and season with some of the vinaigrette.
• Steam the lentils and wheat for 20 min, keeping them
  crunchy. Season with the yogurt and shallots.

PRESENTATION
• Arrange the alfalfa shoots, fenugreek leaves, lettuce, lentils
  and wheat sprouts in a circle on each plate.
• In the centre of each circle, place 4 slices of red tomato.
• Surround with 4 slices of green tomato alternated with
  dollops of the mint yogurt.

SADDLE OF ROAST YOUNG LAMB

Serves 4 • 345 Cal • 23.92 g protein • 8.25 g carbohydrate • 23.88 g fat per serving

1.2 kg (2.6 lb) saddle of lamb,
  400 g (14 oz) per person
Purée of celery, as required
50 g (1¾ oz) onion, thinly
  sliced
200 g (7 oz) aubergines
400 g (14 oz) Crimean
  old-style black tomatoes
1 clove garlic
12 g (½ oz) savory
Olive oil as required
Salt and pepper to taste

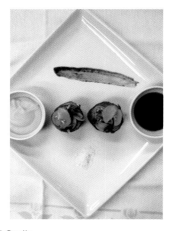

PREPARATION
Aubergines, Tomatoes and Garlic
- Heat the oven to 180 °C (350 °F).
- Peel the aubergines and cut into cubes. In a cast-iron casserole pan, sweat the slivers of onion in olive oil, add the aubergine cubes, season with salt and pepper, and flavour with savory.

- Bake in an oven for about 80 min until the aubergines are well cooked.
- Wash and dry the tomatoes. Bake them in the oven with salt and pepper for 15 min.
- Cook the garlic cloves in their skin for 10 min.

Lamb
- Bone the lamb and remove all the fat. Make a stock with the bone. Reduce the stock and set aside.
- Season the lamb with the olive oil, salt and pepper.
- Heat the oven to 180 °C (350 °F). Heat the olive oil in a pan on top of the stove until smoking.
- Place the pieces of flavoured lamb in the pan and sear in the oil on both sides.
- Transfer to the oven and cook for a maximum of 10 min. Leave to rest outside the oven for 5 min.

PRESENTATION
- Place 1 portion of lamb in the centre of the plate, and top with the garlic in its skin. Put the celery purée and reduced lamb stock in matching recipients and place on the plate.
- Serve with the tomatoes and compote of cooked aubergines on the side.

MANGO WITH PASSION FRUIT COULIS

Serves 4 • 33 Cal • 0.3 g protein • 7.38 g carbohydrate • 0.1 g fat per serving

400 g (14 oz) well-ripened mangoes
2 vanilla pods
200 ml (6¾ fl oz/⅞ cup) Evian mineral water
Sugar substitute equivalent to 4 tbsp sugar
80 g (3 oz) passion fruit

PREPARATION
Vanilla Syrup
- Split the vanilla pods in 2. Bring the mineral water to a boil with the vanilla and the sugar substitute.
- Leave to cool, remove the vanilla pods from the syrup, retain them, and strain the syrup.

Passion Fruit Coulis
- Wash the passion fruit, cut it into 2 and remove the pulp with a spoon.
- Mix the pulp into the vanilla syrup.
- Keep this coulis on ice until just before serving.

PRESENTATION
- Peel and cut the mangoes in 2. Remove the stones and cut the flesh into thin slices.
- Fill each plate with a 1-cm (scant 1/2-inch)-thick layer of the passion fruit coulis. Place slices of mango on it and decorate with half a vanilla pod.

GINSENG TEA

Serves 4 • 0 Cal • 0 g protein • 0 g carbohydrate • 0 g fat per serving

40 ml (1⅜ fl oz/⅛ cup) ginseng essence
1 ltr (2 pt 1⅞ fl oz/4¼ cups) Evian mineral water
Ginger, cut into thin strips, as required, for garnish

PREPARATION
- Add the ginseng essence to the mineral water. Decorate with the ginger and serve.

DAY 3 • 4 P.M. SNACK

VEGETABLE 'SANDWICH' WITH BEEF

Serves 1 • 173 Cal • 22.65 g protein • 18.52 g carbohydrate • 6.95 g fat per serving

50 g (1¾ oz) cold roast beef
2 leaves iceberg lettuce
20 g (¾ oz) tomatoes, sliced
5 g (¼ oz) carrots, grated
50 g (1¾ oz) celery, sliced
5 g (¼ oz) flat-leaved parsley,
   chopped
Salt and pepper to taste

125 g (4½ oz/½ cup) *fromage
   blanc*
Unlimited tea
Unlimited Evian mineral water

PREPARATION

- Lay the lettuce leaves flat.
- Arrange the beef, tomatoes, carrots, celery and parsley on each lettuce leaf, and season with the salt and pepper.
- Roll up each lettuce leaf like a sushi, folding in the ends as you go along to prevent the stuffing from falling out.
- Follow with the *fromage blanc*, tea and mineral water.

DAY 3 • DINNER

ATLANTIC MACKEREL IN LIME-BLOSSOM TEA

Serves 4 • 83 Cal • 9.21 g protein • 2.12 g carbohydrate • 6.95 g fat per serving

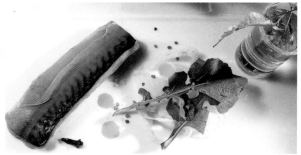

Fish
240 g (8½ oz) Atlantic mackerel
80 g (2¾ oz) fennel
10 g (⅓ oz) roquette sour lettuce

Vinaigrette
2 tsp lemon juice
2 tsp colza (rapeseed) oil
A pinch sea salt
Ground pepper to taste

Sauce
40 g (1½ oz) grey shallots
800 ml (1 pt 11 fl oz/3⅓ cups)
   fish stock
10 g (⅓ oz) lime-blossom
250 ml (8½ fl oz/1 cup) orange juice
1 g (1/16 oz) cloves
4 slivers orange peel
300 ml (10⅛ fl oz/1¼ cups)
   Evian mineral water

PREPARATION

Lime-Blossom Tea

- Clean the mackerel, rinse, cut into fillets and remove the bones. Set the bones and parings aside for making the stock.
- Peel the shallots, then slice them. Place in a pot, cover with water and start to boil, then add the mackerel bones and parings. Cook for 20 min, skim and strain.
- Reduce the fish stock to three-quarters of its volume. Remove from heat and leave to brew with sprigs of lime-blossom for 10 min. Strain and set aside.
- Add the orange juice to the mineral water. Bring to a boil and cook for 15 min.
- Add the cloves and orange peel, boil together for 3 min, and add the reduced fish stock.

Fish

- Salt the mackerel on the skin side, rubbing so that the salt penetrates.
- Heat a Teflon pan for 2 to 4 min. Cook the fish on the skin side only.

Dressing

- Mix the lemon juice and salt until the salt dissolves, and add the colza oil. Add pepper to taste.

PRESENTATION

- Wash and peel the fennel and cut into 4 portions. Remove the large stalks and slice the remaining portions thinly with a mandolin. Season the fennel with some lime-blossom tea sauce.
- Put 1 portion of the fennel in the centre of each plate.
- Place 1 fillet on each plate, and create a circle of vinaigrette around it. Add a good twist of milled pepper and some leaves of roquette lettuce.
- Serve the lime-blossom tea on the side.

CHICKEN FILLETS WITH WILD NETTLE PURÉE

Serves 4 • 407 Cal • 38.28 g protein • 15.6 g carbohydrate • 21.33 g fat per serving

Chicken
4 fillets of free-range chicken,
   each weighing 150 g (5¼ oz)
Tasmanian pepper to taste

Vegetables
2 ltr (4 pt 3¾ fl oz/8½ cups)
   vegetable stock
400 g (14 oz) small vegetables
1 bunch nettles
A few sprigs chervil
A few sprigs tarragon

Stuffing
2 shallots
1 bunch flat-leaved parsley
½ bunch chives
25 g (⅞ oz) *sérac* cheese
1 tsp horseradish, grated
Sea salt to taste

Sauce
150 g (5 oz/1 cup) low-fat cream
20 g (¾ oz/⅓ cup) Dijon
   mustard
Sea salt to taste

PREPARATION

Stuffing

- Peel and mince the shallots. Wash, sponge and chop the parsley.
- Dissolve the shallots in a small saucepan. Add the parsley, incorporate the *sérac* cheese and stir.
- Add the chives, salt and some horseradish. Set aside.

Vegetables

- Peel and cut the small vegetables into small pieces. Cook in the vegetable stock for 15 to 20 min. Remove the vegetables, strain and keep hot. Reserve the stock for cooking the chicken.

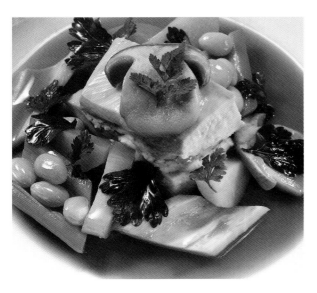

Nettle Purée
- Sort and wash the nettles and boil them in the stock for 5 min.
- Strain and cool, then mince very finely in a liquidiser.

Chicken
- Cut each fillet into 2. Lay the chicken fillets down flat.
- Place the stuffing between 2 fillet halves, and wrap up each stuffed fillet in cling film.
- Bring the vegetable stock to the boil and plunge the chicken fillets into it. Let them cook for 15 min, then remove from the heat and let them rest for 10 min in the stock. Remove the cling film.

Sauce
- Make a gravy by reducing 500 ml (1 pt 1 fl oz/2⅛ cups) of the cooking stock almost to a glaze.
- Add a small amount of additional stock, the cream, the Dijon mustard and blend.

PRESENTATION
- Place the nettle purée in the centre of each plate and place 1 stuffed fillet on top of each mound of nettle purée.
- Divide the vegetables among the plates and pour the sauce around the chicken. Decorate with the chervil and tarragon.

WHITE CALVILLE APPLES WITH CIDER AND APPLE JUICE

Serves 4 • 84 Cal • 0.4 g protein • 19.3 g carbohydrate • 0 g fat per serving

5 apples, preferably with a leaf
100 ml (3⅜ fl oz/⅜ cup) apple juice
1 tsp pectin
8 sprigs fresh thyme
40 ml (1⅜ fl oz/⅛ cup) untreated cider

PREPARATION
- Wash and dry 4 apples. Slice a 'lid' off each, and scoop out the fruit and core, keeping a 1.5-cm (1-in) thick 'wall' on each apple. Keep the lids.
- Put 4 apples with their lids into a saucepan with the cider, apple juice and pectin. Bring to a boil, then leave to cook for about 20 min on low heat.

- Remove the apples from the saucepan, and reduce the juice by three-quarters of its volume. Put the apples back into the juice and leave to crystallise for 5 min on low heat. Keep the cooking liquid.
- Peel the last apple, remove the core and cut the flesh into small cubes. Brown the apple cubes for 5 min in a non-stick pan. Then add 4 sprigs of thyme.
- Preheat the oven to 210 °C (410 °F). Fill the crystallised whole apples with the apple cubes. Put the covers back on, arrange the fruit in an ovenproof dish and top with the reserved cooking liquid. Bake for 20 min, basting at regular intervals.
- Put one apple on each plate and surround with a little ring of juice. Decorate with a sprig of fresh thyme.

MATCHA UJI TEA

Serves 4 • 0 Cal • 0 g protein • 0 g carbohydrate • 0 g fat per person

4 tsp matcha uji powder
1 ltr (2 pt 1⅞ fl oz/4¼ cups) Evian mineral water

PREPARATION
- Brew as you would normal tea and serve.

DAY 3 • EVENING TEA

FRÊNE TEA

Serves 4 • 0 Cal • 0 g protein • 0 g carbohydrate • 0 g fat per serving

8 tsp frêne tea leaves
1 ltr (2 pt 1⅞ fl oz/4¼ cups)
  Evian mineral water

PREPARATION
- Brew as you would normal tea and serve.

CUISINE MINCEUR
Les Prés d'Eugénie

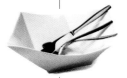

While watching dieters miserably pushing minute portions of carrots around their plates in the mid 1970s, Chef Michel Guérard hit upon the idea of *cuisine minceur* (slimming cuisine). This low-caloried, yet flavourful and nutritious approach to cooking—conceived after extensive nutritional study and experimentation—is constantly evolving as more is discovered about the healing effects of food, and its ability to keep problems such as heart disease, hypertension and cancer at bay.

Eschewing the often unhealthy culinary traditions of French fare such as butter and cream with flour, Guérard—considered the father of spa cuisine—advocates the use of healthier, but no less flavourful alternatives such as olive oil and colza (rapeseed) oil. His sauces are rich in yogurt (also a source of calcium and protein), his oils seasoned with aromatic herbs, and his calcium-enhanced broths prepared from fish bones. Fish—especially fatty fish such as sardines, tuna, salmon and mackerel—are rich in Omega-3 fatty acids and should feature in your diet at least every other day. Ingredients used should be as natural as possible: use natural fructose as a sugar substitute, for example.

Cuisine minceur makes generous use of fruit, fresh vegetables and cereals which are rich in antioxidants and vitamins A, C and E. Dried vegetables, rich in vegetal proteins, glucosides and fibre, slow down the process of hunger while providing energy. Combining dried vegetables with cereals in the right proportion—for example, 50 g (1 ½ oz) of dried vegetables with 100 g (3 oz) of cereal—provides the perfect balance of amino acids.

Cuisine minceur, however, advocates the French love for good wine. Drink a glass of red wine with lunch (the tannin and flavonoids have excellent antioxidant properties), and enjoy one glass of white wine with dinner (to help digestion).

While Guérard uses thermal water to cook those ingredients that require boiling at the 3-Michelin-star restaurant in Les Prés d'Eugénie which he and his wife own, he suggests that you can equally well use mineral water.

On the following pages, you will find Chef Michel Guérard's one-day lunch and dinner programme of delicious 1,200-calorie meals that reflect his healthy approach.

Bon appétit and *bonne santé*!

LUNCH

EGGS WITH CAVIAR

Serves 4 • 123 Cal • 14 g protein • 1 g carbohydrate • 7 g fat per serving

4 very fresh eggs
2 x 30 g (1 oz) pots Iranian
  Sevruga caviar
1 tbsp onion, finely chopped

1 tsp chives, chopped
2 tsp *fromage blanc*
1 tsp salt
A pinch pepper

PREPARATION

- Use a fine saw-edged knife to slice each egg delicately about 1 cm (½ in) above the widest part. Empty 3 of the eggs into a bowl and put the 4th aside (the 4th will not be used in the recipe). Carefully wash the eggshells in hot water and place on a cloth to dry. The shells will be used for serving eggs.
- Beat the 3 eggs. Strain through a wire sieve to remove any shell fragments and stringy portions of egg white.
- Pour the strained eggs into a small heavy-based saucepan. Cook gently over very low heat while beating vigorously with a small whisk, until the eggs start to form a light cream.
- Remove the pan from heat. Season the eggs with salt and pepper. Still stirring, add the *fromage blanc*, chopped onion and chives. Taste for seasoning.
- Place the larger eggshell halves into 4 egg cups. Fill each shell three-quarters full with the egg and cheese mixture. Top with 15 g (½ oz) of caviar, and cover with the top previously cut off. You can just see the caviar under these little bonnets.

Serving these creamed eggs with the traditional accompaniments of caviar—finely chopped onion and chives—adds an enjoyable Eastern European flavour to the dish.

PARSLEY CHICKEN

Serves 4 • 282 Cal • 46 g protein • 2 g carbohydrate • 10 g fat per serving

Chicken
1 chicken, weighing 1 kg (2¼ lbs)
5 tbsp parsley, chopped
1 tbsp chives, chopped
1 tbsp tarragon, chopped
2 shallots, chopped
50 g (2 oz) button mushrooms,
  chopped
1 tbsp *fromage blanc*

1 tsp groundnut (peanut) oil
½ tsp salt
A pinch pepper

Gravy
180 ml (⅓ pt/¾ cups) concentrated chicken stock from 4 g (½ oz)
  chicken essence powder or cube
1 tbsp parsley, chopped
1 clove garlic, unpeeled

PREPARATION

- Preheat oven to 240 °C (465 °F).
- Combine the chopped parsley, chives, tarragon, shallots and mushrooms in a bowl. Add the *fromage blanc*, salt and pepper. Use a fork to work the ingredients together into a smooth paste.
- Lift the skin away from the chicken's breast and legs by sliding your fingers between the skin and flesh. Insert the parsley mixture under the skin. Pat into an even layer over the chicken's breast and thighs.
- Season the chicken inside with salt and pepper. Brush the skin with groundnut oil. Place the chicken in a roasting pan, and cook in the oven for 40 min.
- When cooked, remove the chicken from the pan and keep hot.
- Flatten the garlic clove and add to the hot juices in the roasting pan. Add the chopped parsley. Then add the chicken stock and bring to a boil, scraping the bottom of the pan with a fork to detach caramelised juices. Reduce this gravy by one-third and taste for seasoning.
- Carve the chicken into 4 serving pieces. Place on a heated dish and pour gravy over each piece, using a conical strainer.

This recipe is also suitable for guinea fowl or pheasant.

PARIS-BREST COFFEE RING

Serves 4 • 133 Cal • 3.2 g protein • 7.5 g carbohydrate • 10 g fat per serving

Choux Pastry
1 tsp skimmed milk powder
60 ml (2 fl oz/4 tbsp) water
25 g (1 oz) butter
Sugar substitute equivalent to 1½ tsp sugar
A pinch salt
35 g (1¼ oz/¼ cup) flour
1 egg, beaten
1 egg, beaten (for brushing pastry)
1 tbsp icing sugar (optional)

Filling
Crème Chantilly (see boxed recipe on p123)

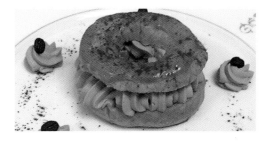

Choux pastry is more easily made if you double the quantities. Make a larger amount, put it all into a piping bag, and use it to make as many rings as you can. Bake what you need and keep the rest in the freezer for another day.

PREPARATION
Choux Pastry
- Put the skimmed milk powder, water, butter, sugar substitute and salt in a small heavy-based saucepan. Bring to a boil.
- When boiling, remove from heat. Stir in the flour with a wooden spatula. Return the mixture to the fire and cook, stirring constantly for 1 min to dry the mixture.
- Transfer the mixture to a warmed bowl. Mix in half an egg, and beat lightly with a fork for a few sec. Then add the other half of the egg. Stop beating when the pastry is supple and smooth.

Paris-Brest Coffee Ring
- Preheat the oven to 220 °C/425 °F.
- Lightly grease a baking sheet, or cover with baking paper.

- Mark a 20-cm (8-in) circle on the baking sheet or paper.
- Fill a piping bag with the choux pastry mixture. Pipe it on to your mark to create a circular ring of pastry. Brush the ring with a light glaze of beaten egg to give it a golden colour.
- Bake the pastry ring in the hot oven for 15 min, with the oven door propped slightly open with a spoon. When the pastry has risen well, reduce the oven heat to 200 °C (400 °F), and bake 15 min longer with the oven door closed.
- Remove the ring from the oven and let cool.
- Cut the ring horizontally into two circular halves.
- Fill the bottom half of the ring with Crème Chantilly. Place the upper ring on top, and powder with a light cloud of icing sugar if desired. Serve on a round dish.

DINNER

LIGHT AND FROTHY CREAM OF SORREL SOUP

Serves 4 • 50 Cal • 4.5 g protein • 2 g carbohydrate • 2.75 g fat per serving

120 g (4¼ oz) fresh sorrel, chopped
2 cloves garlic
1 ltr (1¾ pt/4¼ cups) chicken stock from chicken essence powder or stock cubes
10 ml (⅜ fl oz/2 tsp) olive oil
1½ tsp salt
1½ tsp pepper
2 eggs

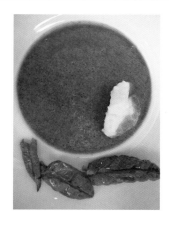

PREPARATION
- Heat the olive oil in a saucepan.
- Peel the garlic cloves, crush them whole with the flat blade of a knife, and brown lightly in oil. Add the chopped sorrel, salt and pepper, and stir.
- Add the chicken stock. Bring to a boil and simmer gently for 15 min.
- Pour the mixture into a liquidiser. Blend for 2 min until the liquid is smooth.
- Return the soup to the saucepan. Heat until the soup starts to simmer.
- With a wire whisk, whisk the eggs in a bowl until light and fluffy. Now add the hot (but not boiling) soup gradually, whisking constantly. The frothy eggs, aerated by whisking, will set on contact with the hot liquid to make the soup light, airy and velvety.
- Serve preferably in white porcelain soup bowls, to set off the soup's attractive green colour and velvety texture.

SAFFRON-STEAMED TURBOT WITH ANCHOVIES

Serves 4 • 80 Cal • 9 g protein • 2 g carbohydrate • 4 g fat per serving

Fish
1 young turbot or halibut, weighing about 1.2 kg (2½ lbs), skinned, cleaned and de-finned
2 whole salted anchovies or 8 tinned anchovy fillets
1 ltr (1¾ pt/4¼ cups) fish stock made from 4 g (½ oz) fish essence cube
A pinch whole saffron

Sauce
1 tbsp mushroom purée (see boxed recipe on p123)
1 tsp fresh cream
4 fresh spinach leaves

PREPARATION
Sauce
- Pour 250 ml (a scant ½ pt/1 cup) of the cooking liquid into a liquidiser. Add the mushroom purée and fresh cream and blend. Transfer to a saucepan and heat.

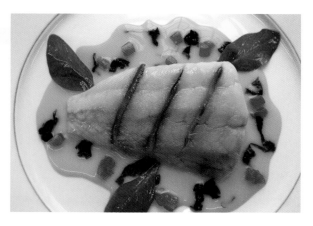

- Wash the spinach leaves carefully, and remove the stalks. Cut the leaves into wide ribbons. Poach in a pan of boiling water for 1 min, drain and add to the sauce.

Saffron-Steamed Turbot with Anchovies

- Leave the whole anchovies under running water for 10 min to desalt them. Remove the bones and divide into fillets. Cut each fillet in half lengthwise, and then across, to produce 16 small anchovy slivers. If using tinned anchovies, simply cut each fillet in half.
- With the point of a sharp kitchen knife, make small deep incisions on both sides of the turbot. Insert an anchovy sliver into each incision.

- Add the saffron to the fish stock. Pour the stock into a fish kettle with a rack and lid, to a level just below the rack. Place the turbot on the rack above the liquid so it cooks in the steam, and does not poach. Cover the kettle and cook the fish gently for 35 min. After cooking, remove the turbot and keep hot.
- Using a metal spatula or palette knife, lift the turbot's flesh away from the backbone. Remove the 2 upper fillets. The backbone now comes away in 1 piece, and the lower fillets can be easily removed.
- Have 4 heated plates ready. Cover each plate lightly with the sauce and place a turbot fillet on each plate.

LITTLE PEAR SOUFFLÉS

Serves 4 • 68 Cal • 7 g protein • 3.6 g carbohydrate • 2.8 g fat per serving

Pear Soufflé
3 pears (very ripe), each weighing about 120 g (4 oz)
½ tsp *eau-de-vie de poire* (pear brandy)
Sugar substitute equivalent to 3 tbsp sugar
2 egg yolks

5 egg whites
15 g (1 oz) butter, softened

Syrup
500 ml (1¼ pts/2⅛ cups) water
Sugar substitute equivalent to 4 tbsp sugar
1 vanilla pod, cut in half length-wise

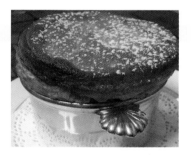

PREPARATION

- Put the ingredients for the syrup in a saucepan. Bring to a boil.
- Peel the pears with a potato peeler, cut into quarters and core them. Poach in the syrup for 15 min.
- Drain the pears, and blend in a liquidiser with the sugar substitute and pear brandy.
- Pour the purée into a bowl and add the egg yolks.
- Use the softened butter to brush the insides of 4 individual soufflé dishes, 9 cm (3½ in) across by 4 cm (1½ in) deep.
- Preheat the oven to 220 °C (400 °F).

- With a balloon whisk, beat the egg whites until soft and snowy. Mix one-quarter into the pear purée. Gradually add the remaining egg whites to the purée mixture, folding in carefully with a spatula.
- Fill the soufflé dishes up to the top with the mixture. Level the surface of each dish with the back of a knife or a palette knife.
- Push the mixture away from the edges of each dish with your thumb to help the soufflés rise.
- Cook for about 8 min in the hot oven. Remove the soufflés from the oven and serve immediately.

CRÈME CHANTILLY

Serves 4

1½ egg whites
Sugar substitute equivalent to 4 tbsp sugar
1 tbsp instant coffee powder

1 drop vanilla essence
6 tbsp whipping cream or 4 tbsp double cream stirred with 2 tbsp iced water

PREPARATION

- Put the egg whites, sugar substitute (pounded to a powder if necessary) and instant coffee powder into a large bowl. Place the bowl over a pan of just simmering water, and whisk for 10 min. The mixture will thicken and then become a stiff meringue. Place the meringue in the refrigerator.
- Flavour the cream with vanilla essence. Whisk in a large bowl. Beat gently at first, and then briskly to incorporate more air. Stop whisking when the cream stiffens.
- Remove the meringue from the refrigerator. With a spatula, gently fold the whipped cream into the chilled meringue.

MUSHROOM PURÉE

Serves 4

420 g (15 oz) button mushrooms
125 g (4½ oz/1 cup) skimmed milk powder
1.25 ltr (2¼ pts/5¼ cups) water

15 ml (½ fl oz/1 tbsp) lemon juice
1 heaped tsp salt
A pinch pepper
A pinch grated nutmeg

PREPARATION

- Trim the mushrooms, cutting off the earthy parts of the stalks.
- Wash the mushrooms thoroughly and drain. Cut them in half and toss quickly in lemon juice to keep them white.
- Dissolve the skimmed milk powder in the water. Put in a saucepan and bring to a boil. Add the mushrooms and season with the salt, pepper and nutmeg. Simmer uncovered for 20 min.
- Remove the mushrooms from the cooking liquid. Purée very finely in a liquidiser. Add 150 ml (¼ pt/⅝ cups) of the cooking liquid, and taste for seasoning.

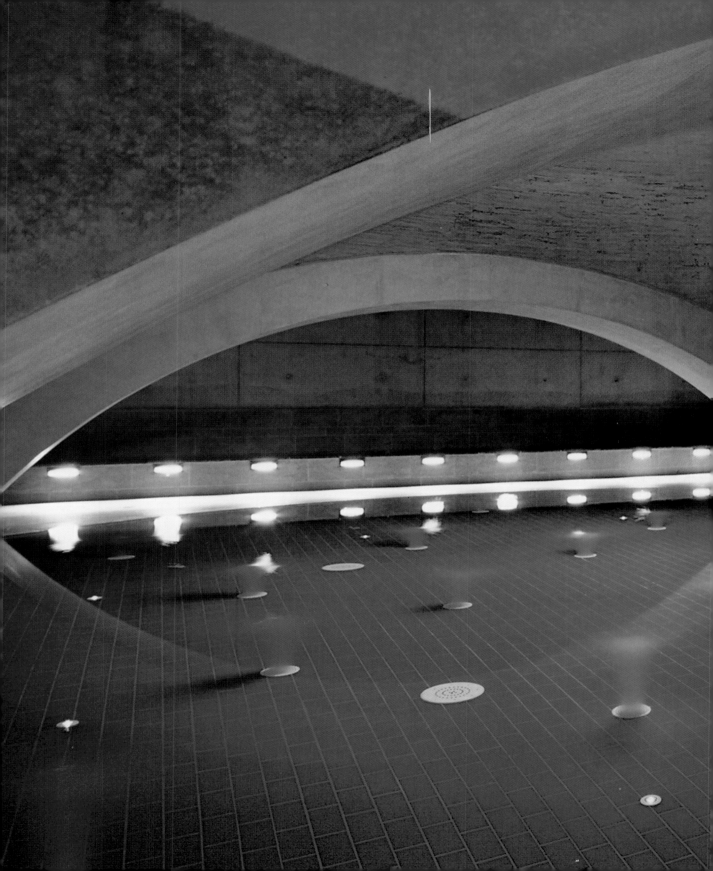

Austria 126   **Finland** 130   **France** 132   **Germany** 154   **Greece** 162
Hungary 164   **Iceland** 166   **Italy** 168   **Monaco** 176   **Portugal** 178
Russia 180   **Spain** 182   **Switzerland** 186   **Turkey** 196   **United Kingdom** 200

SPA DIGEST

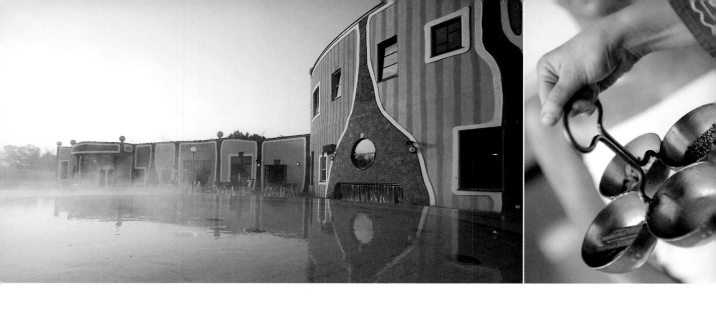

Rogner-Bad Blumau, Hotel & Spa
Styria, Austria

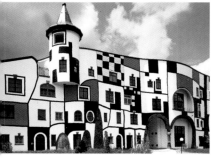

One of the many colourful façades that distinguish the award-winning Rogner-Bad Blumau, Hotel & Spa. Opened in 1997, it is situated in the green heart of the Styrian landscape.

The Rogner-Bad Blumau, Hotel & Spa, designed by Austrian architect Friedensreich Hundertwasser, has the kind of architecture that evokes in adults a child's delight. One is reminded of the fantastic creations of Gaudi, setting the mood for a holiday of unrivalled cheeriness.

The multi-coloured hotel occupies a 40-hectare (100-acre) area. A spacious 2,500-square metre (26,910-square foot) spa offers a variety of unique spa experiences ranging from therapeutic thermal water pools, a sunbathing island, and even the spa's very own volcano lake! Called 'Vulkania', this fantasy spa world is designed to combine the elements of water, fire, air and earth to create the ultimate rejuvenation experience.

The spa also operates Europe's leading holistic health centre—FindeDich. Here professionally trained practitioners introduce you to a comprehensive array of Ayurveda secrets in colourful and exotic surroundings, where the scent of joss sticks and Indian spices permeates the air. The emphasis is on the authentic application of Ayurvedic massages and treatments specially prescribed by an Ayurvedic doctor from India. The philosophy behind Ayurveda calls for the incorporation of nutrition, herbs, plants and spices into the system of massages and treatments. At the restaurant IssDichFit, chefs schooled in Ayurvedic cuisine prepare organic courses for you to complete your Ayurvedic experience.

Discover a variety of other spa treatments harmonising the best of the old and the new. Take, for instance, sound therapy: a holistic treatment developed by Dr Wolfgang Kölbl, which has its roots in the healing traditions of Tibet. This combines the synthesis of tones from instruments such as the Tibetan singing bowls, with playing techniques and trance work. This symphony of sounds lulls you into a deeply relaxed state to attain the apex of self-healing.

Pampering sessions can also be booked at the Wunderschön, the spa's beauty centre. Recently expanded to incorporate more facilities for couples, Wunderschön offers

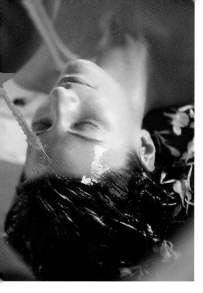

OPPOSITE LEFT: *The spa pool is filled with waters from the Melchior spring, at a temperature of 36 degrees Celsius (97 degrees Fahrenheit).*

OPPOSITE RIGHT, AND LEFT: *Ten professionally trained practitioners and two medical doctors offer a range of traditional Ayurvedic treatments at the health centre, including Shirodhara (pictured).*

BOTTOM: *The spa has extensive indoor and outdoor features including a freshwater wavepool and the Vulcano lake with underwater music.*

aromatic whirlpool sessions for two, his-and-hers anti-stress treatments, and aroma-algae packs that transform unwinding and pampering into a romantic escapade.

The Rogner-Bad Blumau, Hotel & Spa is situated some 90 minutes from Vienna, the city of musical greats. A stay at the Rogner-Bad Blumau, Hotel & Spa promises an intoxicating experience that will surely provide enchantment and music for your soul.

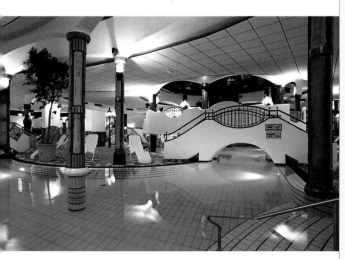

Spa Statistics

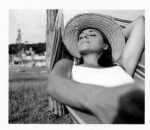

Relax in a pasture filled with the blooms and fluttering leaves of the aspen trees, and enjoy dips in the indoor and outdoor pools fed by the healing waters from the Caspar, Melchior and Balthasar springs.

TYPE OF SPA
Hotel spa

SPA AREA
2,500 sq m (26,910 sq ft)

FACILITIES
2 double treatment rooms, 18 single treatment rooms, 1 outdoor treatment pavilion; 2 consultation rooms; 1 meditation room, various relaxation areas throughout the resort; 3 jacuzzis, 2 whirlpools; 6 saunas, 9 solariums; 2 indoor thermal water pools, 2 outdoor thermal water pools, 1 natural thermal water lake with underwater music for swimming; 1 cold plunge pool, 1 freshwater wave pool; beauty centre, health and mind centre, institute for holistic treatments; 1 hair salon; 2 gymnasiums; 4 outdoor sand tennis courts; 1 beach volleyball court; equestrian facilities nearby; 45-hole golf circuit nearby; 3 spa boutiques

SIGNATURE TREATMENTS
Ayurveda facials with neck and head massage, Ayurvedic treatments; body cocoons with hay, mare's milk, honey and evening primrose oil; Esalen Bodywork, Lomi Lomi Nui Massage, Shiatsu and Intuitive Sensitive Massage, skin and body peeling, Sound Therapy, 'Trester' (draff) or Thalasso (algae) Exclusive Anti-Stress beauty treatments, Thai Yoga Massage, Tui-Na

TREATMENTS & THERAPIES
Acupuncture, anti-ageing treatments, anti-cellulite treatments, aqua therapy, Ayurvedic treatments, Bach Flower Remedies, baths, body bronzing, body scrubs, colonic irrigation and enemas, electrotherapy, eye treatments, facials, firming and slimming treatments, hand and foot treatments, heat treatments, holistic treatments, homeopathy, hydrotherapy, inhalation therapies, life-coach counselling, lymphatic drainage, make-up services, manicures and pedicures, massages, movement therapies, naturopathy consultations, pre- and post-natal treatments, purifying back treatments, reflexology, salon services, scalp treatments, sound meditation and sound therapies, Thai therapies, thalassotherapy, waxing

SPA CUISINE
The organic restaurant IssDichFit offers a selection of spa cuisine and meets various dietary requirements. All the resort restaurants also serve beverages and meals made by ingredients from purely organic sources. Guests can request for special Ayurvedic cuisine. Professional nutrition analysis and advice are also provided.

ACTIVITIES & PROGRAMMES
Fitness checks, healthy spine video screening; aerobics, aquaerobics, belly dancing, biking, golf, hiking, horse riding, inline skating, *qi gong*, spinning, *tai qi*, tennis, yoga; meditation and stretching classes; lifestyle management classes, stress management courses; sports instruction

SERVICES
Consultations; personal training; baby-sitting, childcare; corporate programmes; gift certificates; day-use rooms; transfers on request

LANGUAGES SPOKEN BY THERAPISTS
English, German, Hungarian, Italian, Russian

CONTACT
Rogner-Bad Blumau, Hotel & Spa
A-8283 Bad Blumau
Austria
T: +43 (0)3383 5100 0
F: +43 (0)3383 5100 808
E: spa.blumau@rogner.com
W: www.blumau.com

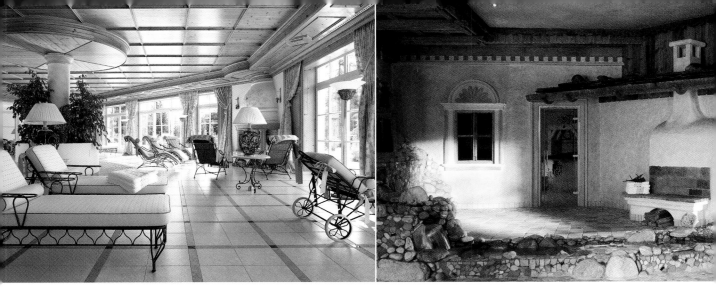

The Spa at the Interalpen-Hotel Tyrol
Telfs-Buchen, Austria

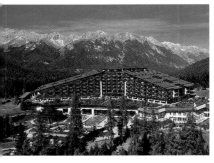

The five-star hotel sits on a high plateau, dwarfed by a mountain range. You will find yourself in a hub of activity whatever time you visit. You may attend an inspirational talk in spring to better your health; roar up in your roadster to a musical festival in summer; go on a mountain adventure with your family in autumn; or warm up with a glass of mulled wine while watching a curling game on the hotel's ice-rink in winter.

The largesse of the Alpine area that surrounds the luxurious Interalpen-Hotel Tyrol is reflected in its spacious interior, which is decorated with Venetian chandeliers, valuable carpets and works of art. The five-star hotel reflects the mantra 'more in every way' expounded by Dr Hans Liebherr, the hotel's founder.

This extravagance extends to The Spa, an expansive two-level area dedicated to beauty, wellbeing, relaxation and vitality. Even the spa menu is expansive, with treatments old and new from the East and West. The staff are able to help tailor a treatment programme geared towards your needs, and can arrange for consultations with physicians, fitness experts and nutritionists.

Massages range from Shiatsu-Massage to Sport Massage—the most exotic being the Pantai Luar, a deeply relaxing treatment from East Asia in which a herbal pack of lime and spices, heated in oil, is applied in rapid strokes to your body, removing old cells and encouraging the growth of new ones.

Besides classic baths such as the Whey Bath, Mud Bath or Herbal Essence Bath, more esoteric ones include the balancing Crystal-Sound-Bath that combines music and light therapy, and the invigorating Hydroxeur-Royal-Bath that combines jets of air with water, scents, colours and sounds. You can also opt to enjoy the Hammam treatment—a soap massage in a lavishly decorated steam room—with a partner.

Dry flotation treatments in which your body is coddled in luxurious substances while you float on a waterbed include the reviving Hay-Bath, the cleansing Cleopatra Bath (with milk, honey and oil), the hormone-regulating Oenothera Biennis-Oil-Bath (with evening primrose), and the moisturising Trester Bath (with wine, earth and calcium carbonate).

Extensive heat facilities and baths are clustered in what resembles a rustic Tyrolean village. These include a Tyrolean Bakehouse (a laconicum of mild heat in which bread is baked), a Stone Bath (in which a hand-forged wheel dips glowing hot stones into water,

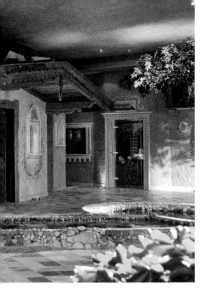

OPPOSITE, LEFT: *Unwind in the relaxation room, which leads out into the garden.*

LEFT: *The Tyrolean Sauna Village comprising a series of heat facilities and a Kneipp stream reflects the rustic surrounds of the region.*

BOTTOM: *You can swim into the outdoor pool (pictured) via a channel from the 50-metre (160-foot) indoor Panorama Pool. In the large outdoor pool, you can be gently massaged on stimulating bubble loungers. The adjacent glass relaxation lounge has a breathtaking view of the Alps.*

releasing a pleasant, cleansing warmth), a Grotto of Precious Stones (a steam bath with crystals) and an Old Salt Room (a flotation pool with sound and light therapy).

The property's emphasis on indulgence is carried over to the spa's 'fitness cuisine': gourmet healthy dishes created with fresh ingredients from Tyrolean farms and cooked in a way to maximise their nutrients. You can watch your dish prepared before your eyes at an open-air kitchen in the Spa-Restaurant. Meals are designed to be easily digested and to boost your body's energy. Indulging in the name of health *is* possible, after all.

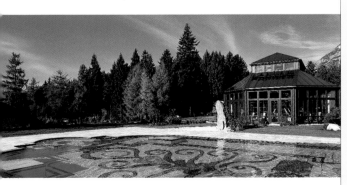

Spa Statistics

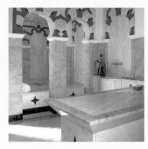

The traditional Hammam treatment brings to Austria a real traditional Turkish delight.

TYPE OF SPA
Hotel spa

SPA AREA
5,000 sq m (53,820 sq ft)

FACILITIES
24 treatment rooms, 1 physio-therapy room; 1 salt grotto; 1 hammam; Tyrolean sauna village comprising 1 alpine sauna, 1 bakehouse, 1 laconicum, 1 stone bath, 1 gem grotto, 1 herb bath, 1 salt pool and 1 Kneipp stream; 1 glass relaxation pavilion; 1 meditation room, 1 relaxation lounge; 1 doctor's room, 1 consultation room; 3 solariums; 1 hair salon; 1 cardio studio, 1 fitness room, 2 Gymnastik rooms, 1 gymnasium; 1 indoor swimming pool, 1 outdoor swimming pool with massage nozzles; 2 indoor tennis courts, 3 outdoor tennis courts

SIGNATURE TREATMENT
Pantai Luar

TREATMENTS & THERAPIES
Anti-ageing treatments, anti-cellulite treatments, aqua therapy, aromatherapy, baths, body bronzing, body wraps, Chinese therapies, depilation, electro-therapy, facials, hand and foot treatments, heat treatment, inhalation therapies, kinesiology, lymphatic drainage, manicures and pedicures, massages, movement therapies, physiotherapy, thalassotherapy; spa packages

PROVISIONS FOR COUPLES
Hammam; Wellbeing Package For Two

SPA CUISINE
'Fitness cuisine', easily digested and energy providing, is available at the Vollkorn Bio Kalorie Restaurant. Traditional food is available, as is cuisine with an Oriental influence. Provisions for various dietary requirements are available on request

ACTIVITIES & PROGRAMMES
Aerobics, aquaerobics, archery, biking, golf, hiking, horse riding, Pilates, rock-climbing, *tai qi*, tennis, yoga; cooking, dance, make-up, massage, meditation, and stretching classes, sports instruction, talks and workshops on health, diet and beauty by visiting consultants

SERVICES
Life-coach counselling; health care, skincare and nutrition consultation; body fat analysis, assessment, personal training; baby-sitting, childcare

LANGUAGES SPOKEN BY THERAPISTS
Dutch, English, French, German, Italian

ADMISSION
Exclusively for hotel guests

CONTACT
Interalpen-Hotel Tyrol
Dr-Hans-Liebherr-Alpenstraße 1
A-6410 Telfs-Buchen
Austria
T: +43 (0)5262 606
F: +43 (0)5262 606 190
E: interalpen@interalpen.com
W: www.interalpen.com

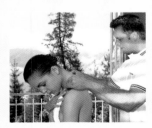

For quick relief, opt for one of the 25-minute massages that include the Migraine Massage, which releases tension from your head and neck; the Acupressure Massage, which regulates your internal energies; and the Aromatic-Oil Massage, which invigorates, soothes or refreshes, depending on your choice of oils.

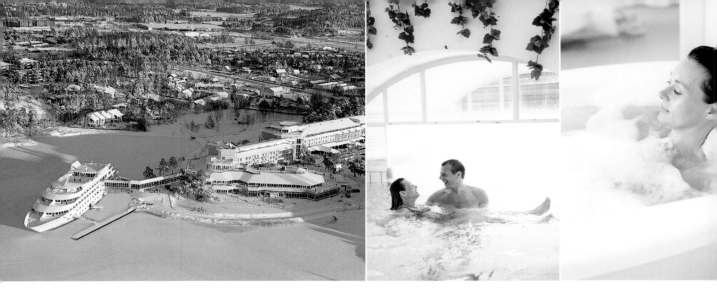

Naantali Spa at Naantali Spa Hotel & Resort
Naantali, Finland

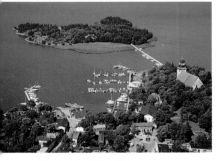

TOP AND ABOVE: *The scenery around the resort complex takes on a different feel with each season. The main hotel and the yacht offer a total of 350 rooms and suites. In the interest of health, guests can opt for allergen-free rooms equipped with wooden floors and dedicated to non-smokers.*

Naantali, 'the official holiday city of Finland', faces the Baltic Sea on the country's southwest coast. In the 18th century, it hosted aristocrats and courtiers from the Russian Empire, and it has welcomed ruling presidents over the last 100 summers. Visitors have been enjoying the waters of the Viluluoto Spring and the clays of Luolalanjärvi Lake since 1732.

In keeping with the area's rich bathing heritage, Naantali Spa is a fully qualified member of the Royal Spas of Europe. The spa is located within the Naantali Spa Hotel & Resort complex, which incorporates a luxury cruiser—the Sunborn Princess Yacht Hotel—as a permanent feature in its bay, together with an arcade of shops and restaurants, convention facilities and comprehensive fitness centres. Naantali Spa packages in conjunction with accommodation are available.

The spa, with its modern up-to-date facilities, offers a wide range of treatments. Many of these are based on European traditions and revolve around the use of marine-derived products from French brand Phytomer and German Lipogen facial products.

The spa is especially famous for its 60-minute Natural Clay Treatment that uses the traditional local blue clay that has been kept pure by the region's prevailing winters. The clay, which has no scent or taste, is heated, then mixed, applied to your skin, and left for 30 to 40 minutes. This relaxing, stress-relieving treatment helps to detoxify, relieves pain, and stimulates the circulation.

Your skin should feel softer, and your mind refreshed after this uniquely restorative treatment. Clay packs and peat treatments are also available. (However, if you are not at the peak of health, you are advised to enquire about the suitability of clay treatment.)

The spa also offers a special selection of 15-minute baths. Perhaps the most unusual of these is the Polar Night Bath—a uniquely invigorating bath with essential oils, integrated with light therapy, that is especially designed to enhance your mood on dark winter evenings. During your bath, you will also be

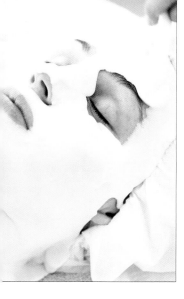

OPPOSITE, CENTRE: *The indoor swimming complex is romantically linked to an outdoor area that overlooks the bay.*

OPPOSITE, RIGHT: *Water treatments include the Bath With Peat Extracts From Arctic Plants which can be stimulating or relaxing.*

LEFT: *Over 12 face treatments feature on the menu. The most popular is the 60-minute Facial Treatment Based On Skin Type Analysis in which you are given the facial that is most appropriate for your skin's needs.*

given a special herbal brew to drink, available in relaxing or stimulating versions.

A small selection of therapies from the East includes Shiatsu (Japanese Treatment Method) during which the vital energy points on your body are massaged.

Another favourite massage is Zone Therapy (Chinese Treatment Massage). During this treatment, the therapist will concentrate on specific zones of your feet—this is believed to balance the functions in the corresponding organs of your body.

Reflecting the town's bathing heritage, the spa boasts a lavish water complex that includes saunas, jacuzzis, and indoor and outdoor swimming pools. All these, combined with the scenic unspoilt beauty of maritime Naantali and its surrounding islands, makes your visit here an unforgettable experience.

Guests can also participate in one of the region's amusing local traditions on the morning of Sleepyhead Day, 27 July—by throwing a person recognised for his or her outstanding contributions to the community into the sea.

Spa Statistics

TYPE OF SPA
Hotel spa

SPA AREA
2,000 sq m (21,530 sq ft)

FACILITIES
20 single massage rooms; 5 consultation rooms, 1 relaxation lounge; 10 bath rooms, 2 jacuzzis, 2 reflexology pools; 5 saunas, 2 steam rooms; 1 solarium; 1 hair salon, 1 make-up room, 4 nail rooms, 4 pedicure rooms; 1 aerobics studio, 1 gymnasium; 1 indoor swimming pool, 1 outdoor swimming pool; 3 golf courses (10–15 min drive); 1 tennis court; 1 spa boutique

SIGNATURE TREATMENT
Natural Clay Treatment

TREATMENTS & THERAPIES
Anti-ageing treatments, anti-cellulite treatments, aromatherapy, baths, body scrubs, body wraps, Chinese therapies, electrotherapy, eye treatments, facials, firming and slimming treatments, hair analysis/ treatments, hand and foot treatments, heat treatments, lymphatic drainage, make-up services, manicures and pedicures, massages, movement therapies, purifying back treatments, reflexology, scalp treatments, thalassotherapy, waxing

SPA CUISINE
Low calorie, low-fat options are available at Paviljonki. A light buffet of dishes of seafood and local ingredients is available at Café Roma, and the Sunborn Princess à la carte (on the yacht) serves delicious meals made

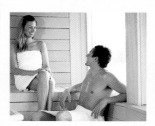

In a nod to the Finnish sauna tradition, the resort boasts five saunas on the property including one on the yacht.

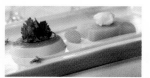

Healthy dishes are created from fresh seafood and Icelandic ingredients from the area.

of Finnish and international ingredients. Provisions for various dietary requirements are available on request at all of the property's restaurants.

ACTIVITIES & PROGRAMMES
Aerobics, aquaerobics, biking, golf, hiking, sailing, *tai chi,* tennis, yoga; cooking, dance, lifestyle enhancement, make-up, stretching and wardrobe-planning classes; sports instruction, talks by visiting consultants

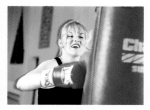

The property offers a good mix of restful as well as more active pursuits.

SERVICES
Body composition analysis; life-coach counselling; personal training, skincare and nutritional consultations; baby-sitting; corporate programmes; day-use rooms

LANGUAGES SPOKEN BY THERAPISTS
English, Finnish, Swedish

ADMISSION
Membership is available but not required for admission.

CONTACT
Naantali Spa Hotel & Resort
Matkailijantie 2
FIN-21100 Naantali
Finland
T: +358 (0)2 44 550
F: +358 (0)2 445 5101
E: info@naantalispa.fi
W: www.naantalispa.fi

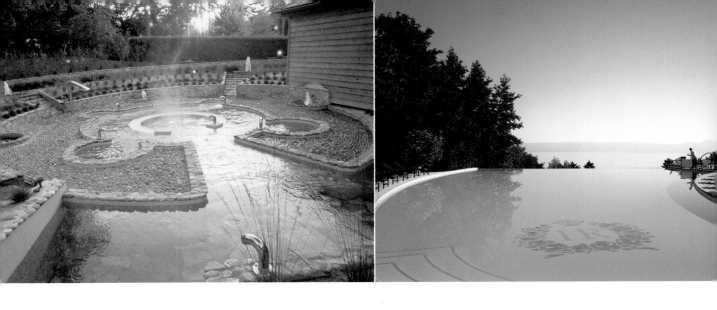

Better Living Institute at Hotel Royal – Royal Parc Evian
Evian-les-Bains, France

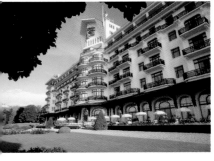

ABOVE: *Hotel Royal is nestled between the French Alps and Lake Geneva in the beautifully landscaped Royal Parc Evian, which includes a forest of century-old trees and over 200 varieties of roses. Besides enjoying a leisurely stroll through this parkland, other pursuits favoured by guests include winning at the baccarat tables at the waterfront casino and hitting the bulls-eye at the archery range.*

OPPOSITE, BOTTOM: *Many of the treatments designed to awaken your energies revolve around the use of ingredients nurtured by the earth, such as the Massage With Oils, Soothing Flower Bath, or Mud Treatment With Trace Elements (pictured).*

The Hotel Royal, situated within the 17-hectare (42-acre) grounds of Royal Parc Evian, is an elegant establishment that was built in 1909 in honour of a regular visitor to Evian, Edward VII, Prince of Wales and subsequently King of England. A visit to Evian follows in the steps of fashionable members of high society who have visited the famous source of mineral waters in the centre of town since 1789. A more recent tradition is to visit the Better Living Institute, located on the ground floor, and accessible from all floors of the hotel via a private lift.

Treatments revolve around the spa's concept of 're-energy', which aims to rebalance your body and mind, and enhance your energy reserves. The Re-Energise Plan involves five hours of treatment per day for five consecutive days. The first day revolves around helping you eliminate toxins and negative energies; the second, releasing tension and encouraging relaxation; the third, renewing your physio-psychological energies; the fourth, stimulating your energies; and the fifth,

re-energising your entire being. Packages or plans for 2- and 6-day stays are also available, and these are tailored according to your length of stay, personality, and goals, which may include increasing your vitality, getting fit, slimming down, easing gracefully into middle age, getting back in shape, or bonding with your new baby.

Treatments include a comprehensive range of Asian therapies, as well as European classics such as fangotherapy and manual lymphatic drainage. Treatments may also be enjoyed on an à la carte basis.

A nutritional programme known as La Cuisine Synergique® is designed to complement your desired plan. This is a low-calorie but creative gastronomic feast influenced by nutritherapy, phytotherapy and Chinese medicine. A balanced selection of herbs, spices and ingredients, and a specific method of preparation are essential in ensuring that the dishes—designed to address your needs, such as balance and energy, over the course of your stay—are high in flavour, texture and

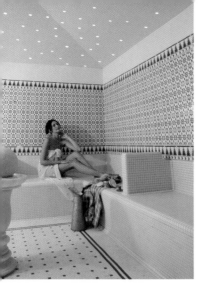

OPPOSITE, LEFT: *The flower-shaped hydro-contact trail, which offers hydro-massages through a symphony of fountains and underwater jets, is at once playful and therapeutic.*

OPPOSITE, RIGHT: *Swim towards the edge of the infinity pool to enjoy one of the property's most breathtaking views of Lake Geneva.*

LEFT: *The exotically tiled steam room with twinkling starlights on the ceiling and a fountain in the centre resembles a resplendent Moroccan palace.*

nutritional value. To further complement La Cuisine Synergique® and your treatment objectives, you will be prescribed essential waters—of rosemary, sage, juniper, artemisia, lavender or mint—to drink.

With your energy restored after a course of treatment at the spa, you can take home a better appreciation of balancing your health and wellness, as well as the experience of having made a pilgrimage to one of the most famous historical spa towns in Europe.

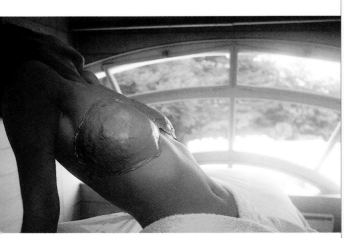

Spa Statistics

TYPE OF SPA
Resort spa

SPA AREA
1,600 sq m (17,220 sq ft)

FACILITIES
34 single treatment rooms; 1 relaxation lounge; 1 cold plunge pool, 1 hydro-contact trail, 1 jacuzzi; 1 sauna, 1 steam room; 1 solarium; 1 hair salon, 1 nail salon; 1 aerobics studio, 1 gymnasium; 1 indoor swimming pool, 1 outdoor swimming pool, 1 outdoor children's pool; 1 private golf course (Evian Masters Golf Course, 1 km/0.6 miles from the hotel); 1 squash court, 5 tennis courts; 1 climbing wall; 1 spa boutique

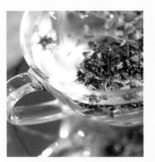

Before and after your treatment, you can sip rare teas, infusions (pictured), as well as essential waters derived from the distillation of aromatic plants.

SIGNATURE TREATMENT
Re-Energise Plan

TREATMENTS & THERAPIES
Acupuncture, anti-ageing treatments, anti-cellulite treatments, aqua therapy, aromatherapy, baths, Ayurvedic treatments, body bronzing, body scrubs, body wraps, bust treatments, Chinese therapies, electrotherapy, eye treatments, facials, firming and slimming treatments, hair treatments, hand and foot treatments, hydrotherapy, jet lag treatments, lymphatic drainage, manicures and pedicures, massages, movement therapies, pre- and post-natal treatments, purifying back treatments, reflexology, scalp treatments, Thai therapies, waxing; 2-, 5- and 6-day packages,

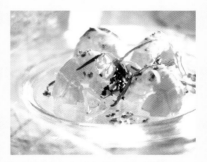

La Cuisine Synergique® includes these Dublin Bay Prawns, gently cooked to retain a maximum of amino acids.

6-day Mother-Baby Companion Programme for mothers and fathers (which includes spa treatments, use of facilities, participation in activities for baby between 3 to 9 months of age, and free baby-sitting at the crèche)

SPA CUISINE
La Cuisine Synergique®, based on elements from Chinese and Indian philosophies, developed by head chef Michel Lentz, is available exclusively at Le Jardin des Lys. Provisions for various dietary needs are available on request. (See also 'Spa Cuisine', pp106–119.)

ACTIVITIES & PROGRAMMES
Aerobics, aquaerobics, archery, biking, golf, hiking, horse riding, rock-climbing, sailing, stretching, tennis, yoga; cooking classes

SERVICES
General healthcare, skincare, and nutritional consultations, naturopathic consultation; body composition analysis, personal training; free transfers to Evian city centre, the Casino and the Golf course

LANGUAGES SPOKEN BY THERAPISTS
English, French, German, Italian, Russian, Spanish

CONTACT
Hotel Royal – Royal Parc Evian
South Bank of Lake Geneva
74500 Evian-les-Bains
France
T: +33 (0)4 5026 8500
F: +33 (0)4 5075 6100
E: reservation@royalparcevian.com
W: www.royalparcevian.com

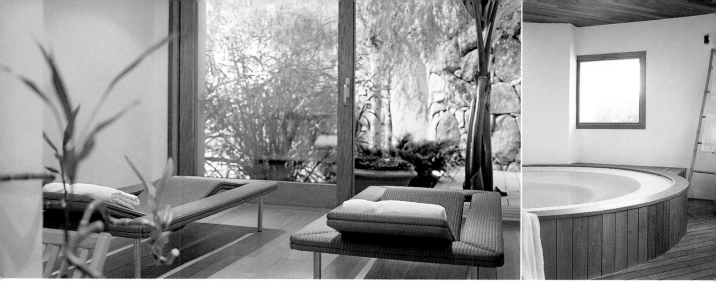

Cala Rossa Spa at Grand Hotel de Cala Rossa
Corsica, France

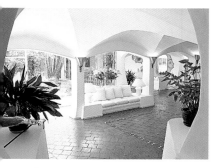

The hotel's interior is a play on textures: white stone arches, teak loungers, Juniper woodcarvings and earthenware.

The Grand Hotel de Cala Rossa, nestled in a garden between the mountains and the sea, is a quintessential Mediterranean home with lovely nooks and crannies, and individually decorated rooms that inspire daydreams and lazy days. Being among the green pines that line the red rocks, white sand and turquoise sea will give you a sense of oneness with nature.

You can also reconnect with nature at the Cala Rossa Spa. The spa area overlooks a lush garden, which creates the effect of bringing the outdoors indoors. Treatments are based on Phytomer and Kanebo products comprised of ingredients derived from Father Neptune; the latter also incorporates Mother Earth's bounty with colour therapy and the Chinese concept of energy. The space dedicated to relaxation, beauty and fitness also reflects a chic, modern Oriental ethos in its music and minimal décor.

Discover the healing energies of colour in the Full Coloured Clay Facial And Body Care, a treatment in which different coloured clays are applied to your face and body; the colours are chosen according to your personal biological rhythm and the time of treatment. This is followed by a Chinese Massage to remove any energy blockages within your body.

Saveur Du Marquis is an appropriately invigorating treatment, given the spa's close proximity to the sea. It includes an exfoliation using salt harvested from the area, followed by a massage with myrrh oil to regenerate the skin, leaving it silky smooth.

Chinese Massage, a vigorous massage to your back and legs performed by an osteopath, is one of the spa's most popular massages. It is especially sought after during the months of May, June, September and October when you can enjoy it in a treehouse between the hotel and the sea.

The spa's selection of body treatments and massages—which include Shea Butter Relaxation Massage and Aromatic Massage With Essential Oils—is augmented with a wide range of beauty and grooming

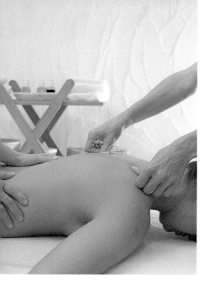

OPPOSITE, LEFT: *Relax and put your feet up on these sleek loungers, and enjoy the sight of a lush green garden.*

OPPOSITE, RIGHT: *Even the jacuzzi area is an oasis of calm with its chic simplicity.*

LEFT: *Four-Hand Modelling is an extra pampering massage which is performed in tandem by two therapists, with options for relaxation or slimming.*

BOTTOM: *The sleek indoor swimming pool opens out into a lush garden.*

treatments for men and women to rebalance the body, mind and spirit.

The spa's quietude invites you to linger after your treatment to sip a fresh mint tea or a green tea with lemon, as you look out on to the lush garden and contemplate all the wonders of nature.

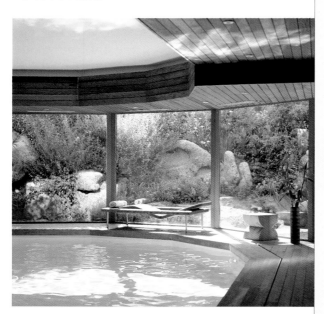

Spa Statistics

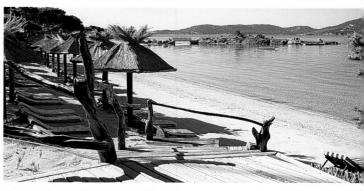

The surrounding seaside is a place for quiet reflection.

TYPE OF SPA
Hotel spa

SPA AREA
500 sq m (5,380 sq ft)

FACILITIES
6 single indoor treatment villas,
1 outdoor treatment pavilion;
1 relaxation lounge; 1 jacuzzi,
1 sauna, 1 steam room;
1 outdoor solarium; 1 hair salon;
1 nail salon; 1 aerobics studio,
1 cardio studio, 1 gymnasium;
1 indoor swimming pool;
1 spa boutique

SIGNATURE TREATMENTS
Full Coloured Clay Facial And
Body Care, Saveur Du Marquis

TREATMENTS & THERAPIES
Anti-ageing treatments, anti-cellulite treatments, aromatherapy, body bronzing, body scrubs, body wraps, bust treatments, eye treatments, facials, firming and slimming treatments, hair treatments, hand and foot treatments, heat treatments, lymphatic drainage, manicures and pedicures, massages, reflexology, salon services, scalp treatments, waxing; half-, 1-, 3- and 6-day spa packages

SPA CUISINE
Not available, but provisions for various dietary requirements are available on request.

ACTIVITIES & PROGRAMMES
Aerobics, aquaerobics, biking, sailing, snorkelling, tennis, yoga; stretching classes, sports instruction

SERVICES
Life-coach counselling;
baby-sitting

LANGUAGES SPOKEN BY THERAPISTS
English, French, Italian

CONTACT
Grand Hotel de Cala Rossa
20137 Porto-Vecchio, Corsica
France
T: +33 (0)4 9571 6151
F: +33 (0)4 9571 6011
E: info@hotel-calarossa.com
W: www.hotel-calarossa.com

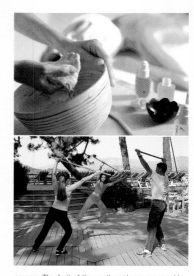

CENTRE: *The fruit of the earth and sea are used in luxurious treatments.*

ABOVE: *Stretching exercises are extra invigorating, as they take place outdoors on the deck with the scent of roses, pine trees and sea air.*

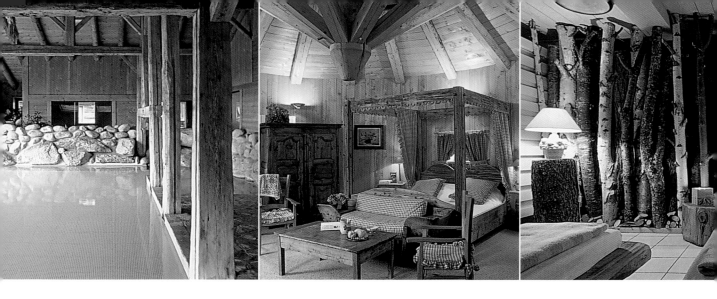

La Ferme de Beauté at Les Fermes de Marie
Megève, France

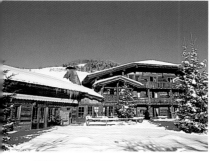

Winter makes the area seem even more picturesque. During the ski season, the King and Queen of Sweden are known to rent a private chalet at Les Fermes de Marie.

Stroll around the hamlet of alpine farms that surrounds Les Fermes de Marie, and you will see that this hotel, with its wooden walls and French farmhouse antiques, exudes a similar warmth and old-world charm. Both in summer and winter, a sophisticated crowd feels comfortably at home in this cosy hotel.

La Ferme de Beauté, also known as The Beauty Farm, radiates the same aura of rustic chic, with a décor that incorporates the earthy textures and elements found in nature, including walls of raw wood or smooth stone and cosy open wood fireplaces. Even the indoor swimming pool with its open rafters suggests a stylish barn. Glaciated boulders feature prominently in the décor; these are believed to emit healing properties to enhance the well-being of health-seeking spa-goers. Within these surroundings, you can regain the sense of harmony so lacking in a busy life.

The spa's relaxing and restorative therapies focus on the use of Les Fermes de Marie line of products, derived from pure and natural alpine plants and local herbs. The star ingredient is the edelweiss—a hardy plant that can withstand the extremes of UV rays and winters, and is prized for its remineralising and moisturising properties. Most popular is the Edelweiss Cream No. 1, a luxurious velvety cream that hydrates and restores suppleness to your skin. Among the other unique products is Cereal Flakes Exfoliating Care, aptly described as 'muesli for your skin'; it contains wheat to remove dead cells and restore radiance and softness to your complexion.

To obtain the glow of rosy cheeks without having to hike through the mountains, lie back and enjoy the 90-minute Mountain Energetic Facial Care. This treatment begins with a back massage, after which you lie on basalt pebbles to ease tension and help you to relax. A facial is then followed by a scalp and face massage with semi-precious stones or a jade roller, a facemask, and a gentle mist of flower water to awaken you.

To keep your body smooth and moisturised, select the one-hour Snow Cream

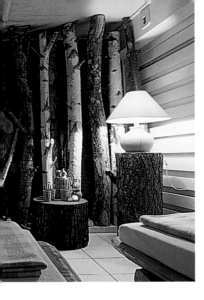

OPPOSITE, LEFT: *The indoor swimming pool has a laid-back alpine feel with its open rafters, wood panelling and smooth granite boulders. It overlooks a herbal garden.*

OPPOSITE, CENTRE: *Rooms are decorated with traditional fabrics and furnishings, each room with a distinct character. The Tower Suite (pictured) is an unusual circular space.*

LEFT: *A wall of raw logs contributes to the warmth and intimacy of the relaxation area.*

Care. Your skin is first prepared for the treatment with a loofah scrub to boost circulation. It is then exfoliated with a blend of salt and conifer essential oils, and a slight tinge of honey. The treatment concludes on a relaxing note with a fragrant herbal body wrap.

Boost your vitality and strength, and in the process, leave your skin satiny smooth with the 50-minute Mineral Elixir Body Care. It begins with Snow Cristal Exfoliating Care using three types of minerals (rhodochrosite extract, malachite and quartz), known for their regenerative, antioxidising and detoxifying qualities. A Pink Clay Body Pack further detoxifies and moisturises your body. This treatment is also a good antidote to stress.

In addition to the ever-popular massages (which include mechanical versions such as the G5) and facials, you can also enjoy a variety of water treatments such as jet showers and warm mud baths. However, by far the most exhilarating session must be a dip in the outdoor jacuzzi—especially during winter when the snow is falling.

Spa Statistics

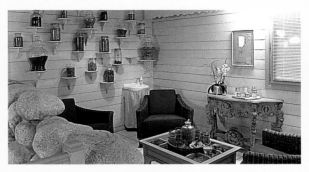

Jars of herbs decorate the white wooden walls in the reception area where you can start to unwind with a cup of Anis-Réglisse, a special homemade liquorice and anise herbal tea.

TYPE OF SPA
Hotel spa

SPA AREA
200 sq m (2,150 sq ft)

FACILITIES
16 single treatment rooms; 1 indoor jacuzzi, 1 outdoor jacuzzi, 1 reflexology pool; 1 sauna, 1 sunbed; 1 hair salon; 1 gymnasium; 1 indoor swimming pool; 1 spa boutique

SIGNATURE TREATMENTS
Mineral Elixir Care, Mountain Energetic Facial Care, Snow Cream Care

TREATMENTS & THERAPIES
Anti-ageing treatments, anti-cellulite treatments, aromatherapy, baths, body scrubs, body wraps, bust treatments, Chinese therapies, eye treatments, facials, firming and slimming treatments, foot treatments, hair treatments, heat treatments, hot stone therapies, jet lag treatments, lymphatic drainage, massages, movement therapies, osteopathy, pedicures, reflexology, Thai massage, thalassotherapy, waxing; introductory, full-, 2- and 6-day packages

SPA CUISINE
Not available, but provisions for various dietary requirements are available on request.

ACTIVITIES & PROGRAMMES
Yoga; massage and stretching classes, sports instruction

SERVICES
Private spa parties

LANGUAGES SPOKEN BY THERAPISTS
English, French

CONTACT
Les Fermes de Marie
Chemin de Riante Colline
74120 Megève
France
T: +33 (0)4 5093 0310
F: +33 (0)4 5093 0984
E: contact@fermesdemarie.com
W: www.c-h-m.com

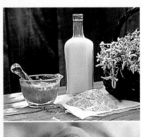

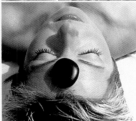

CENTRE: *Your skin benefits from the pure and active ingredients derived from plants grown at high altitudes.*

ABOVE: *Stone therapies (pictured), Chinese therapies and Thai therapies add a touch of the exotic to the spa experience.*

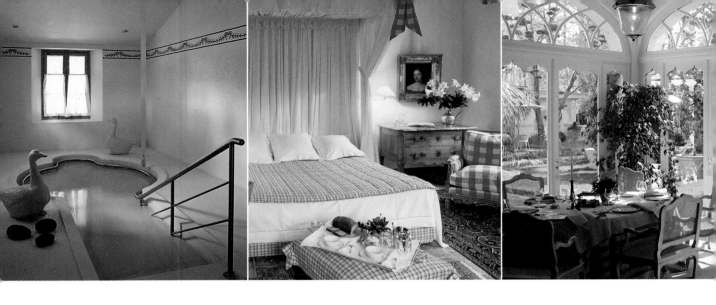

La Ferme Thermale® Minceur Spa at Les Prés d'Eugénie
Landes, France

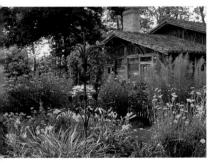

ABOVE: *La Ferme Thermale® Minceur Spa has been called 'Europe's most sensual spa'. The farmhouse faces east to avoid the summer heat and the prevailing west wind. In this house, spacious galleries open to the treatment cabins and windows look out to the countryside.*

TOP LEFT: *The signature Thermal White Kaolin Mud Bath envelops bathers in a pasteurised clay that provides a state of weightlessness, thereby facilitating free movement and relaxation.*

The Landes countryside may not have the reputation and glamour of Paris or the vivacity of Venice; yet what it lacks in celebrity, it more than makes up for with its charm and refinement. The landscape of lush cornfields and pine forests is home to the town of Eugénie, named after Empress Eugénie, wife of Napoleon III, and patroness of the baths. In the 19th century, the imperial couple gave this area its position as a sophisticated spa, where the chic and regal came to take their mineral baths in a natural, rustic setting.

More than a century later, another couple of prominent social standing is continuing in this tradition at Eugénie. Michel and Christine Guérard own and run Les Prés d'Eugénie, a deluxe complex comprising four hotels, two restaurants and La Ferme Thermale® Minceur Spa—altogether a 15-hectare (37-acre) getaway where the weary come to eat, enjoy the spa and indulge themselves in the French definition of tasteful luxury.

The original spa, built in the mid-1800s, specialises in medicinal treatments for long-term curists. The modern La Ferme Thermale® Minceur Spa sits close to this period-architecture building and is housed in a stunning 18th-century style Landes farmhouse. It is set in gardens replete with old varieties of roses, fruit and vegetables. Its 20 treatment rooms epitomise the best of Gallic spa luxury—and here too, the culinary genius of Michel Guérard and the decorative brilliance of Christine Guérard come into play.

In this traditional atmosphere where comfort and style are paramount, even the robes you slip into once you enter the spa are designed by Christine and made by Edith Mezard, one of France's top makers of intimate apparel. You will know that you are stepping into bliss as you prepare your senses for the treat ahead.

The spa's signature treatment is the Thermal White Kaolin Mud Bath. First concocted by Michel Guérard in his own kitchen, this unique emulsion of kaolin and thermal water has the consistency of a pastry cream and is known for its detoxification effects.

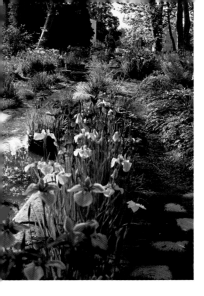

OPPOSITE, CENTRE: *The Couvent des Herbes was an 18th-century nunnery built during the reign of Louis XV. One of the most charming rooms in Les Prés d'Eugénie is found in this hotel. Called Le Temps des Cerises (pictured)—or Cherry Time—it is on the ground floor overlooking the Parson's Garden.*

OPPOSITE, RIGHT: *Christine Guérard's sophisticated touch is evident everywhere in the hotels.*

LEFT: *Many of the rooms open up to views of blooming gardens which fill the air with exotic fragrance.*

You immerse in it without sinking, gently floating, your head in the clouds. This treatment can be followed by the Penetrating Hydro-Massaging Thermal Shower, in which your body is showered with thermal water through oscillating jet sprays while you recline on a heated white marble table.

Post-treatment, you can refresh yourself sipping herbal teas made from thyme, lemon, eucalyptus and honey in the reception salon. Then make your way to Le Jardin des Quatre Saisons (the spa's relaxation room) for restful dreams while sprawled out on Louis XV-inspired sleigh beds.

No visit to Les Prés d'Eugénie is complete without a trip to Michel's three-Michelin-star restaurant. Michel is considered the innovator of *cuisine minceur*, and his culinary creations achieve the seemingly impossible—he makes dieting enjoyable. At Les Prés d'Eugénie, the French have perfected the arts of pleasurable living, fine dining and spa regeneration, and combined them into a superb ensemble that you will never forget.

Spa Statistics

TYPE OF SPA
Resort spa

SPA AREA
1,000 sq m (10,760 sq ft)

FACILITIES
20 single treatment rooms (including mineral water baths, mud baths, medicinal pools, 2 mineral underwater massage rooms); 5 consultation rooms (1 for dietician, 4 for medical consultation); 1 meditation room, 1 relaxation room; 2 whirlpools with mineral water; 2 steam rooms; 1 natural outdoor solarium; 1 nail salon; 1 cardio studio, 1 gymnasium, 1 Pilates studio; 1 outdoor swimming pool; 1 golf course; 2 tennis courts; 1 spa boutique selling herbs, home and table linen, linen tunics and beeswax candles

SIGNATURE TREATMENTS
Penetrating Hydro-Massaging Thermal Shower, Thermal White Kaolin Mud Bath

TREATMENTS & THERAPIES
Anti-ageing treatments, anti-cellulite treatments, aqua therapy, aromatherapy, Bach Flower Remedies, baths, body scrubs, body wraps, bust treatments, eye treatments, facials, firming and slimming treatments, flotation on white kaolin mud bath, hair treatments, hand and foot treatments, heat treatments, hydrotherapy, inhalation therapies, lymphatic drainage, make-up services, manicures and pedicures, massages, post-natal treatments, purifying back treatments, reflexology, rheumatology, waxing

SPA PACKAGES
Beauté Nature package includes 5 treatments combining the virtues of mineral water and medicinal plants; Pure Spa package includes a 7-day stay at the Relais and Chateaux with slimming cuisine

SPA CUISINE
Michel Guérard's restaurant at the original Les Prés d'Eugénie hotel seeks to make dieting a breeze. Olive oil replaces butter and cream, and lots of vegetables, fresh fruit and cereals are used for their anti-oxidising properties. Yet Cuisine Minceur Active® serves up 1200-calorie meals that still manage to excite the most discerning taste buds. (See also 'Spa Cuisine', pp120–123.)

SERVICES
Consultation on dieting, nutrition and skin care; baby-sitting; private spa parties; gift certificates; free transfers to airport as part of Pure Spa package

LANGUAGES SPOKEN BY THERAPISTS
English, Flemish, French, German, Italian, Portuguese, Spanish

ADMISSION
Les Prés d'Eugénie is closed from January to mid-February. Contact the hotel for cookery lessons in spring and autumn.

CONTACT
Les Prés d'Eugénie
40320 Eugénie-les-Bains
France
T: +33 (0)558 050 607
F: +33 (0)558 511 010
E: reservation@michelguerard.com
W: www.michelguerard.fr

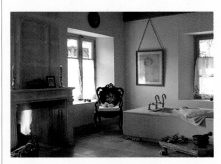

The spa is decorated with 18th- and 19th-century paintings and furnishing. Terracotta flooring, pristine white marble and French country chic define its interiors.

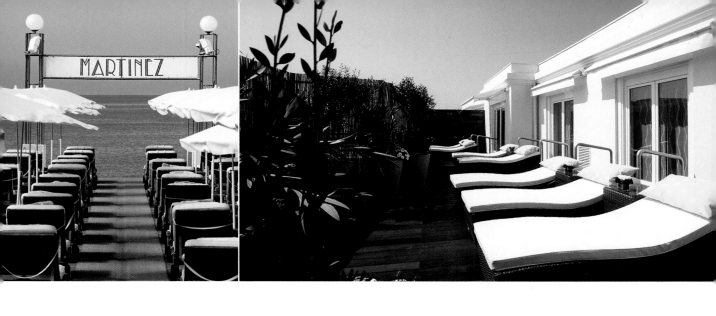

Martinez Givenchy Spa at Hotel Martinez Cannes
Cannes, France

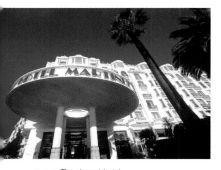

ABOVE: *The elegant hotel, a symbol of Cannes, has been immortalised in films such as* Festival in Cannes *starring Anouk Aimée.*

OPPOSITE, BOTTOM: *Guests staying in a penthouse apartment have their own slice of heaven—a private deck with a breathtaking view of the French Riviera.*

The handsome 1930s façade of the Hotel Martinez Cannes is an icon on the seafront of La Croisette. When the rich and famous visit the French Riviera, they are likely to frequent its two-Michelin-star restaurant, La Palme d'Or. Like the annual Cannes Film Festival, the hotel rolls out the red carpet for a star-studded cast of guests including director Francis Ford Coppola and actor Sean Connery, and also royalty such as Archduke Franz Josef of Vienna.

Awards bestowed on the property include one by UK's *Tatler* magazine (January 2003), which dubbed its apartments on the penthouse level, the 7th floor, 'the most beautiful suites with a view'. With butler service, a generously sized bathtub with a view, and a private deck overlooking the bay and the islands beyond, you may be tempted to spend your entire stay in the two apartments or 11 junior suites on the rooftop. But while you can request to enjoy certain massage treatments in your room, most guests prefer to enjoy theirs at the Martinez Givenchy, a sanctuary of health and beauty devoted to the use of hotel guests and members, located just across the hallway.

The view from this centre alone has sent even the most jet set to seventh heaven, as have its popular pampering European treatments that focus on enhancing your youth and beauty. Treatments use Swisscare Givenchy products, and revolve around hydrotherapy, phytotherapy, thermal mud, herbal wraps and classic European massages.

Exclusively Givenchy, the spa's self-styled ultimate treatment, comprises a body scrub to exfoliate and oxygenate your skin, a luxurious bath with Givenchy oils, and a hydrating wrap that involves lying on a waterbed while being buffeted by water jets.

Treatments on the spa menu are also influenced by cultures from various corners of the globe. The most hedonistic of these is the Four Hand Massage, a synchronised massage performed by two therapists working in tandem using ylang-ylang oils derived from flower blossoms from Mauritius. The most

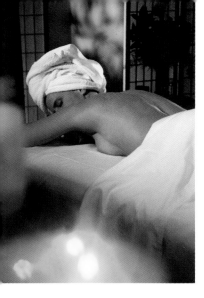

OPPOSITE, LEFT: *The hotel's pier (pictured) along the private beachfront and its swimming pool are the most glamorous places to be seen bronzing your body.*

OPPOSITE, RIGHT: *The teak deck of the outdoor relaxation area, framed by olive trees, has a distinct Mediterranean air, while the indoor relaxation area is a picture of repose.*

LEFT: *Treatment rooms are spacious yet intimate, elegantly screened yet bathed with natural light.*

Spa Statistics

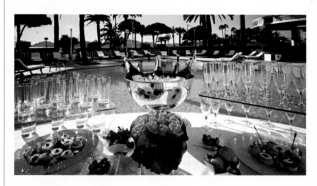

TYPE OF SPA
Hotel spa

SPA AREA
900 sq m (9,690 sq ft)

FACILITIES
8 single treatment rooms; 1 relaxation room; 1 sauna; 1 solarium; 1 hair salon; 1 cardio studio; 1 outdoor heated swimming pool; 4 golf courses nearby, 7 tennis courts nearby

SIGNATURE TREATMENTS
Exclusively Givenchy, Four Hand Massage, The Canyon Love Stone Massage

TREATMENTS & THERAPIES
Baths, body scrubs, body wraps, facials, firming and slimming treatments, hair treatments, hand and foot treatments, hot stone therapies, hydrotherapy, lymphatic drainage manicures and pedicures, massages, reflexology, thalassotherapy, waxing; spa packages

SPA CUISINE
Not available, but provisions for various dietary requirements are available on request.

ACTIVITIES & PROGRAMMES
Sports available on request

SERVICES
Baby-sitting and childcare available on request

LANGUAGES SPOKEN BY THERAPISTS
English, French

ADMISSION
The spa is exclusively reserved for hotel guests and members of the hotel's Givenchy Health Club.

CONTACT
Hotel Martinez Cannes
73 La Croisette
06406 Cannes
France
T: +33 (0)4 9298 7490
F: +33 (0)4 9339 6782
E: martinez@hotel-martinez.com
W: www.hotel-martinez.com

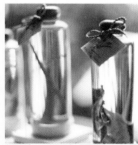

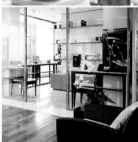

TOP: *Cannes enjoys 300 days of sunshine a year, but the swimming pool (pictured), in the shade of century-old palm trees, is always heated to a comfortable 28 degrees Celsius (82 degrees Fahrenheit).*

CENTRE: *Bottles of essential oils resemble gifts from Mother Nature.*

ABOVE: *Perfumes, skincare creams, and Givenchy handbags are the most popular items with spa-goers looking for a memento of their visit.*

exotic treatment is The Canyon Love Stone Massage during which your body is stroked and your energies balanced with special stones—warm and chilled—collected from rivers in the American West.

After a pampering session like this, you may want to schedule an appointment with the hotel's Parisian hairdresser, like many immaculately coiffed spa-goers.

Given its following with the fashionable crowd, a visit to the spa and hotel is becoming as much of a part of Cannes as are the limousines, convertibles and private yachts.

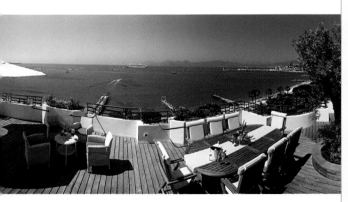

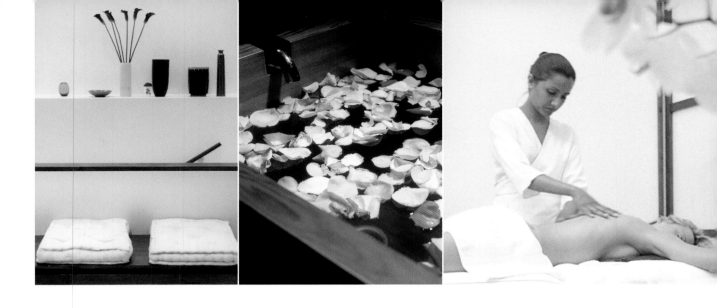

Spa Cinq Mondes
Paris, France

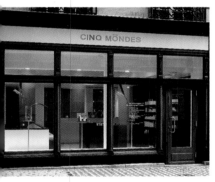

Spa Cinq Mondes is located within a cobble-stone pedestrian square shared by restaurants and galleries. Parking is conveniently located underground.

When Jean-Louis Poiroux and his wife took a year off to travel around the world in search of the best beauty and wellbeing rituals, they brought back to Paris their own brand of beauty and face and body rituals inspired by healing philosophies they encountered and the great masters they studied under.

These rituals are served up at their Spa Cinq Mondes, a sleek Japanese-inspired haven within the cultural and artistic heart of the French capital. Cinq Mondes, which stands for 'five worlds', pays homage to Japanese, Chinese, Indian, Thai and Mediterranean influences in its treatments, along with other rituals springing from countries in other parts of the globe.

The rituals, personalised according to your needs, were created in conjunction with Soin du Spa Cinq Mondes products: in-house professional preparations created under dermatological control. These are free of silicon, artificial colours and animal ingredients, and are not tested on animals. Even the

essential oils stem from sources that are strictly controlled. The products, although developed with modern technology, remain true to their philosophical or historical origins. Likewise, treatments are designed to be relevant to the lifestyles of chic Parisians; but the therapists are continually trained by masters in the relevant fields to ensure that the treatments remain true to their roots.

The warming herbal and spice *boreh* which Indonesian farmers apply to sore muscles after a hard day's work, for example, has been translated into the Aromatic Scrubbing Massage—a scrub comprised of sea salt, almond powder, nutmeg, vertiver and vanilla oil. It gently coats your skin with aromatic moisture and produces a warm, tingly feeling.

The toned derrieres of Brazilian dancers in Bahia inspired the exclusive Crème De Café treatment, in which a cream comprised of pure caffeine, kola nut and green coffee bean extracts is applied to your body with firm, rapid strokes. After this stimulating massage, performed in quick and slow rhythmic

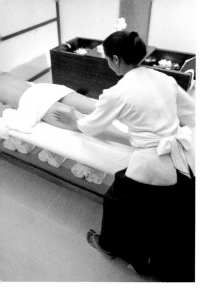

OPPOSITE, LEFT: *Details within this Zen-like waiting area change every few months: a visual feast for the eyes.*

OPPOSITE, CENTRE AND RIGHT: *After luxuriating in a Traditional Japanese Bath With Flower Petals and Essential Oils, adjourn for a facial or massage within the Pluie de Fleurs ('rain of flowers') room.*

LEFT: *The therapists' stylish yet practical robes of natural silk are a modern take on the Japanese kimono and wide-legged* tae kwon do *(martial arts) trousers.*

phases like a dance, your body is wrapped in red clay and laminaire algae which helps purify, remineralise and beautify your skin and aids the slimming, toning process.

Couples who wish to share the spa experience together can book a double treatment room and ask for the Felicity Package. This includes a steamy session in the hammam followed by an Ayurvedic Massage.

Travellers and people who spend long hours bent over a computer can relax sore muscles through a medium-pressured Ayurvedic-styled massage known as the Special 'Hunched Shoulders' Massage.

All the treatments in the spa are deliberately high on touch and performed without the use of electrical beauty equipment: an antidote to the modern world we live in.

The low resonance of a Balinese gong marks the beginning and the end of each session. This exotic touch helps you let go to enjoy your session, and gently brings you back to the present when your treatment is over, with your body, mind and spirit fully balanced.

Spa Statistics

TYPE OF SPA
Day spa

SPA AREA
450 sq m (4,840 sq ft)

FACILITIES
1 double treatment room,
8 single treatment rooms,
1 single treatment room
with bath (Pluie de Fleurs);
1 yoga and *tai chi* room;
1 relaxation room; 1 hammam;
1 spa boutique

SIGNATURE TREATMENTS
Aromatic Scrubbing Massage
With Spices And Sea Salt Body
Scrub, Crème De Cafe

TREATMENTS & THERAPIES
Anti-ageing treatments, anti-cellulite treatments, aromatherapy, Ayurveda, baths, body scrubs, body wraps, Chinese massage therapies, facials, firming and slimming treatments, hand and foot treatments, heat treatments, Indonesian therapies, jet lag treatments, lymphatic drainage, Oriental waxing, pre- and post-natal treatments, reflexology, Thai therapies

PROVISIONS FOR COUPLES
1 double treatment room,
1 hammam; Felicity Package;
discounts for couples having
certain treatments together

ACTIVITIES & PROGRAMMES
Massage classes for couples;

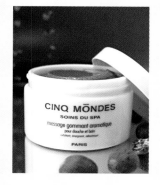

tai chi and yoga classes;
talks by visiting consultants

SERVICES
Private spa parties;
gift certificates

LANGUAGES SPOKEN BY THERAPISTS
English, French

ADMISSION
Membership is available but not required for admission. Members have access to classes and can bring guests.

CONTACT
Spa Cinq Mondes
6 Square de l'Opera
75009 Paris
France
T: +33 (0)1 4266 0060
F: +33 (0)1 4266 0570
E: contact@cinqmondes.com
W: www.cinqmondes.com

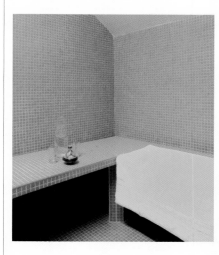

TOP: *Soin du Spa Cinq Mondes products used during the spa rituals can also be used to enjoy a spa experience at home; each comes with visual instructions on application techniques to help enhance the treatment's efficacy.*

LEFT: *The hammam incorporates aromatherapy and colour therapy which allow you to select your choice of colours and scents. For a complete session in the hammam, book The Maghreb Ritual which can be enjoyed solo or with a partner.*

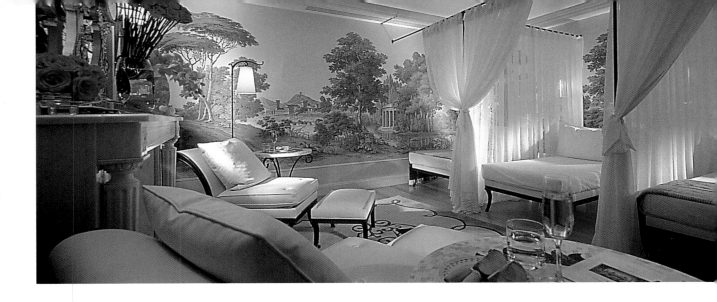

Le Spa at the Four Seasons Hotel George V
Paris, France

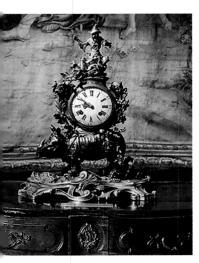

The hotel, owned by Prince Al Waleed of Saudi Arabia, is decorated with classical French furnishings, Art Deco details, antique tapestries and objets d'art. It is also thoughtful and functional—7 of its 245 rooms and suites are fitted for disabled guests.

Located off the Champs-Elysées in Paris' Triangle d'Or, the Four Seasons Hotel George V has commanded several historical roles since opening in 1928. In 1929, the Young Plan outlining war repatriation agreements was signed on the site; and in 1944, it was the headquarters of General Dwight Eisenhower during the Liberation of Paris. This epitome of Parisian style is a favourite site for society parties and seasonal couture collection launches.

The property has garnered several awards including three Michelin stars for its restaurant, Le Cinq, and four awards for excellence in *The Gallivanter's Guide* 2002 ratings. Its spa and health club was voted the sixth top hotel spa outside the United States and Canada in 2002 by readers of *Travel + Leisure*.

Located on the lower level of the hotel, the spa was designed by French interior designer Pierre-Yves Rochon, who fully refurbished the hotel for its reopening in 2000. Many of its cosmopolitan range of treatments, that marry French essential oils and Eastern energy philosophies, cater to glamorous Parisian lifestyles.

To loosen back, neck and shoulder muscles after browsing the boutiques at Saint Germain des Près or Avenue Montaigne, opt for the 30-minute deep tissue Shopping Massage, or the 2-hour License To Shop package, which offers an additional reflexology, Vitamin A Facial and Spa Paradise cocktail.

Thirty-minute express treatments are available, but if you can only spare half that time, ask for the Amma Massage—a relaxing chair massage. The spa also offers special treatments for male spa-goers; these include a Herbal Back Cleansing Treatment.

The spa's signature treatments include the Four Seasons George V Massage, an anti-stress massage that uses a different essential oil for each season. The massage incorporates Korean relaxation techniques in which the therapist applies vibrational movements—quick left-right moves—and sways various parts of your body. Other unique treatments include Fasciapulsology, in

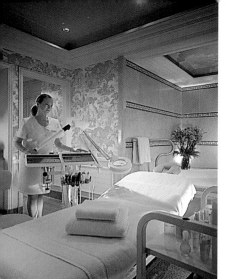

OPPOSITE: *In the serene setting of the relaxation room, you can listen to a choice of CDs on your personal headset while sipping a cup of green tea.*

LEFT: *The spa offers 11 facials that include European favourites such as the Restructuring Seaweed Facial And Lifting Treatment (both for mature skins); energy-balancing treatments such as Eye Ritual With Energising Stones (in which crystals chosen for your needs are used); and Relaxing Green Tea Facial (which balances your skin and your mind).*

which the therapist focuses on your acupoints and your fascia to relieve pain and stress, and bring about harmony within your body.

Two unique treatments developed by the spa's sister property in Mexico include the Margarita Body Scrub, in which lemon, salt and tequila are applied to your body in circular movements to stimulate circulation. The scrub leaves your skin velvety-soft, and your legs feeling lighter. The Punta Mita Massage With Tequila is a fragrant, warming massage that banishes aches with tequila and sage oil. The therapist uses her hands and forearms instead of fingers: a tradition practised by Native American Indians to help sustain the pressure.

Around 14,000 blooms are used every week in the floral sculptures that adorn the spa and hotel. To remember the floral themes that change each week, you can purchase the book *Les Fleurs de Jeff Leatham* by the hotel's Artistic Director, along with Ambre du Népal—the spa's signature fragrance—and products from Grasse, Provence that are used in the spa treatments.

Spa Statistics

TYPE OF SPA
Hotel spa

SPA AREA
750 sq m (8,070 sq ft)

FACILITIES
1 double treatment room, 10 single treatment rooms; 1 relaxation lounge with tea service; 2 jacuzzis, 3 saunas, 3 steam rooms; 2 hair salons, 1 nail salon; 1 cardio studio, 1 gymnasium; 1 indoor swimming pool; 1 spa boutique

SIGNATURE TREATMENTS
Fasciapulsology, Four Seasons George V Massage, Margarita Body Scrub, Punta Mita Massage With Tequila

TREATMENTS & THERAPIES
Acupuncture, acoustic acupuncture, anti-ageing treatments, anti-cellulite treatments, aromatherapy, baths, body bronzing, body scrubs, body wraps, bust treatments, Japanese therapies, electrotherapy, eye treatments, facials, firming and slimming treatments, hair treatments, hand and foot treatments, hair treatments, heat treatments, hot stone therapies, jet lag treatments, lymphatic drainage, make-up services, manicures and pedicures, massages, movement therapies, osteopathy, purifying back treatments, reflexology, salon services, scalp treatments, waxing; full- and half-day packages

PROVISIONS FOR COUPLES
1 VIP double treatment room with jacuzzi, sauna, steam room and shower; Romance Forever package in VIP room includes a facial and a massage for each person; Couples Massage (50-min shiatsu for two)

SPA CUISINE
A healthy and light selection of dishes created by Chef Philippe Legendre can be ordered at the spa lounge in addition to fresh fruit, cocktails and herbal teas. Vegetarian dishes are available on the menu or on request.

ACTIVITIES & PROGRAMMES
Aqua gym, *ashtanga* yoga; swimming lessons

SERVICES
Personal training; baby-sitting; complimentary shoeshine and tea service; gift certificates; day-use rooms

LANGUAGES SPOKEN BY THERAPISTS
English, French

ADMISSION
In-house guests are given priority. Treatments are available to non-residents only from Mondays to Fridays, from 10 A.M. to 4 P.M..

CONTACT
Four Seasons Hotel George V
31 Avenue George V
75008 Paris
France
T: +33 (0)1 4952 7210
F: +33 (0)1 4952 7939
E: spa.par@fourseasons.com
W: www.fourseasons.com

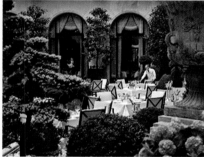

CENTRE: *During the summer months, light meals can be enjoyed al fresco at the Marble Courtyard next to the three-Michelin-star restaurant, Le Cinq.*

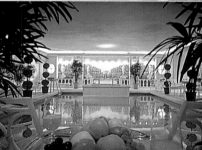

ABOVE: *You can imagine yourself relaxing or exercising in the gardens of Versailles, thanks to the trompe l'oeil murals by the swimming pool that bring the outdoors indoors. The spa's quintessential French décor contributes to its tranquil and refined ambience.*

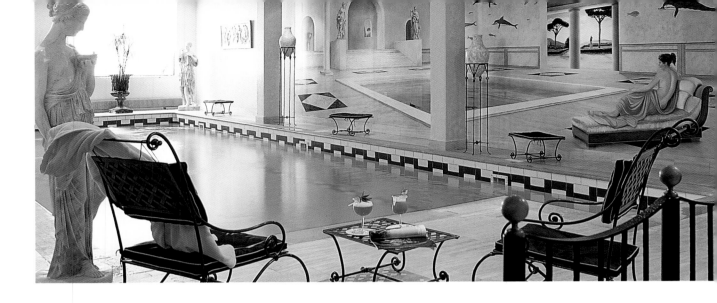

Spa Le Lana at Hotel Le Lana
Savoie, France

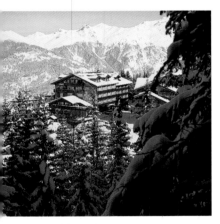

ABOVE: *The area is especially picturesque during winter's blue hour when the hotel's chandeliers and candles are lit, casting a romantic glow against the white coat of snow.*

OPPOSITE, BOTTOM: *Fitness buffs can tone their bodies in the gymnasium.*

After hurtling down the surrounding ski slopes, the four-star Hotel Le Lana is an ideal base to return to. It offers home-styled warmth and intimacy where you can indulge in an intimate tête-à-tête by the fireplace, and later retire to a luxurious and spacious suite or apartment to enjoy sweet dreams for the night.

If you wish to rest, relax or beautify yourself, make your way to the hotel's Spa Le Lana, a small but attractive spa. The peaceful aura of this spa is enhanced by the soothing sounds of nature—the twitter of birds and a cascade of falling water.

The spa's mantra, 'beauty is health made visible', is reflected in its selection of treatments that help to maintain your youthful appearance, health and overall wellbeing. These treatments, which can be ordered à la carte or as a package, are influenced by the healing effects of chromatherapy, principles of Chinese medicine, the Eastern concept of energetic rebalancing, and the Western concept of lymphatic drainage. Each treatment is

highly personalised, with the techniques and products used determined by your own individual energy characteristics.

This personalised approach is best reflected in the spa's signature treatment—the 45-minute Chromo Therapeutic Wrappin menu—in which different-coloured clays are applied to your body; the clay colours are chosen according to the month and year of your birth. The treatment also includes a massage with essential oils and a hot bath.

Interestingly, this innovative chromatherapy method, also used in the 90-minute Facial Chromo Lifting and the 30-minute Chromo Therapeutic Eye Treatment, was awarded the 'Prize for Innovation' at the Paris Beauty Trade Show in April 1998.

Classic European treatments include a 45-minute Sport Massage which helps your body recover after strenuous exercise; and a 60-minute Relaxation Massage to transport you into a state of bliss. Another very popular treatment is the 60-minute Treatment of the Bust, which helps maintain the appearance of

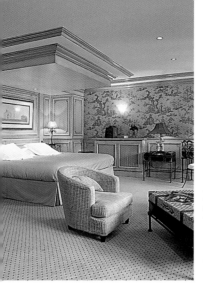

OPPOSITE: *The pool area, the spa's pièce de résistance, is also a soothing space to relax. The columns, arches and statues here echo the architectural details within the hotel.*

LEFT: *Soft fabrics, warm woods, and an eclectic selection of furniture from various eras create a cosy warmth in the hotel.*

your décolletage: one of the first areas of your body to reveal the signs of ageing.

If you are still energised after your day on the slopes, have a workout in the gymnasium. Alternatively, do some laps in the indoor swimming pool under a starlit ceiling—an area that combines elements that are modern and yet evocative of ancient Rome. With its arches, columns, statues and imaginative trompe l'oeil, you may for a moment imagine that you are bathing in an ancient Roman bath.

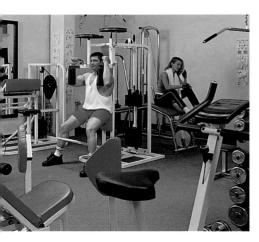

Spa Statistics

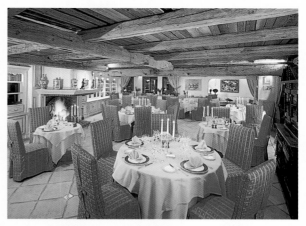

The hotel's interior reflects a cosy alpine ambience.

TYPE OF SPA
Hotel spa

SPA AREA
300 sq m (3,230 sq ft)

FACILITIES
4 single treatment rooms; 1 jacuzzi; 1 sauna, 1 steam room; 1 cardio studio, 1 gymnasium; 1 indoor swimming pool; 1 spa boutique

SIGNATURE TREATMENT
Chromo Therapeutic Wrappin

TREATMENTS & THERAPIES
Anti-ageing treatments, anti-cellulite treatments, aromatherapy, baths, body wraps, bust treatments, facials, firming and slimming treatments, hand and foot treatments, lymphatic drainage, manicures and pedicures, massages, purifying back treatments, reflexology, thalassotherapy, waxing

LANGUAGES SPOKEN BY THERAPISTS
English, French

CONTACT
Hotel Le Lana
BP 95
73121 Courchevel Cedex
Savoie
France
T: +33 (0)79 080 110
F: +33 (0)79 083 670
E: info@lelana.com
W: www.lelana.com

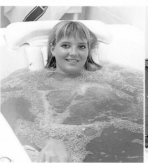 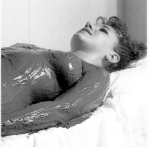

ABOVE LEFT: *Relax after a day on the slopes and treat tired muscles to the luxury of a hot therapeutic spa bath.*

ABOVE RIGHT: *Treatments revolve around the use of Phytobiodermie from Switzerland, which is made from natural ingredients such as algaes, clays, essential oils, plants and trace minerals.*

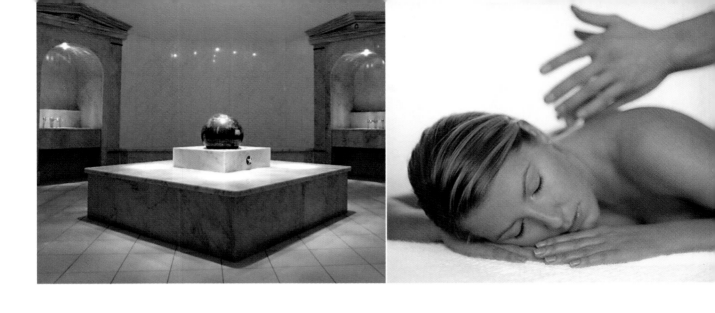

Spa Trianon at Trianon Palace Versailles
Versailles, France

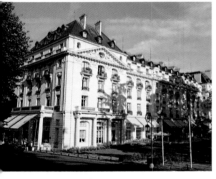

The five-star hotel comprises a total of 192 rooms and suites over two buildings—the five-star Palace (pictured) which dates back to 1910, and the more recently built Pavilion. The main palace, dressed in classical stone architecture, blends harmoniously into 3 hectares (8 acres) of parkland composed of centuries-old trees.

The Trianon Palace has played several starring roles in history. In 1919, the Peace Treaty of Versailles was drawn up in its Salon Clemenceau, and since opening its doors in 1910, the hotel has hosted a constellation of luminaries including silver screen legend Marlene Dietrich, former American president Dwight D. Eisenhower, and royalty such as Queen Elizabeth II. Located at the edge of Louis XIV's royal domain, the hotel is just 20 minutes from downtown Paris. Yet the tranquillity within the grounds hints at the estate's provenance as a cloister for Capuchin friars.

Reflecting the classic elegance of the hotel and the serenity of the estate, the Spa Trianon, a member of the Starwood Spa Collection, is a generous three-storeyed space dedicated to beauty, fitness, wellbeing and relaxation, and is one of the leading spas in the Paris area. Grand Roman pillars flank the entrance of the spa, while expansive windows allow natural daylight into this serene space, and allow you to soothe your eyes by admiring the view of the splendid park of Versailles. The spa also overlooks the indoor swimming pool, its white walls a calming contrast to the blue ripples of water.

Many of its treatments, reflecting classical European spa traditions, revolve around the use of water and therapeutic ingredients derived from the sea. Popular options include body scrubs, facials and massages. Products used in the treatments include the French marine-based brand Phytomer, and Japanese brand Kanebo.

Certain packages make reference to the life of the hotel's illustrious former neighbour, Louis XIV. These include The Athenais Program, which is named after a mistress of Louis XIV. This programme, which is designed to make you feel like royalty, includes a multi-jet bath, a 50-minute body massage and a luxurious hydrating facial. The Trianon Program, named after a small retreat where Louis XIV found peace and quiet, will calm you with a body treatment (select from a seaweed or marine-mud wrap, vibrosauna session, or

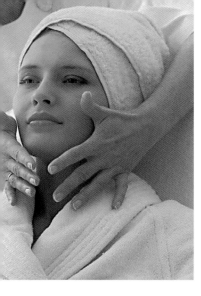

OPPOSITE, LEFT: *Relax your body within the grand marble hammam.*

OPPOSITE, RIGHT: *It is easy to feel like royalty under the expert hands of the therapists.*

LEFT: *Looking good is one step towards feeling good, which is one of the mantras of the spa.*

pressure therapy), a multi-jet bath and a 50-minute body massage. The Venus Program will make you feel like the goddess of love and beauty with three body treatments (a scrub, vibrosauna or pressure therapy, and hydrojet), a multi-jet bath, a 50-minute body massage, and a 30-minute facial massage.

Therapies from the East include Shiatsu, Foot Reflexology, and AromaVedic Esthetic Massage: an aromatic massage for the face and body inspired by Indian Ayurveda. Another languid way to spend a day would be to relax in the indoor swimming oasis, or bask in the sun on the terrace of the outdoor solarium. Alternatively, you can have a light meal by the poolside, or enjoy a healthy meal on the terrace at The Café Trianon overlooking the park of the palace of Versailles.

You can request to close the spa for your private party, and a special pampering selection of spa programmes can be arranged for a group of up to 30 people. Or simply enjoy a relaxing weekend escape with the weekend golf and spa, or bank holiday packages.

Spa Statistics

TYPE OF SPA
Hotel spa

SPA AREA
2,800 sq m (30,140 sq ft)

FACILITIES
26 single treatment rooms; 1 relaxation room; 2 dry flotation beds, 2 whirlpools; 2 saunas, 1 steam room; 1 external solarium; 1 hair salon; 1 cardio studio, 1 gymnasium; 1 indoor swimming pool, 2 tennis courts; 1 spa boutique

SIGNATURE TREATMENTS
AromaVedic Esthetic Massage, The Athenais Program, The Trianon Program, The Venus Program

TREATMENTS & THERAPIES
Anti-ageing treatments, anti-cellulite treatments, aqua therapy, aromatherapy, Ayurvedic treatments, baths, body scrubs, body wraps, Chinese treatments, dry flotation treatments, electrotherapy, eye treatments, facials, firming and slimming treatments, hair treatments, hand and foot treatments, heat treatments, hydrotherapy, jet lag treatments, lymphatic drainage, manicures and pedicures, massages, pre- and post-natal treatments, purifying back treatments, reflexology, vibrosauna, waxing;

spa packages including 1- and 3-night packages with accommodation and spa treatments

SPA CUISINE
A healthy and light selection of low-calorie options is available at The Café Trianon restaurant which serves French food. These can be ordered in-room 24 hours a day. Vegetarian options are available.

ACTIVITIES & PROGRAMMES
Aquaerobics, tennis; cooking classes

SERVICES
Baby-sitting; concierge

LANGUAGES SPOKEN BY THERAPISTS
English, French

ADMISSION
Membership is available but not required for admission (non-hotel guests are required to be members in order to use the swimming pool area).

CONTACT
Trianon Palace Versailles
1 Boulevard de la Reine
78000 Versailles
France
T: +33 (0)1 3084 5000
F: +33 (0)1 3084 5001
E: spa.trianon@westin.com
W: www.westin.com/trianon-palace

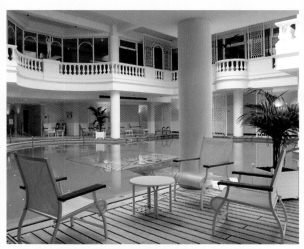

The spa area, overlooking the indoor pool, resembles a temple of wellbeing.

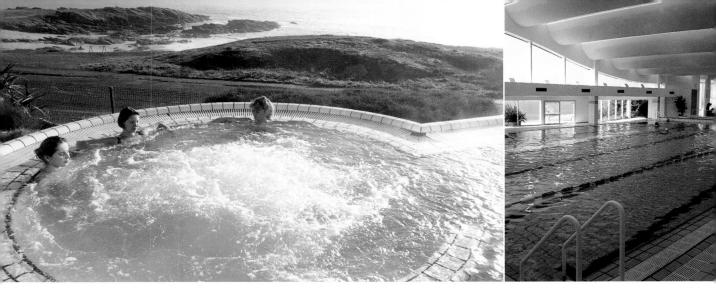

Thalassa Quiberon at Sofitel Thalassa Quiberon and Sofitel Diététique Quiberon
Quiberon, France

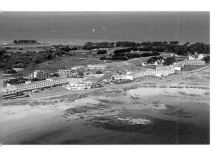

The view is also a drawcard at Thalassa Quiberon, which perches dramatically on the far end of the Quiberon peninsula that runs 14 kilometres (9 miles) out to sea.

After seawater therapy helped cyclist Louison Bobet recover from a serious accident in the 1960s, the Tour de France champion began promoting similar cures in the Quiberon peninsula, turning the once sleepy fishing village into a key destination for modern thalassotherapy. Despite the attention the village now receives from international visitors, it still retains an intimate charm evident in the small abodes, and absence of high-rise buildings.

Visitors looking to fine-tune their health and rejuvenate themselves after the strains of daily life check into the Thalassa Quiberon, which offers a series of classical thalassotherapy treatments derived from seawater and algae delivered through a variety of baths, jets and wraps. The emphasis these days is less on rehabilitation, but more on wellbeing. Guests are encouraged to stay for a minimum of 6 days to benefit fully from a course of treatment, but it is possible to experience the centre over one or two days. You are encouraged to see the centre's physician on arrival, though you may instead produce a certificate of health from your general physician.

Programmes comprising four treatments a day over six days focus on different areas of concern. These include Vitality, to counter problems stemming from overwork, and stress and fatigue; Young Mother, to help new mothers get back into shape 3 to 8 months after giving birth (the spa can arrange for a baby-sitter to look after your little one); Marine Beauty, for wellbeing; and Masculine Tonic, a fitness and grooming programme for men that also aims to correct any metabolic problems stemming from poor eating habits. If you have heavy, swollen or painful legs, opt for the Leg Tonic programme, and if you are looking to recover from a muscular problem or injury, the Health programme will help you.

The focal point of the spa is the Aquatic Course in which two physiotherapists guide

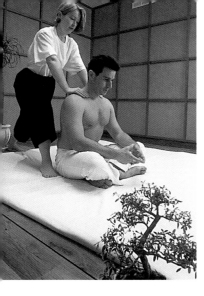

OPPOSITE, LEFT: *Breathe in the sea air, enjoy the mild climate, and take in the panorama of the Atlantic Ocean and island of Belle Ile en Mer from the outdoor jacuzzi that is linked to the indoor Aquatic Course.*

OPPOSITE, RIGHT: *Other water facilities include indoor pools for doing some laps or aquaerobics.*

LEFT: *Complementary therapies from the East include Massage Thai, Yoga, and Vibrations Japonaises.*

you through a course of underwater jets that will help relax, stimulate and oxygenate your body. The seawater, heated to 34 degrees Celsius, contains minerals and trace elements that are essential to rebalancing your body.

The centre also offers complementary treatments and therapies such as the gentle Californian Massage to bring about physical and psychological balance. In Sophrology, you learn relaxation and other techniques to lower your stress levels; athletes also use this to help enhance their performance.

Guests visiting the institute will typically stay at one of two affiliated four-star hotels: your choice is influenced by your goals. If you are seeking to shed some kilos, book into the 78-room Sofitel Diététique Quiberon where meals are geared towards this purpose. Others may opt for the 133-room Sofitel Thalassa Quiberon. Like the thalassotherapy centre, both hotels overlook the sea, the area's source of healing.

Spa Statistics

TYPE OF SPA
Destination spa/thalasso centre

SPA AREA
7,000 sq m (75,350 sq ft)

FACILITIES
24 massage rooms, 61 seawater treatment rooms; 5 consultation rooms; 1 meditation room, 5 relaxation rooms; 3 jacuzzis; 1 sauna, 2 steam rooms; 2 solariums, 1 sunbed; 1 hair salon, 1 nail salon; 1 gymnasium; 1 indoor Aquatic Course with outdoor jacuzzi, 2 indoor pools for aquaerobics, 2 indoor pools for rehabilitative exercises; 1 golf course (20 km/12 miles from the spa), 2 tennis courts; 1 spa boutique

SIGNATURE TREATMENTS
Marine Beauty, Masculine Tonic and Young Mother programmes

TREATMENTS & THERAPIES
Acupuncture, anti-ageing treatments, anti-cellulite treatments, aqua therapy, baths, body bronzing, body scrubs, body wraps, bust treatments, Chinese therapies, electrotherapy, eye treatments, facials, firming and slimming treatments, hair treatments, hand and foot treatments, heat treatments, hydrotherapy, lymphatic drainage, manicures and pedicures, massages, mechanical massages, postnatal treatments, pressotherapy, reflexology, scalp treatments, Thai therapies, thalassotherapy, waxing; 6-day programmes

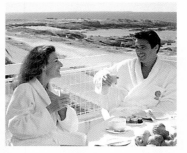

Soak up the seaside atmosphere from many areas of the property.

SPA CUISINE
A light lunch is available at Café Jardin at the Thalassa Institute where you can enjoy the view of the sea from the large terrace. Imaginative low-calorie meals created by Chef Patrick Jarno are available at L'Océan Saveurs at Sofitel Diététique. During a full-board stay, a dietician will guide you in your choice of meals. 'Welbeing' options created by Chef Angélo Oriliers, which are low in calories, are available at Le Thalassa at Sofitel Thalassa, which serves gastronomic meals with a focus on seafood.

ACTIVITIES & PROGRAMMES
Aerobics, biking, golf, hiking, horse riding, sailing, Sophrology, tennis, yoga; cooking, massage and nailcare classes, sports instruction

SERVICES
Blood test, body composition analysis, medical consultation, nutritional consultation; babysitting; free transfers to the railway station and airport on certain days at certain times

LANGUAGES SPOKEN BY THERAPISTS
English, French, German

CONTACT
Sofitel Thalassa/
Sofitel Diététique Quiberon
Pointe de Goulvars, BP 10802
56178 Quiberon
France
T: +33 (0)2 9750 2000
F: +33 (0)2 9730 4763
E: h0562@accor-hotels.com
W: www.thalassa.com

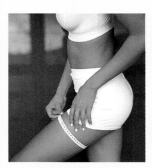

The institute's professionals will administer seawater therapy to help you shed some inches in the Subli-Slimming programme.

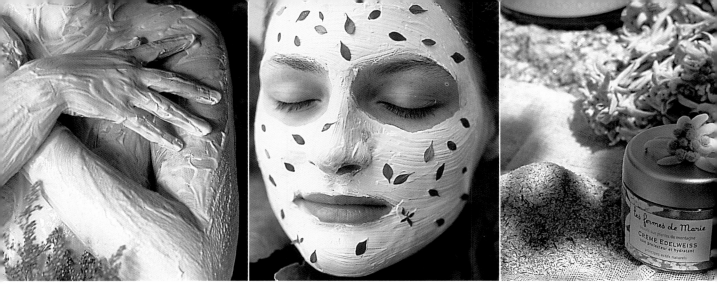

Villa Marie Spa at Villa Marie Ramatuelle St Tropez
St Tropez, France

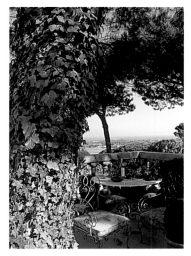

ABOVE: *The gardens are made for intimate talks with a loved one, writing one's journal, or simply daydreaming away.*

OPPOSITE, BOTTOM:
Balancing your body and mind is even more restful and pleasurable when it takes place out of doors.

Lovers and nature lovers can lose themselves within the grounds of Villa Marie Ramatuelle St Tropez as they explore its themed gardens of aquatic features, grapevines, palms, cacti, citrus trees and aromatic herbs. Within the garden—which overlooks the Bay of Pampelonne, famed for its beautiful beaches—is an emerald green swimming oasis of natural rocks. You can also daydream as you look out on to the distant sea from the private patio or terrace of your charming pastel-clad room in the small hotel.

The Villa Marie Spa is another oasis where you can pass your days in languid pleasure with relaxing and restorative treatments that are personalised according to your needs. These help you regain a sense of balance that may have been thrown off kilter in the daily grind of a fast-paced lifestyle.

Treatments harness the pure yet active ingredients of alpine plants and herbs from Les Fermes de Marie line of products, the key ingredient being the edelweiss reknowned for its remineralising, moisturising qualities. While the line may be alpine inspired, the treatments also incorporate ingredients and fragrances that embody the spirit and scents of the Mediterranean and the French Riviera.

After soaking up the sun on the nearby beaches, you may want to nourish your sun-kissed skin with a 25-minute After-Sun Repairing Jasmine Care with moisturising products. A soothing and revitalising medley of edelweiss, meadowsweet, blueberry and arnica, it melts into your body and face.

Some of the treatments smell delicious enough to eat. The 50-minute Mediterranean Care, for instance, is an exfoliating treatment of light brown sugar, honey, crushed nuts and orange flower essential oils, which leaves your skin moisturised and perfumed with a lingering fragrance that typifies the south of France.

This is followed by a Rassoul Body Pack of detoxifying natural clay from the desert combined with restorative geranium oils that nourish your skin. After your body is sufficiently soothed with Argan oil from North Africa, you can sip an orange flower herbal tea.

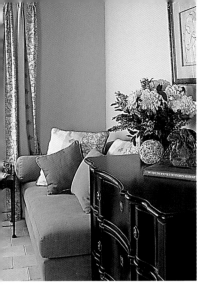

OPPOSITE, LEFT: *Your skin is slathered with luxurious clay from the desert during Mediterranean Care.*

OPPOSITE, CENTRE AND RIGHT: *The edelweiss, the symbol of Les Fermes de Marie range, features prominently as a key ingredient in all products.*

LEFT: *The hotel is intimately sized with 35 rooms and 4 suites, each with its own character. Soothing pastels combine with modern touches and chic flea market finds add to the eclectic feel.*

Spa Statistics

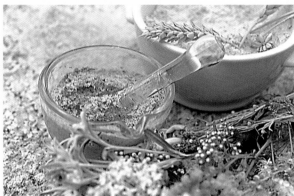

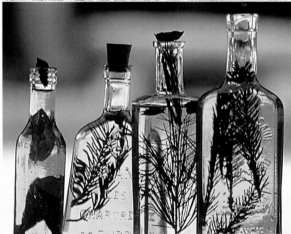

TOP: *Treatments harness pure yet potent all-natural ingredients from alpine regions.*

ABOVE: *Beautifully bottled gifts from Mother Nature enhance the healing experience, and remind you of the spa's connection to the earth.*

If you are seeking an antidote to stress, opt for the 50-minute Mineral Elixir Body Care. This includes a Snow Cristal Exfoliating Care using three types of minerals (rhodochrosite extract, malachite and quartz) that leaves your skin feeling silky smooth and your body energised. A Pink Clay Body Pack detoxifies and further moisturises your body.

The spa menu also includes massages, reflexology, facials and stone therapy. Certain treatments can be enjoyed in one of two cabins which overlook the Côte d'Azur and the horizon. These cabins are enveloped in the fragrance of the garden and shaded by the cover of the pine grove.

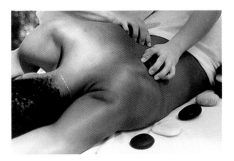

TYPE OF SPA
Hotel spa

SPA AREA
50 sq m (540 sq ft)

FACILITIES
4 single treatment rooms, 2 outdoor pavilions; 1 outdoor swimming pool; 1 spa boutique

SIGNATURE TREATMENTS
After-Sun Repairing Jasmine Care, Mediterranean Care, Mineral Elixir Care

TREATMENTS & THERAPIES
Body scrubs, body wraps, facials, fasciatherapy, firming and slimming treatments, hot stone therapies, massages, reflexology

ACTIVITIES & PROGRAMMES
Massage classes

SERVICES
Private spa parties

LANGUAGES SPOKEN BY THERAPISTS
English, French

CONTACT
Villa Marie Ramatuelle St Tropez
Route des Plages
Chemin Val de Rian
83350 Ramatuelle
France
T: +33 (0)4 9497 4022
F: +33 (0)4 9497 3755
E: contact@villamarie.fr
W: www.c-h-m.com

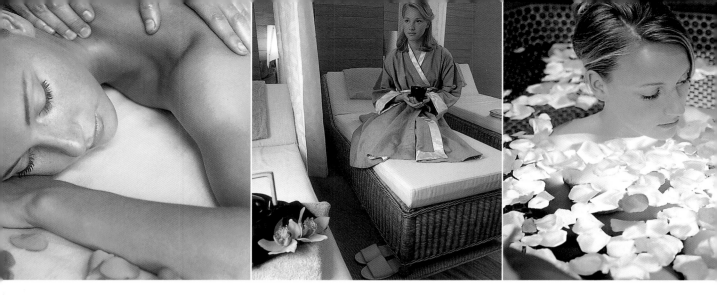

Amrita Spa at Raffles Hotel Vier Jahreszeiten
Hamburg, Germany

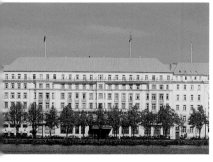

ABOVE: *Since opening its doors in 1897, the hotel has grown from just 11 rooms to 156 luxurious and individually decorated rooms and suites, many with a lakefront view.*

OPPOSITE, BOTTOM: *The spa's small size allows therapists to be in tune with each guest's needs.*

Guests (known as 'residents') of the luxurious Raffles Hotel Vier Jahreszeiten, on the western bank of the Inner Alster Lake, include luminaries from politics, business and entertainment. The elegant landmark within Hamburg's prestigious business and retail districts has been consistently rated as one of the World's Best Places to Stay in the *Condé Nast Traveler's Gold List* from 1997 to 2001.

The hotel's timeless charm and personalised attention are echoed in Amrita Spa on the fifth floor. In this intimate healing space, residents and members relax, recharge and rejuvenate their bodies, minds and spirits through classic European *kur* therapies and treatments based on Eastern philosophy. The spa sees itself as a total wellness centre; in Sanskrit, 'Amrita' means 'elixir of youth'.

Guests seem to instinctively seek out the Thermal Kur during winter and the Thalasso Kur during summer. The former warms the muscular system with a moor mud wrap, while the latter nourishes and cleanses with a

spirulina algae wrap. Both treatments continue with a hydro-massage with thermal salt and algae respectively; the bubbles that buffet the body rinse off the substances at the same time. These *kur* conclude with deeply relaxing full-body massages.

The Oxygen De Luxe Facial, the spa's most expensive facial, is also its most popular among female and male guests for its complexion-clarifying and line-smoothening effect.

The spa's signature treatments—the Amrita Elixir Of Youth, Samezen Hot Stone Massage and the Amrita Ayurvedic Massage—are also its most exotic. The latter takes place entirely with you lying supine, without the interruption of turning over. After a grounding foot and head massage, the therapist pours copious amounts of hot herbal and sesame oils on your body and uses effleurage strokes over your energy channels. Using graceful movements, the therapist then semi-cradles you as she massages your back. The session ends with a calming Shirodara. This nurturing treatment fosters mental clarity

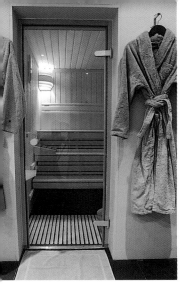

OPPOSITE, LEFT: *Body massages available include Swedish Massage, Sports Massage and Aromatherapy Massage.*

OPPOSITE, CENTRE: *Relax in between treatments in this rest area. You can also listen to music channels—ranging from soothing classics or rousing rock—via a private headset by each chaise lounge.*

OPPOSITE, RIGHT: *The spa is a pampering oasis where you can relax and recharge in a luxurious setting.*

LEFT: *The sauna (pictured) and cold plunge pool—the male and female changing rooms each have a set—can be used as a relaxing treatment in itself, or to prepare the body for a massage.*

and provides a sense of peace, and is best enjoyed in the morning, which will allow your body time to balance itself.

Guests who have more time to spend at the spa can opt for well-rounded day packages that focus on Ayurvedic or herbal treatments.

Besides receiving the benefits of marine-, mineral- and plant-based ingredients used in the spa's rituals, guests may choose to work out in the gym, or achieve body-mind fitness through personal training.

A delicious complement to the spa experience is a healthy spa breakfast or lunch which can be ordered into the spa or your room—and served course by course if you so desire.

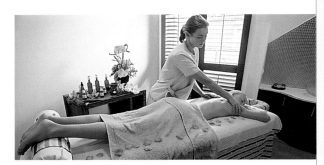

Spa Statistics

TYPE OF SPA
Hotel spa

SPA AREA
500 sq m (5,380 sq ft)

FACILITIES
5 treatment rooms; 1 consultation room; 1 meditation room, 1 relaxation room; 2 cold plunge pools, 2 reflexology pools; 1 Hydro-massage tub; 2 saunas, 2 steam rooms; 2 sunbeds; 1 hair salon; 1 gymnasium; 1 spa boutique

SIGNATURE TREATMENTS
Amrita Ayurveda Massage, Amrita Elixir Of Youth, Samezen Hot Stone Massage, Amrita Spa Body Treatment

TREATMENTS & THERAPIES
Anti-ageing treatments, anti-cellulite treatments, aromatherapy, baths, body bronzing, body masks, body scrubs, body wraps, bust treatments, Chinese therapies, eyebrow shaping and colouration, facials, firming and slimming treatments, hair treatments, hand and foot treatments, head and scalp treatments, hot stone therapies, hydrotherapy, jet lag treatments, make-up services, manicures and pedicures, massages, movement therapies, permanent make-up, pre- and post-natal treatments, reflexology, thalassotherapy, waxing; spa ritual packages, spa weekend packages

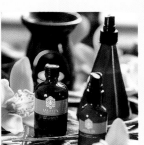

The spa's all-natural range from its Amrita Spa Private Label (pictured) may be purchased for home use. The spa also uses products from Kerstian Florian.

PROVISIONS FOR COUPLES
2 double treatment rooms; treatments for couples. The Amrita Spa Weekend Package

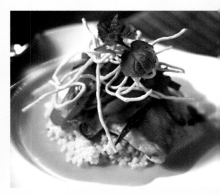

Like its sister spas worldwide, Amrita's spa cuisine emphasises delicious—and attractive—meals that are nutritiously balanced and low in fat, sodium and cholesterol.

for two in a deluxe double room includes meals and treatments for a personal spa programme.

SPA CUISINE
Low-fat and vegetarian meals are available on request. A breakfast and lunch menu of spa cuisine may be enjoyed at the Café Conde restaurant and Jahreszeiten Grill, or ordered in-room or into the spa area.

ACTIVITIES & PROGRAMMES
Autogenic training, martial arts, meditation, *tai qi*, yoga

SERVICES
Nutrition consultation; life-coach counselling; ergometric assessment, fitness assessment, personal training; gift certificates

LANGUAGES SPOKEN BY THERAPISTS
English, French, German, Swedish, Japanese

ADMISSION
Residents and members have exclusive use of the spa facilities. Treatments are available to non-residents and non-members at certain times.

CONTACT
Raffles Hotel Vier Jahreszeiten
Neuer Jungfernstieg 9-14
20354 Hamburg
Germany
T: +49 (0)40 349 40
F: +49 (0)40 349 426 00
E: amrita-spa.hvj@raffles.com
W: www.amritaspas.com

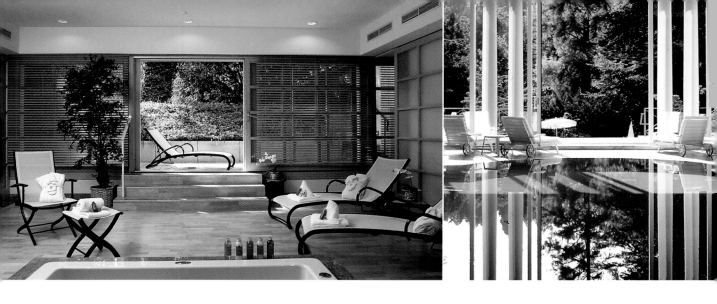

Brenner's Spa at Brenner's Park-Hotel & Spa
Baden-Baden, Germany

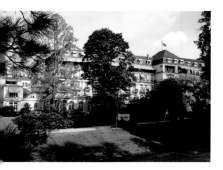

The grand hotel, dating back to 1872, retains a Parisian charm, resplendent with antiques and chandeliers.

'I fully believe I left my rheumatism there', wrote Mark Twain of the famous thermal baths in Baden-Baden that were built in the late 1800s. Modern-day visitors to the area take to the waters just as eagerly as did the American author and other international visitors—who also befriended Lady Luck in 'the loveliest casino in the world', according to famous actress Marlene Dietrich.

These attractions are but a short walk from Brenner's Park-Hotel & Spa, tucked within 6 hectares (15 acres) of parkland, where under the shade of the cypress and beech trees and surrounded by the scent of magnolias, you will enjoy a oneness with nature.

To revitalise your body, mind and spirit, pay a visit to Brenner's Spa, where you may imagine that you have stepped back into Roman times as you float in the Roman styled swimming pool. You may also imagine taking a trip to far-flung corners of the globe through innovative massage rituals developed by its therapists, or new treatment trends brought to you by guest therapists from foreign lands.

Exotic massage rituals include Thai Treatment (performed by therapists trained by specialists from Thailand), Bali Treatment (an exfoliating treatment with aloe vera pearls and hot oil), and Maharaja Massage Mystics (inspired by pampering ceremonies enjoyed by Indian princesses). The Caribbean Caress (a gentle massage with oils from the Caribbean) and African Alignment (a firm massage and therapeutic exercise which makes you feel reborn) are available together as a two-hour package known as Black and White. Despite its name, Body Torture—a massage with strong pressure inspired by techniques from the Orient—is very revitalising.

For a total pampering experience, book the Spa Suite which can hold a close circle of up to four friends. Within this private space, you can baste in a Japanese blossom steam bath, relax on the green quartzite heated benches in the laconicum, or refresh yourself under a shower of water, mist, light and aromas. A spa butler will attend to your refreshments and coordinate your treatments.

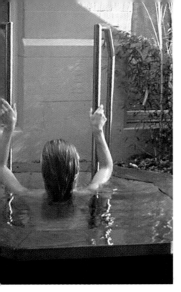

OPPOSITE, LEFT: *The spa suite is described as a spa within a spa. On a warm day, imagine you are in the tropics as you enjoy an Asian influenced Thai Treatment or Bali Treatment on its private terrace. Its décor is a fusion of elements from Europe and Asia.*

OPPOSITE, RIGHT: *The indoor swimming pool of ionised water resembles a Roman bathing temple with its high vaulted ceilings, tall columns and painted frescoes. In summertime, soak up some rays on the adjacent private terrace overlooking the lush private park.*

LEFT: *Literally chill out in this outdoor cold plunge pool made of slate encircled by bamboo.*

The Bvlgari Suite focuses on treatments of the eponymous luxury product line. Its Inner Illumination programme offers the ultimate in pampering and is an excellent way to initiate yourself into the delights of the spa. It includes a sensuous body wash with green tea extract, an exfoliation using a lime scrub with yogurt cream, and a relaxing full body massage.

If you are a gourmand, there is a unique Brenner's Spa programme specially designed to cater for you. Book the two-night Park Restaurant Meets Spa Suite package, and you will enjoy not only the spa, but fine dining as well at the hotel's award-winning Park Restaurant. For golf enthusiasts, there is another tailor-made package: the Golf, Spa & Drive programme. Men can also select combinations of treatments designed specifically for their needs from a separate menu.

The spa's private label Spirit of Jaipur comprises a luxurious range of bath and body products, allowing you to continue a pleasing personal ritual of pampering, relaxation and rejuvenation when you return home.

Spa Statistics

TYPE OF SPA
Hotel spa

SPA AREA
2,000 sq m (21,530 sq ft)

FACILITIES
1 private spa suite (for a group of up to 4 friends), 1 double treatment room, 1 Bvlgari luxury treatment room, 18 single treatment rooms; 4 consultation rooms; 1 meditation room; 1 relaxation lounge; 1 cold plunge pool, 2 whirlpools; 1 Biosauna, 1 Finnish sauna, 1 aroma steam room, 1 steam room; 1 solarium; 1 hair salon; 1 aerobics studio, 1 cardio studio, 1 gymnasium; 1 indoor swimming pool; golf courses nearby (on German and French side), 10 tennis courts (at a private club nearby); 1 spa boutique. Second Beauty Spa opening December 2003.

SIGNATURE TREATMENTS
Arabian Soap Rough Cleansing Massage, African Alignment, Bali Treatment, Body Torture, Caribbean Caress, Maharaja Massage Mystics, Thai Treatment; Black & White package

TREATMENTS & THERAPIES
Anti-cellulite treatments, aqua therapy, aromatherapy, baths, body bronzing, body scrubs, body wraps, bust treatments, electrotherapy, facials, firming and slimming treatments, hair treatments, hand and foot treatments, heat treatments, hydrotherapy, Indonesian therapies, jet lag treatments, lymphatic drainage, make-up services, manicures and pedicures, massages, movement therapies, purifying back treatments, reflexology, salon services, scalp treatments, Thai therapies, waxing; half-, full-, 2- and 5-day spa packages, 2-night spa packages

PROVISIONS FOR COUPLES
1 spa suite, 1 double massage suite

SPA CUISINE
Light, calorie-reduced dishes made from fresh produce are available at the conservatory-styled Wintergarten restaurant

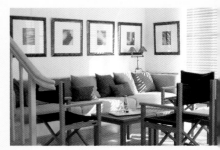

Feel right at home in this fitness lounge in your bathrobe after a spa session, or in your exercise gear after a workout. Enjoy a light snack, vitamin drink or fitness cocktail at the adjoining sports bar.

which offers informal all-day dining. The classical cuisine incorporates a Mediterranean touch that is young and unconventional. Provisions for various dietary requirements are available on request, or in conjunction with a consultation with a dietician.

ACTIVITIES & PROGRAMMES
Aerobics, aquaerobics, biking, golf, hiking, rock-climbing, tennis; cooking, make-up, massage, meditation, nailcare, lifestyle management and stretching classes, sports instruction; talks by visiting consultants

SERVICES
Body composition analysis; general healthcare consultation, nutritional consultation, skincare consultation; life-coach counselling; personal training; baby-sitting; corporate programmes; gift certificates; personal butler service

LANGUAGES SPOKEN BY THERAPISTS
Arabic, English, French, German, Russian

ADMISSION
Membership is available but not required for admission.

CONTACT
Brenner's Park-Hotel & Spa
Schillerstrasse 4-6
76530 Baden-Baden
Germany
T: +49 (0)72 219 000
F: +49 (0)72 2138 772
E: info@brenners.com
W: www.brenners.com

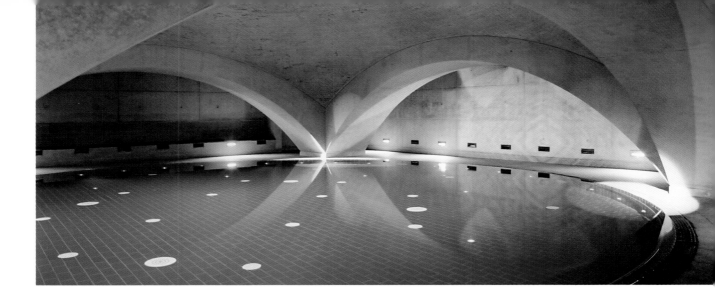

Liquidrom Therme at the Tempodrom
Berlin, Germany

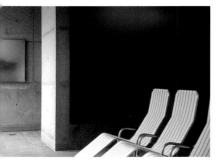

In this seating area you can relax, listen to the music and enjoy a good view of the Liquidrom.

Berlin has been described as a city addicted to change. While its many parks, canals, and forest-lined lakes remain its most decorative real estate, Berlin is never afraid to add new forms of expression to its cityscape. The Tempodrom—Berlin's ultramodern multi-media centre—is one of the boldest statements in modern architecture. Its tent-like structure is reminiscent of the forms drafted by the Expressionist architects of the 1920s. Under the Tempodrom's gigantic circus roof are three separate arenas: two providing the space for events as diverse as plays, concerts, circus performances and sporting events, and the third housing Liquidrom—a unique German reinterpretation of the spa experience.

The Liquidrom is the aquatic stage of the Tempodrom. About 20 years ago, multi-media artist/writer/entrepreneur Micky Remann became fascinated with the question of what a whale's song would sound like underwater. This fascination led to the invention of Liquid Sound—a sensuous new bathing experience that envelopes bathers in a collage of coloured lights, music and nature sounds. Liquid Sound enhances the water's therapeutic benefits—effectively making Micky Remann the world's only 'musical director of a spa'.

The entire Liquidrom experience has been fittingly described as being in a holistic concert hall. The indoor swimming pool is a circular water basin covered by a vaulting roof with a window at its peak. Liquidrom's state-of-the-art sound system pumps out music above and below the water surface. In keeping with the pool's salinity and temperature, the system reproduces perfect whale and dolphin sounds in the centrepiece pool.

Bathers can sign up for Aqua Wellness sessions here. Aqua Wellness is a special form of bodywork that takes place in a warm water pool. It combines elements of soft stretching movements, massage and joint release as well as breathing exercises in a unique way above and under water. Specially designed movements aim to improve your

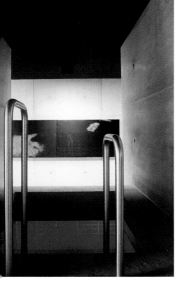

OPPOSITE: *The Liquidrom at the Tempodrom is located in the heart of Berlin, close to the Potsdamer Platz, Brandenbürger Tor, and the famous Tiergarten. Both Liquidrom and Tempodrom are closely associated with music. In August, Tempodrom attracts thousands of visitors to the Heimatklange—its world music festival.*

LEFT: *After a sauna, a dip in the plunge pool (pictured) stimulates and reawakens your entire body.*

BOTTOM: *The Liquidrom's innovative design extends even to the showers, with their avant-garde lighting and original artwork.*

spine's agility while releasing a calming flow of energy through your body. The body experiences a whole new sensation of movement as you float weightless in the water. A session leaves you with a heightened sense of awareness while helping to ease away physical and emotional tensions.

Besides being a city of change, Berlin is also a city that parties all night. Local legend has it that you're likely to be confronted with a *kneipe*, or pub, around every street corner. With Liquidrom now firmly planted on the local map, you have the opportunity to leave Berlin recharged—even as you try to keep pace with this hectic city.

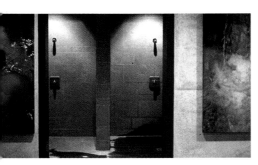

Spa Statistics

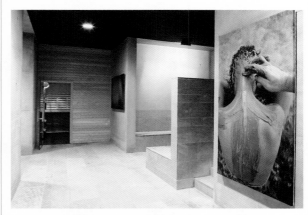

Striking photoart images in concrete by New York artist Linda Troeller greet you everywhere at the Liquidrom, heightening your awareness of being ushered into a unique experience.

TYPE OF SPA
Day spa

SPA AREA
1,000 sq m (10,760 sq ft)

FACILITIES
4 single indoor treatment rooms; 1 cold plunge pool; 1 sauna, 1 steam room; sound-chairs; 1 indoor swimming pool (with saltwater and underwater music), 1 outdoor swimming pool (with hot saltwater of 40 degrees Celsius/104 degrees Fahrenheit); 1 spa boutique

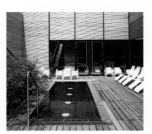

The outdoor Japanese onsen *pool is heated for bathers all year round.*

SIGNATURE TREATMENTS
Aqua Wellness (water therapy), Aqua Wellness Massage, Beauty Face Massage, Cosmic Touch (*reiki*), Deep Relaxation, Energetic Body Work (shiatsu), Energetic Trance Massage, Foot Reflex Zone Massage, Hawaiian Bodywork, Indian Warm Oil Massage, Structural Body Work

TREATMENTS & THERAPIES
Aqua therapy, Ayurvedic treatments, facials, massages

ACTIVITIES & PROGRAMMES
The Liquidrom holds musical nights with different themes on different days of the week, such as jazz on Thursdays and classical music on Fridays. There are also special events such as photography exhibitions, ultraviolet performances and multi-media presentations. Check the Liquidrom calendar for details.

LANGUAGES SPOKEN BY THERAPISTS
English, German

ADMISSION
Spa is opened daily from 10 A.M. to 10 P.M., and from 10 A.M. to midnight on Fridays and Saturdays. Opening hours are extended to 2 A.M. on full moon nights. Bathers are charged on a per-hour basis.

CONTACT
Liquidrom Therme Berlin
Moeckernstrasse 10
D-10963 Berlin
Germany
T: +49 (0)30 7473 7171
F: +49 (0)30 7473 7172
E: liquidromberlin@aol.com
W: www.liquidrom.com

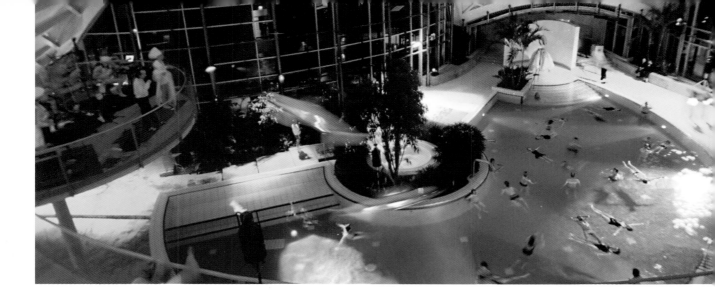

Toskana Therme
Bad Sulza, Weimar, Germany

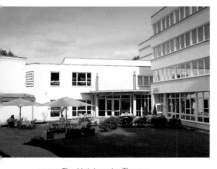

ABOVE: *The Hotel an der Therme is surrounded by rolling vineyards, ancient castles and ruins, rivers and forests—a modern establishment in a landscape of historical interest and natural beauty.*

OPPOSITE, BOTTOM: *The spa opens till midnight on weekends and to 2 A.M. on full moon nights! You can purchase day tickets and family tickets (2 adults, 1 child) that give you at least 2 hours in the pools.*

Bad Sulza, a sleepy East German backwater about 193 kilometres (120 miles) from Berlin, is an old town with only 3,300 inhabitants, set in the verdant hills of Thuringia: an area often hailed as the 'Tuscany of the East'. As early as 1848, spa-goers at Bad Sulza were seeking relief from skin, joint and respiratory diseases in its warm, soothing waters as salty as those of the Dead Sea.

Despite Germany's long history of curative bathing, new spas were a rarity in the country until recently, and old spas reinventing themselves were almost as rare. But in November 1999, a brand-new spa concept was born when the Toskana Therme Spa opened—and Bad Sulza has become a magnet for lovers of the avant-garde.

Though still sparsely populated, the town now attracts a pilgrimage of some 1,000 visitors per day. They come here to 'worship' at a place called the Liquid Sound Temple: the grand centrepiece of the Toskana Therme Day Spa.

The philosophy behind the high-tech Liquid Sound Temple is unique. Seven interconnected pools offer cutting-edge water therapies dramatically merged with music and underwater sound. Bathers in the Liquid Sound Temple, housed in a windowless wooden dome, can soak under the stars in the centrepiece pool while listening to world music or the latest New Age compositions.

Spa-goers can also book Aqua Wellness sessions in the Liquid Sound pools. An 80-minute individual session with a bodyworker begins with a massage on the water surface. This culminates in a symphony of stretching, massaging, rocking, and swaying movements underwater to achieve a natural flow of energy between two persons, resulting in a state of absolute peace and relaxation.

For something even more exotic, treat yourself to a Hawaiian Bodywork session. A bodyworker massages you with warm aromatic oils while your auditory senses are soothed by music from Polynesia's Tiki culture, creating a true symphony for the skin. There is also a unique bio-saunarium for sauna lovers which combines a temperate

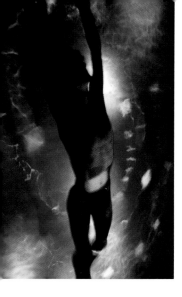

OPPOSITE: *The futuristic design of Toskana Therme prepares one for the odyssey of experience to be savoured within its hi-tech domed structure.*

LEFT: *Some have likened bathing in Liquid Sound to making a return to the mother's womb. During a Liquid Sound experience, the body makes contact with music in the water, and is lured into a state of total relaxation. Tickets for special Friday performances at the Liquid Sound Temple must be booked in advance.*

sauna experience with coloured lights and music. Here, you can also enjoy the inhalation of cold steam from the Bad Sulza saltwater.

The Toskana Therme complex also includes the Hotel an der Therme, where spa-goers can proceed for beauty treatments. This modern facility offers 80 single and double-sized rooms with views of the park, and an additional 60 non-smoking rooms. The hotel is linked to the Toskana Therme spa and guests enjoy private, direct spa access. This spa is truly a wellness waterpark fit for the 21st century, rightly placing Germany firmly back on the world map of futuristic spas.

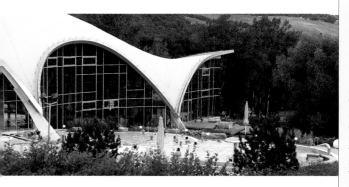

Spa Statistics

TYPE OF SPA
Natural saltwater and mineral spring spa

SPA AREA
3,000 sq m (32,290 sq ft)

FACILITIES
12 single treatment rooms, 2 double indoor treatment rooms; 1 sound therapy room, 1 music therapy room; 2 consultation rooms, 6 medical consultation rooms; 1 meditation room, 2 relaxation rooms; 1 cold plunge pool, 4 whirlpools; 3 saunas, 1 steam room; 2 solariums; 1 hair salon, 1 nail salon; 1 aerobics studio, 1 cardio studio, 3 gymnasiums; 5 indoor pools, 2 outdoor pools with Liquid Sound, 1 Liquid Sound Temple; 1 labyrinth; 1 spa boutique (selling Sothys and Malu Wilz products)

SIGNATURE TREATMENTS
Liquid Sound sessions, Aqua Wellness (floating water movement and massage in Liquid Sound), Hawaiian Massage

TREATMENTS & THERAPIES
Anti-ageing treatments, anti-cellulite treatments, aqua therapy, aromatherapy, Ayurvedic treatments, baths, body scrubs, body wraps, bust treatments, colonic irrigation and enemas, electrotherapy, eye treatments, facials, firming and slimming treatments, hand and foot treatments, heat treatments, holistic treatments, hot stone therapy, hydrotherapy, inhalation therapies, jet lag treatments, life-coach counselling, lymphatic drainage, make-up services, manicures and pedicures, massages, movement therapies, reflexology, salon services, scalp treatments, waxing

SPA CUISINE
The hotel restaurant and the spa restaurant serve vegetarian dishes made from organic products. The ingredients come from local growers, wherever possible. The menu focuses on vegetable and milk products.

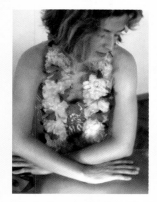

The spa offers several versions of its speciality Hawaiian treatment. There is an Aqua Wellness and Hawaiian combo as well as a Four-Handed Hawaii treatment for double the pampering.

PROVISIONS FOR COUPLES
Aqua Wellness Synchronous Sessions For Two

ACTIVITIES & PROGRAMMES
Hiking, yoga; cooking classes, talks by visiting consultants. Special art performances take place on different days of the week or month at the Liquid Sound Temple. Check with the spa for details on on-going concerts above and below water, underwater musicals, readings, dance, plays, etc.

SERVICES
Consultations on body composition analysis, healthcare, skincare, and nutrition classes; babysitting, childcare; gift certificates

LANGUAGES SPOKEN BY THERAPISTS
English, German

ADMISSION
Overnight accommodation at the hotel includes 2 hours bathing in the Toskana Therme Spring Baths per day. Guests can use a private bridge linking the hotel to the spa.

CONTACT
Toskana Therme
Wunderwaldstrasse 2a
D-99518 Bad Sulza
Germany
T: +49 (0)36 4619 2881
F: +49 (0)36 4619 2095
E: toskana@kbs.de
W: toskana-therme.de

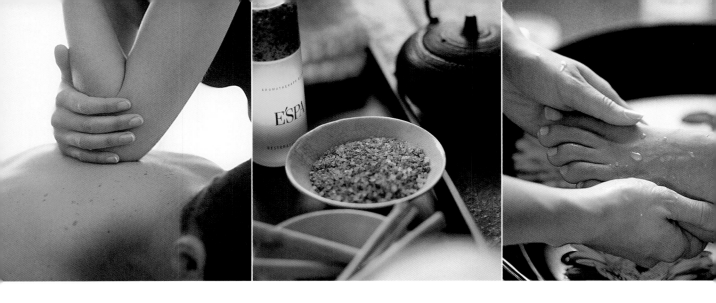

GB Spa at Hotel Grande Bretagne
Athens, Greece

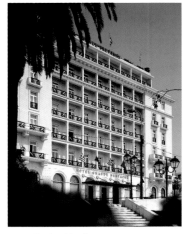

ABOVE: *The hotel, itself a historic landmark, offers views of ancient historic sights such as the Acropolis and the Parthenon from a number of its rooms.*

OPPOSITE, BOTTOM: *Each treatment room is a soothing space that is minimalist in design.*

The former residence of a wealthy Greek expatriate opened its doors as the Hotel Grande Bretagne in 1872, offering a luxurious comfort—that otherwise only existed in grand homes of that era—to guests that included royals, celebrities and artists. The palatial hotel, located in the heart of Athens, is a short walk from museums, the Plaka (the charming old quarter), the business centre and fashionable Kolonaki Square.

The GB Spa, a member of the Starwood Spa Collection, continues the emphasis that ancient Greeks placed on health and wellbeing. At this urban hideaway, you can escape from all the stresses of the modern world. You may also wish to heed the advice of Hippocrates, and have a massage every day.

Allocate some time before your treatment to relax your body in the spa's facilities that include a laconium, herbal steam bath, Amethyst Grotto, Finnish sauna, an ice fountain and reflexology footbaths. Then let yourself be pampered with a range of holistic treatments from ESPA that balance your phys-

ical and mental equilibrium. These therapies, inspired by cultures from both East and West, harness the use of indigenous ingredients.

The spa's signature treatment, The Ancient Greek Ritual, is an intensive 1-hour-40-minute session that nourishes and purifies your body. A footbath, gentle skin brushing and body exfoliation is followed by an ESPA Express Facial. Your body is then cocooned in linen in a warm envelopment of marine algae with the gentle massage programme of the unique Belle Epoque, stimulating circulation and melting away stress and tension.

Another house speciality, the GB Spa Hot Stone Massage, is a 1-hour-40-minute session in which you are massaged with smooth basalt stones, aided by a medley of essential oils chosen to suit to your needs. This treatment brings about a sense of balance, and improves your flow of energy.

The sweetest treatment on the menu is the 1-hour-10-minute Nourishing Yogurt, Honey & Sugar Treatment. After a welcoming footbath, your body is exfoliated with a blend

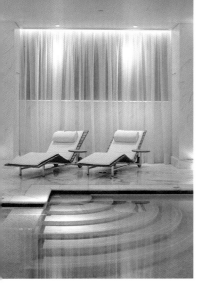

OPPOSITE, LEFT: *Let your stress melt away under the nurturing touch of the therapists.*

OPPOSITE, CENTRE: *The ESPA products used combine the best of aromatherapy and thalassotherapy to benefit your skin, body and mind.*

OPPOSITE, RIGHT: *Most treatments begin with a welcoming Foot Ritual which comprises a relaxing footbath and massage.*

LEFT: *The indoor swimming pool is a sleek area of repose.*

of sugar and olive oil, followed by a Greek Honey & Yoghurt Body Wrap that leaves your skin feeling silky smooth. A deep scalp massage completes the relaxing session, leaving you feeling like a delicious morsel.

To share the spa experience with a loved one or a friend, book the Couples Suite. Alternatively, opt for the half-day ESPA Duet Delight package: a 1-hour-40-minute treatment for two. Within the Serial Thermal Chamber, you can slather mineral-rich muds on each other before basting in a steam bath to nourish the skin; subsequently, retreat to the Couples Suite where you can enjoy any of the treatments together side by side.

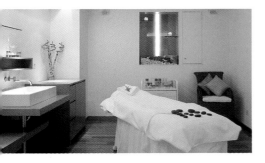

Spa Statistics

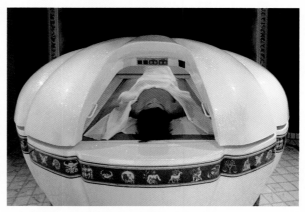

Within the heated confines of this Belle Epoque Wellness Capsule, you will enjoy a warm massage as water rains down on you, combined with aromatherapy and light therapy. Your therapist will select a programme that is suited for you, but the controls can be adjusted by you from within the bed.

TYPE OF SPA
Hotel spa

SPA AREA
840 sq m (9,040 sq ft)

FACILITIES
1 double treatment room, 5 single treatment and wet rooms; 1 relaxation room; 1 sauna, 2 steam rooms; 1 Amethyst Grotto; 1 laconium; 1 herbal bath; 1 hair salon; 1 gymnasium; 1 indoor swimming pool, 1 outdoor swimming pool; 1 spa boutique; 1 juice bar

SIGNATURE TREATMENTS
The Ancient Greek Ritual, GB Spa Hot Stone Massage, Nourishing Yogurt, Honey & Sugar Treatment

TREATMENTS & THERAPIES
Aromatherapy, body scrubs, body wraps, eye treatments, facials, heat treatments, hot stone therapies, jet lag treatments, massages, pre- and post-natal treatments, purifying back treatments, salon services, scalp treatments, waxing; Half Day Retreats include treatments, use of the GB Thermal Suite, swimming pool, relaxation and changing rooms; Full Day Retreats additionally include a light, 2-course spa lunch.

PROVISIONS FOR COUPLES
1 double treatment room known as the Couples Suite; ESPA Duet Delight package

SPA CUISINE
Spa cuisine that is low in calories and fat can be enjoyed at the Atrium. Some options may be ordered in-room. Fresh juices and smoothies can be enjoyed at the GB Spa Juice Bar.

ACTIVITIES & PROGRAMMES
Jogging

SERVICES
Gift certificates; day-use rooms

LANGUAGES SPOKEN BY THERAPISTS
English, Greek

ADMISSION
Membership is available but not required for admission. Annual membership, by approval only, includes 20% off treatments and free entrance to the heat facilities and the pool.

CONTACT
Hotel Grande Bretagne
Constitution Square
105 63 Athens
Greece
T: +30 21 0333 0818
F: +30 21 0333 0200
E: info@grandebretagne.gr
W: www.grandebretagne.gr

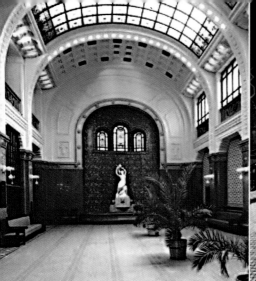
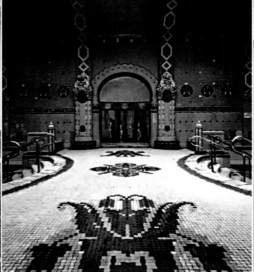
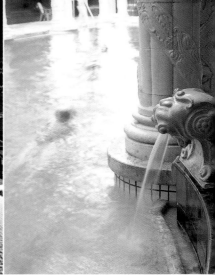

The Saint Gellért Medicinal Bath and Pools at the Danubius Hotel Gellért

Budapest, Hungary

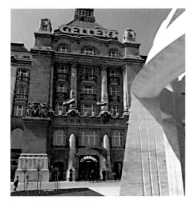

ABOVE: *Built in 1918, the landmark Danubius Hotel Gellért attracts a parade of princes, maharajahs and millionaires who come to absorb the medicinal properties of its famous baths.*

OPPOSITE, BOTTOM: *The Hotel Gellért is named after Bishop St Gellért, who died a martyr's death preaching Christianity to local pagans some 1,000 years ago. Today, spa-goers can experience the best of the twin cities of Buda and Pest here. Situated by the riverbank, major attractions of both cities are within easy access.*

It is easy to see why the Hungarians and visitors love their Danubius. Standing on the riverbank of the River Danube, on the side of the historic city of Buda, the hotel is as historic as they come. Built during the darkest days of World War I, restored after the bombings of World War II, it presents a façade that is at once poised and dignified. Little surprise then that the Gellért is Budapest's most famous hotel.

Just as gypsy music, a sampling of traditional Hungarian fare, a sip of coffee at the chic cafés along Andrassy Avenue, and a visit to the Opera Theatre define a trip to Budapest, no itinerary is complete without a trip to the baths. Though Budapest may be a city filled with old and new baths, the Gellért Bath is the most famous, and some say, the best that the city has to offer.

The Gellért Spa has a history that dates back even further than the hotel itself. During the days of Turkish rule (1526–1678), it was called the Aga Bath or the Bath of Virgins. According to local folklore, the young virgins were hidden away for protection and they lived and bathed in the spa. Today, the baths continue to be a legend in spa history.

The hotel's thermal baths are accessed by a charming, old-fashioned elevator. Original Roman pipes carrying natural spring waters still feed the inside and outside thermal pools, steam rooms, and bubble baths. The baths are housed in a glorious Art Deco temple culminating in a marvellous domed ceiling. The spa complex is made up of thermal baths, steam rooms, a massage hall, a swimming pool, an area for curative massage, a chiropody hall and even a dentistry complex.

The bath's services range from mud treatments and galvanic baths to medical gymnastics. The massage room offers 15-minute and 30-minute sessions that cost little more than a cuppa in some other European cities. Massages here may be

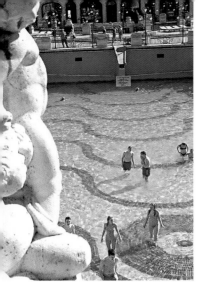

OPPOSITE, LEFT: *The ornate spa has a marble-pillared lobby decorated by bronze statues, leather chairs and richly patterned carpeting.*

OPPOSITE, CENTRE: *The interior of the spa is reminiscent of the Turkish Age, with Art Nouveau style ceramics lending an air of grandeur.*

OPPOSITE, RIGHT: *The indoor swimming pool is a favourite photographic subject.*

LEFT: *This 30-metre (100-foot) outdoor pool with its wave machine is especially popular with young people.*

frills-free, but they hark back to a time when masseurs did what they do best—provide a healing, spirits-restoring good old massage.

Most landmark hotels hold a special place in the hearts of their citizens. Today, foreign guests also seek soothing sanctuary along-side Hungarians in their famous Saint Gellért Medicinal Bath and Pools. Thus, appreciation of these famous baths has become universal.

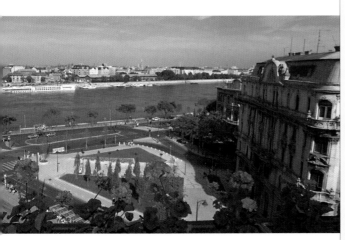

Spa Statistics

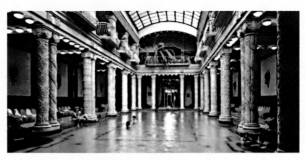

The centre of the building that houses the baths is a spacious hall that is covered by a giant dome. The spa under the dome is reminiscent of the spacious halls of the Roman thermal baths.

TYPE OF SPA
Medical spa

SPA AREA
320 sq m (3,440 sq ft)

FACILITIES
5 medical consultation rooms; 1 cold plunge pool, 1 whirlpool; 1 sparkling bath, 4 thermal baths, 1 wave bath; carbonated mist chambers (for treating arteriosclerosis); 1 sauna, 4 steam rooms; 3 solariums, 80 sunbeds; 1 hair salon; 2 gymnasiums; 1 indoor swimming pool, 1 outdoor swimming pool; 1 spa boutique

SIGNATURE TREATMENTS
Underwater traction bath, underwater jet massage

TREATMENTS & THERAPIES
Anti-ageing treatments, anti-cellulite treatments, aqua therapy, baths, chiropody, hand and foot treatments, heat treatments, hydrotherapy, inhalation therapies (including special treatments for asthma and chronic bronchitis patients), manicures and pedicures, massages, medical massage, movement therapies, rheumath-ology treatment, Thai therapies

SPA CUISINE
Danubius Hotel Gellért offers a wellness menu that has dishes with low fat and low cholesterol levels. The Danubius Wellness menu is available at the Duna Restaurant. Vegetarian and diabetic dishes are also available on request.

ACTIVITIES & PROGRAMMES
The hotel does not offer sports activities or classes on location, but helps to organise biking sessions, cooking and dance lessons for guests.

SERVICES
Body composition analysis; general healthcare, nutrition and skincare consultations; baby-sitting, childcare; corporate programmes; private spa parties; night-bathing on weekends

ADMISSION
Baths are open to the public. Admission to the baths is free for hotel guests.

LANGUAGES SPOKEN BY THERAPISTS
English, French, German, Italian

CONTACT
Danubius Hotel Gellért
1111 Budapest
Szent Gellért Tér 1
Hungary
T: + 361 (0)889 5500
F: + 361 (0)889 5505
E: gellert.reservation@ danubiusgroup.com
W: www.danubiusgroup.com/gellert

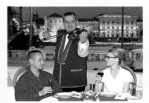

The restaurants at Hotel Gellért are as famous as its baths. They offer a fine selection of Hungarian gourmet dishes.

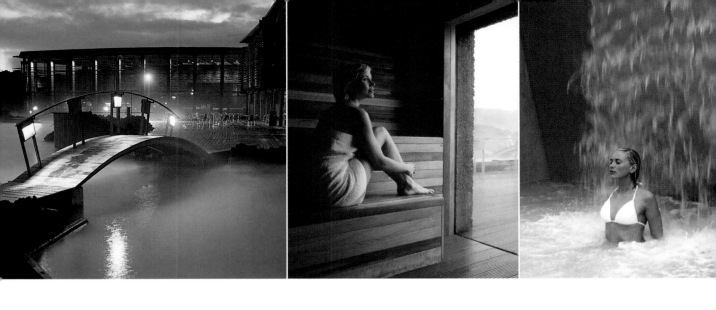

Blue Lagoon Geothermal Spa
Grindavík, Iceland

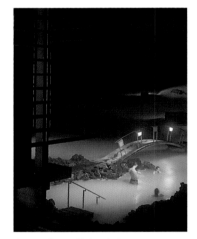

Architect Sigridur Sigthorsdottir used materials such as the lava characteristic of the area, and Jatoba wood from Brazil in designing the futuristic-looking spa area. The robust Jatoba wood has the capacity to age gracefully into a soft grey colour, allowing the building to blend with its natural surroundings.

Blue Lagoon is a natural geothermal spa located less than a 40-minute drive from the capital Reykjavík. The beauty and therapeutic benefits of its waters —one-third fresh water and two-thirds seawater—lure local residents and foreigners alike. The water originates from 2 kilometres (1.2 miles) below the earth's surface, maintains a constant temperature of 36 to 39 degrees Celsius (97 to 102 degrees Fahrenheit), and is piped directly to the geothermal spa where guests enjoy outdoor bathing all year long. As you luxuriate in the waters in your bathing suit, you will marvel at a landscape that appears even more dreamlike in winter when the lifeguards who keep a watchful eye on your safety are tightly wrapped in warm clothes.

With its milky turquoise waters, steam, lava caves and silica mud, Blue Lagoon resembles an other-worldly moonscape. The natural mineral salts (that balance and relax the body), blue green algae (to nourish and soften the skin) and white silica mud (that cleanses and exfoliates) are what give the water its rich

hue and therapeutic properties. These gifts from the earth also feature in the Blue Lagoon range of products used in massages, body and face treatments that take place within a secluded area of the lagoon, as you soak up the water's healing ingredients and are lulled by its rhythmic lapping on your body.

The house speciality, the Blue Lagoon In-Water Massage, comes in variations ranging from a 10-minute Head and Shoulder Massage to a 50-minute Full Body Massage. Silica massage, salt glow, cellulite treatment based on Blue Lagoon silica mud, nourishing treatment based on blue green algae and mineral salts are among the treatments available. Blue Lagoon facial and slimming body wraps based on mineral salt scrubs and wraps are also available.

Modern, spacious changing and shower rooms are on the site and the entrance fee includes the use of Blue Lagoon shower gel, hair conditioner and moisturising cream. Between lagoon bathing sessions, visit a sauna with a view of the lagoon. Enjoy a

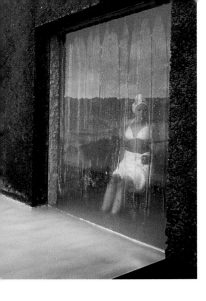

OPPOSITE, LEFT: *The Blue Lagoon appears even more dramatic at dusk when the sun goes down and the lights come up.*

OPPOSITE, CENTRE: *Guests enjoy a view of the lagoon while relaxing in the sauna.*

OPPOSITE, RIGHT: *Enjoy nature's hydro-massage while you stand under the sleek sheet of falling water.*

LEFT: *Blue Lagoon geothermal seawater flows into parts of the steam room.*

unique Blue Lagoon steam bath with white walls that resemble white silica mud, and take a cosy steam bath in a lava cave. Try standing under the Blue Lagoon waterfall for an energising massage. Freshen up by walking through a cold water sprinkle. Guests also have access to the therapeutic white silica mud located in special boxes by the lagoon.

In addition to its positive effects on skin, the Blue Lagoon is known for its healing power as regards psoriasis. An out-patient clinic reserved exclusively for Blue Lagoon guests undergoing treatment lies less than a kilometre (0.7 miles) from the geothermal spa.

To complement picture perfect moments back at the lagoon, sip on a Blue Lagoon cocktail. Then pamper your taste buds at the Blue Lagoon Restaurant with gourmet cuisine as well as fresh Icelandic ingredients and fish. The view of the lagoon through the floor-to-ceiling windows is breathtaking. The food, scenery, fresh air, and healing elements from the earth and water work as one to create an experience that inspires your entire psyche.

Spa Statistics

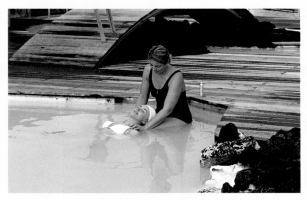

Blue Lagoon massage and treatments take place outdoors and in-water.

TYPE OF SPA
Geothermal spa

SPA AREA
7,700 sq m (82,880 sq ft)

FACILITIES
Geothermal lagoon (5,000 sq m/ 53,820 sq ft), 1 geothermal waterfall, 1 indoor pool, 1 lava cave, 1 water sprinkle; in-water treatment area; 1 sauna, 2 steam rooms; 1 spa boutique

SIGNATURE TREATMENTS
Blue Lagoon In-Water treatments

TREATMENTS & THERAPIES
Anti-cellulite treatments, body scrubs, body wraps, firming and slimming treatments, foot treatments, hydrotherapy, purifying back treatments, silica massage

SPA CUISINE
Light snacks and gourmet meals made from fresh

Icelandic ingredients are available at the Blue Lagoon Restaurant. Seafood features prominently on the menu.

SERVICES
Meeting rooms; gift certificates, coach service between Blue Lagoon and airport, and Blue Lagoon and Reykjavík

LANGUAGES SPOKEN BY THERAPISTS
English, Icelandic

CONTACT
Blue Lagoon
Svartsengi
240 Grindavík
Iceland
T: +354 420 8800
F: +354 420 8801
E: lagoon@bluelagoon.is
W: www.bluelagoon.is

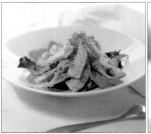

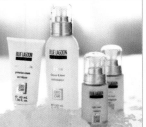

LEFT: *The Blue Lagoon Restaurant serves a mix of local and international dishes.*

RIGHT: *Through Blue Lagoon's on-line shop at www.bluelagoon.is, you can purchase their unique Blue Lagoon products wherever you are in the world.*

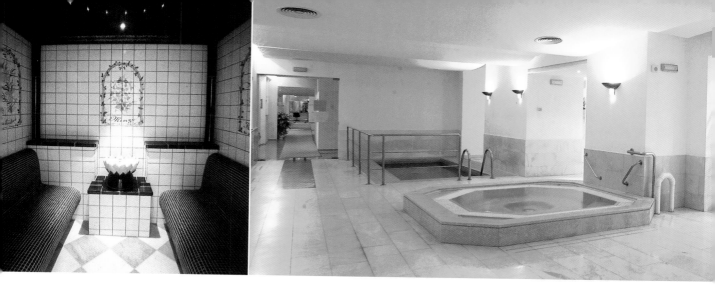

Espace Henri Chenot at Grand Hotel Palace
Merano, Italy

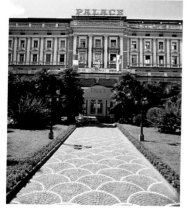

The grand 125-room and 12-suite hotel is set in an oasis of calm against a mountainous backdrop.

German author Franz Kafka was one of many guests who have lavished praise on the elegant Grand Hotel Palace since its opening in 1906. The aristocratic Castle Schloss Maur, housing suites and a peaceful, ancient chapel, stands adjacent to the grand *belle époque* hotel.

Guests in search of tranquillity can find it in a leisurely breakfast on the terrace overlooking the park, lying in the sun beside the outdoor pool, playing chess in a shady corner of the garden, accompanied by the rustling of palm leaves and the scent of pine trees, or admiring the sunset with a loved one.

Those who seek to regain their mental and physical equilibrium find respite in Espace Henri Chenot, the hotel's health and beauty centre located on the Garden Floor, which is run by husband and wife team Henri and Dominique Chenot along with their team of physicians and therapists. Treatment in the centre is focused on the concept of 'biontology': a term coined by Henri to mean 'the study of the essence of life and its evolution'.

Biontology reflects Henri's researches into bio-energetic psychology, naturopathy and Chinese medicine. Its holistic approach combines the use of energising treatments, hydrotherapy, phytotherapy, diet and lifestyle changes to detoxify the body in order to slow down the signs of premature ageing typically brought about by fatigue and the effects of pollution. This synthesis of Western science and Eastern healing energy benefits the harmony of the body's biological rhythm.

Ideally, treatment should take place over a period of six days. Six-day treatment/seven-night healthcare packages focus on anti-ageing, anti-stress or slimming. Treatment includes accommodation, a recommended diet, group exercise in the gym or pool, lectures on health, and consultancy with the centre's physician. Energizing Treatments, involving low-intensity electrical impulses being sent through the meridians to stimulate the organs and balance the body's flow of vital energy, are also included. Shorter four-night

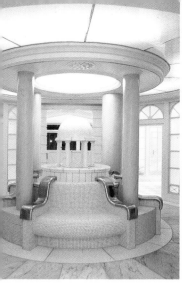

OPPOSITE, LEFT: *Inhalation therapy takes place in this ornate, starlit herbarium, also known as the aromatic cave.*

OPPOSITE, RIGHT: *Hydrotherapy, one facet of biontology, helps improve blood and lymph circulation, aiding the removal of toxins.*

LEFT: *Unwind in between treatments in this heated relaxation area that resembles a white palace.*

weekend packages are available, and treatments can be taken on an à la carte basis.

On arrival at the centre, you are encouraged to undergo a Bio-Test/Bio-Energetic Check-Up so that a physician can prescribe a course of treatments to suit your needs. The checkup analyses the areas of energy imbalance in your body, revealing your energy state in graph form. A Bio-Check Stabilometry, an analysis of your posture and your audio, visual and masticatory functions, is also available.

The centre also offers sophisticated medical cosmetic treatments to beautify your body. These treatments include the revitalising and wrinkle-reducing Cosmetic Toning-Up Treatment and the Cellulitis Treatment that remodels fatty tissue deposits with an oxygen-ozone injection.

Henri Chenot Sources de la Santé products that are used in the treatments may be purchased from the spa boutique, as can their perfume line. You can also bring home advice on how to lead a more balanced life from talks on wellbeing given by the centre.

Spa Statistics

TYPE OF SPA
Hotel spa

SPA AREA
2,000 sq m (21,530 sq ft)

FACILITIES
25 single treatment rooms; 2 relaxation rooms; 1 Kneipp pool, 2 saunas, 2 steam rooms; 2 solariums; 1 hair salon; 1 gymnasium; 1 indoor swimming pool, 1 outdoor swimming pool; 1 spa boutique

SIGNATURE TREATMENTS
Energizing Treatments; treatments revolving around Henri Chenot Method Biontology

TREATMENTS & THERAPIES
Anti-ageing treatments, anti-cellulite treatments, firming and slimming treatments, aqua therapy, aromatherapy, body wraps, bust treatments, energising treatments, facials, hydrotherapy, inhalation therapies, lymphatic drainage, manicures and pedicures, medical cosmetic treatments, movement therapies, reflexology, scalp treatments, waxing; healthcare packages

SPA CUISINE
A detoxifying Bio-Light diet is served at a dining area reserved for guests on the cure plan. It can also be ordered in-room.

ACTIVITIES & PROGRAMMES
Aerobics, aquaerobics; conferences on the philosophy of health

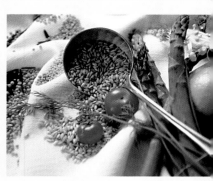

The purifying Bio-Light diet includes a generous amount of fresh fruit, fruit juices, and raw and cooked vegetables. You will not find proteins and carbohydrates served together in the same meal. The diet is free of salt and saturated fat.

SERVICES
Bio-Test/Bio-Energetic Check-Ups, Bio-Check Stabilometry, impedenziometrie (body fat analysis); personal training; baby-sitting; ergometric assessment, fitness assessment, nutritional consultation; baby-sitting; childcare; gift certificates

LANGUAGES SPOKEN BY THERAPISTS
English, French, German, Italian

CONTACT
Grand Hotel Palace
Via Cavour 2-4
39012 Merano
Italy
T: +39 0473 271 000
F: +39 0473 271 100
E: info@henrichenot.com
W: www.henrichenot.com

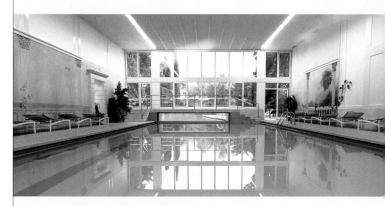

The hotel's outdoor pool is located against a backdrop of majestic mountains. There is also an indoor pool (pictured) that can be enjoyed year-round in all weather.

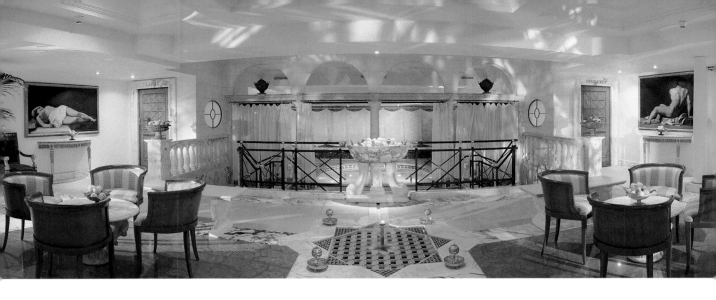

Health & Fitness Centre at Rome Cavalieri Hilton
Rome, Italy

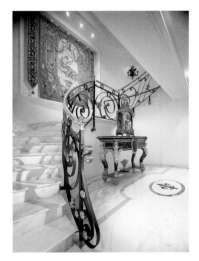

Art connoisseurs will feel at home in this hotel, which houses a large collection of French Louis XV and First Empire French furniture, old masters' paintings, rare tapestries and artefacts, and Italian modern art in the public spaces and suites. Many were obtained through Christie's and Sotheby's.

The opulent Rome Cavalieri Hilton, nestled in 6 hectares (15 acres) of private parkland in a residential district, offers commanding views of the city from the balcony of each of its 372 rooms and suites. Travellers who want extra privacy and luxury should book a suite on the Executive Floors (the hotel was the first in Rome to provide these); the ultimate being the Imperial and Presidential Suites furnished with antiques and significant pieces of furniture—including sofas that once graced Karl Lagerfeld's Paris home—and equipped with their own gazebo, solarium, and private hydro-massage pool behind bullet-proof glass. Even discerning four-legged companions of hotel guests are coddled with an in-room dining menu for pets.

The hotel has garnered a clutch of awards, including those for its rooftop garden restaurant, La Pergola. Its spa, known simply as the Health & Fitness Centre, was ranked among the world's top 100 by German *Vogue* magazine in 1998, and Best Fitness Centre 2001 by *Gala*, a German weekly magazine.

The centre, designed around a series of lavish sunken pools complete with ornate columns, mosaics and sculptures, recalls the grand baths that typified the heyday of ancient Rome. The *pièce de résistance* is the indoor swimming pool where you can bask by the comforting warmth of a pinewood fire after a daily swim. Adjoining it is a smaller pool divided into a hot section and a cold section, linked by a narrow stone path dubbed the Japanese Walk. Alternating between the hot and cold pools boosts your body's circulation.

Unknot tired muscles with body treatments, or enhance your complexion with a series of anti-ageing treatments from La Prairie, a brand that marries luxury with scientific advancements. The centre's most indulgent treatments, using La Prairie's top-of-the-line Caviar Collection of skin products, revolve around the delicacy of kings—caviar. Caviar extracts—prized for their lifting, illuminating and moisturising properties—and seaweed proteins are used in Skin Caviar, a 90-minute facial that brightens and freshens the skin,

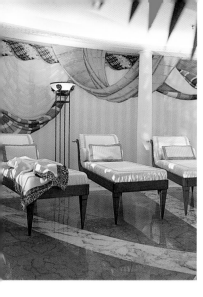

OPPOSITE: *Rome's ancient bathing heritage is reflected in the centre's sunken hot and cold baths. Bathing in them is to heed the saying, 'when in Rome, do as the Romans do'.*

LEFT: *The Roman-styled relaxation and meditation area overlooks the Turkish baths.*

BOTTOM: *At the indoor pool, you can soak up some sun under the glass cupola, get a hydro-massage under the spouted waterfall, or warm up by the antique fireplace.*

and Caviar Skin Toning, a 90-minute firming body treatment described as extreme luxury.

To complement your pursuit of health and beauty, feed your body with a light, healthy selection of Mediterranean food and fresh juices at the centre's Health Bar, or tone it in the gym, cardio room or Life Circuit. While working your way through the latter—an 800-metre (875-yard) route that winds through the hotel's park with fitness stations at intervals—you can feast your eyes on and feed your soul with the beauty of the natural surrounds and a view of the Eternal City.

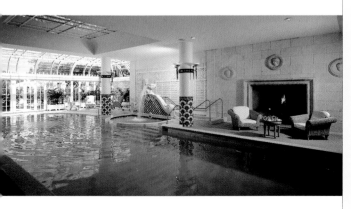

Spa Statistics

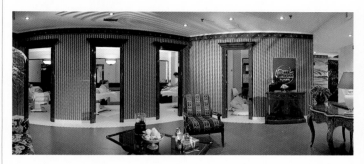

TYPE OF SPA
Hotel spa

SPA AREA
2,100 sq m (22,600 sq ft)

FACILITIES
6 single indoor treatment rooms; 1 consultation room; 1 meditation/relaxation room; 1 cold plunge pool, 2 jacuzzis, 2 whirlpools; 2 saunas, 1 steam room; 1 solarium, 2 sunbeds; 1 nail salon; 1 aerobics studio, 1 cardio studio, 1 gymnasium, 1 Pilates studio; 1 indoor swimming pool, 2 outdoor swimming pools; 1 spa boutique

SIGNATURE TREATMENT
Caviar Skin Toning, Skin Caviar

TREATMENTS & THERAPIES
Anti-ageing treatments, anti-cellulite treatments, body bronzing, body scrubs, bust treatments, eye treatments, facials, firming and slimming treatments, hand and foot treatments, lymphatic drainage, make-up services, manicures and pedicures, massages, movement therapies, purifying back treatments, reflexology, waxing; spa packages

SPA CUISINE
A healthy and light selection of Mediterranean dishes (low in calories, cholesterol, fat and sodium), vegetarian meals, energy-giving fruit juices and other refreshments are available at the Health Bar in the spa centre.

ACTIVITIES & PROGRAMMES
Aerobics, aquaerobics, golf, Pilates, spinning, tennis; massage and stretching classes

SERVICES
Medical consultation, nutritional consultation; personal training; baby-sitting, childcare; corporate programmes; gift certificates; day-use rooms; free shuttle bus to city centre

LANGUAGES SPOKEN BY THERAPISTS
English, French, Italian

ADMISSION
The centre is for the exclusive use of hotel guests and members.

CONTACT
Rome Cavalieri Hilton
Via Cadlolo 101
00136 Rome
Italy
T: +39 06 350 91
F: +39 06 3509 2241
E: info@cavalieri-hilton.it
W: www.cavalieri-hilton.it

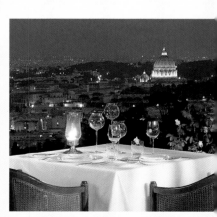

TOP: *Within the opulent spa, you can enjoy a cosmopolitan range of treatments including a Shiatzu Massage, Ayurvedic Massage and Lymph-Drainage Massage.*

ABOVE: *At La Pergola, diners can gaze at St Peter's dome while savouring the Michelin-starred cuisine.*

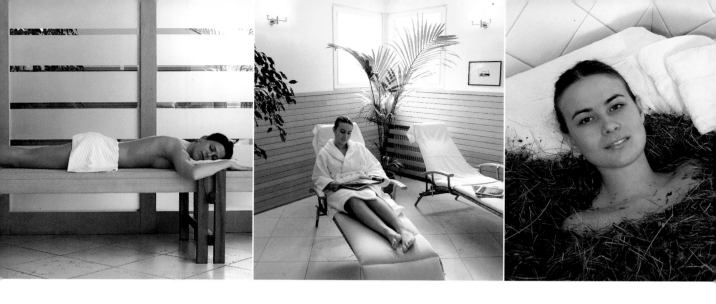

Heubad at Hotel Heubad
South Tyrol, Italy

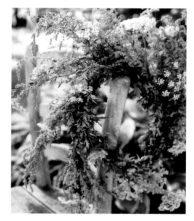

ABOVE: *Guests can enjoy the fresh air and fragrance of the blooms around the 80-bed hotel, which is situated at the foot of the Schlern mountains.*

OPPOSITE, BOTTOM: *The elegant indoor swimming pool offers a panoramic view over a church tower and beyond, and is especially beautiful at sunset. You can catch some rays from its sun terrace, though on a lazy summer day, you may want to enjoy the outdoor pool that is encircled by a floral garden.*

Nature lovers and history buffs are among the guests drawn to the Hotel Heubad (German for 'hay bath') which is set among the picturesque pastures, forests and mountains of northern Italy's south Tyrol region. Visitors to the area can enjoy the fresh air and the calming songs of nature on long walks and hikes, and admire quaint cottages as well as Prösels Castle, a medieval fortress that is renowned for its weapons collection. Like its surrounds, the 43-room hotel retains much of its rustic character. The hotel also possesses the intimacy and warmth only possible in a family-run establishment.

Approaching the hotel, you are likely to notice the fragrance of fresh hay—a clue to the hotel's provenance as the home of the hay bath. The property was founded over a century ago in 1903 when Anton Kompatscher (the forefather of its current owners), together with Dr Josef Clara, a local doctor who provided medical and financial backing, began a guest house and hay bath station. The surrounding meadows of the Dolomites, some 2 kilometres (1 mile) above sea level, offered the ideal conditions for growing the ingredients needed in the hay bath. Here at altitude, the fresh air and sunshine nourished the right combination of beneficial flowers and herbs.

The Hay Bath remains the establishment's signature treatment. Today, this takes place at Heubad, the hotel's modern spa, connected to the indoor swimming pool. In Anton's time, the hay bath could only be enjoyed briefly after the July harvest. However, in 1991, Marie Kompatscher, Anton's granddaughter-in-law, developed a method for the hay bath to be enjoyed hygienically and attractively year-round.

To benefit fully from the hay bath, guests are recommended to have a hay bath and a massage each day for a week. Other treatments available in the spa include lymphatic drainage, underwater massage, and a range of beauty and grooming treatments. A beauty treatment package—which includes two hay baths, two massages, a facial, a pedicure and use of the solarium, swimming pool, sauna and steam bath—is also available.

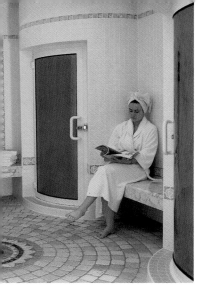

OPPOSITE, LEFT: *The spa area, screened by frosted glass panels, is bathed in natural light.*

OPPOSITE, CENTRE: *In between treatments, rest at the relaxation lounge, or flip through some magazines.*

OPPOSITE, RIGHT: *To have a hay bath at Heubad is to experience a tradition that has been practised onsite for over 100 years. The hay used is gathered only in July, the prime time for harvest. It is then stored in barns until it is required for use.*

LEFT: *The sauna and two steam baths are situated next to the indoor pool.*

Spa Statistics

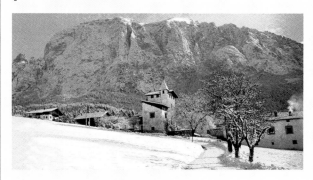

TYPE OF SPA
Hotel spa

SPA AREA
300 sq m (3,230 sq ft)

FACILITIES
7 single treatment rooms; 1 relaxation lounge; 1 cold plunge pool; 1 sauna, 2 steam rooms; 1 solarium; 1 nail salon; 1 gymnasium; 1 indoor swimming pool, 1 outdoor swimming pool; 1 spa boutique; 1 library

SIGNATURE TREATMENTS
Hay Bath

TREATMENTS & THERAPIES
Anti-ageing treatments, anti-cellulite treatments, aromatherapy, baths, body bronzing, body scrubs, eye treatments, facials, hair treatments, hand and foot treatments, heat treatments, hydrotherapy, lymphatic drainage, manicures and pedicures, massages, reflexology, waxing; beauty treatment package

SPA CUISINE
A healthy selection of Mediterranean and local cuisine is available in the restaurant and dining room. Vegetarian meals are available on request.

ACTIVITIES & PROGRAMMES
Biking

SERVICES
Gift certificates

LANGUAGES SPOKEN BY THERAPISTS
Italian, German

ADMISSION
Membership is available, but not required for admission.

CONTACT
Hotel Heubad
Schlernstrasse 12
I-39050 Völs am Schelrn (BZ)
Italy
T: +39 0471 725 020
F: +39 0471 725 425
E: info@hotelheubad.com
W: www.hotelheubad.com

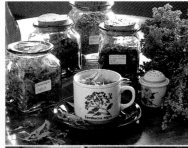

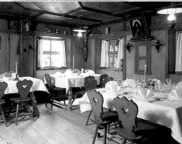

TOP: *A popular activity is climbing the Schlern mountains, pictured here with an old farm house in the foreground. The climb takes about 4 hours.*

CENTRE: *Before and after your spa treatment, you can enjoy special hay bath herbal tea brewed with herbs and wildflowers from the surrounding region.*

ABOVE: *Little pepper and salt are used in the dishes, so you can virtually taste the freshness of the local ingredients. Organic products harvested in South Tyrol are emphasised during a special culinary week in June. The other special culinary week held in October focuses on traditional local fare.*

Mementos available from the spa boutique include herbal teas and Italian cosmetic products made from natural ingredients. The cookbook *Die Küche in Südtirol*, containing recipes by Anneliese Kompatscher, sister of the current owner, is an ideal culinary memento of your stay. Linen bags of hay are undoubtedly the most popular souvenirs; their lingering fragrance a reminder of a bath that is steeped in both nature and history.

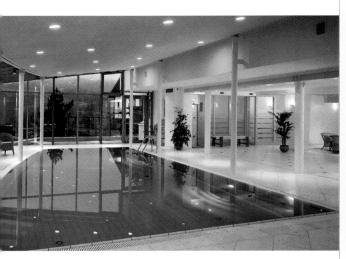

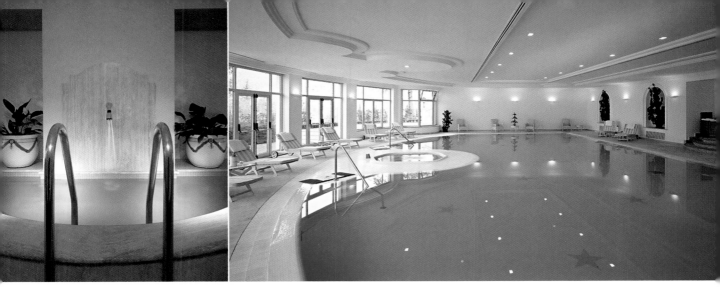

Medical Beauty Center
at Grand Hotel Palazzo della Fonte
Fiuggi, Italy

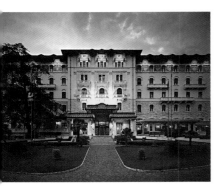

Behind the liberty-style façade (pictured) is an English-style manor resplendent in brocade curtains, antique carpets and Murano glass lamps. The 153 individually decorated rooms and suites are clad with wooden floors and floral wallpaper and boast over-sized marble bathrooms.

The elegant Grand Hotel Palazzo della Fonte is nestled between chestnut and oak trees in 6 hectares (15 acres) of private parkland 700 metres (2,300 feet) above sea level. Royalty and luminaries—who have included silver screen legend Ingrid Bergman and artist Pablo Picasso—are among those who have taken refuge in this sanctuary, 50 kilometres (31 miles) from Rome. The choice suite is the one inhabited by the King of Italy, Vittorio Emanuele III, in 1914, two years after the hotel opened its doors.

The history of the region is inextricably connected with healing waters in the area which cured Pope Bonifacio VIII of his kidney stones in the Middle Ages. Two centuries later, the great Italian artist Michelangelo Buonarotti famously quipped that its waters could 'crack open stone'.

The region's tranquillity, reflected in its name—which is derived from *'fiugy'*, dialect for the ferns that bring such freshness to the

area—extends to the Medical Beauty Center. Within this pastel-hued refuge on the lower ground floor of the hotel, you can refresh your body and mind with a range of tactile Oriental treatments and enhance your beauty with medical European therapies.

The treatment menu revolves around anti-ageing, de-stressing, slimming, toning, relaxing and beautifying. Packages range from two to seven nights, and focus on different goals. Treatments may also be enjoyed on an à la carte basis. The centre's wellness experts will be able to advise you on a course of treatments that best suits your needs, and personalise a diet according to your goals.

For treatments high on touch, opt for exotic massages such as the rejuvenating Ayurvedic Massage (which improves your body's defences and balances the body, mind, and spirit) and Shirodhara (a 'massage for the mind' which enhances the body's healing power, helps improve memory, and relieves

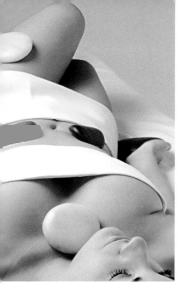

OPPOSITE, LEFT: *A cold plunge pool takes centrestage at the heat treatment area.*

OPPOSITE, RIGHT: *Various magazines have named the outdoor swimming pool, built in 1936, as one of the finest in Europe; you can enjoy a refreshing swim from the end of May to the end of September. The heated indoor pool (pictured) can be enjoyed all year round.*

LEFT: *The spa's signature Stone Therapy uses warm basalt stones and hot essential oils to gently massage your body, harmonising your chakras, and balancing your emotional, mental and physical energies.*

mental tension and headaches). Classical European treatments include Mud Therapy and Thalassotherapy; each comprises a scrub using Apoterm (with clays and thermal water) from the Spanish Germaine de Capuccini range, a body wrap using Spa Marine products, and a massage with essential oils.

Treatments based on Western science include Dermosonic Body Treatment (a non-invasive ultrasound and subdermic therapy to reduce cellulite, stretch marks and scars). Other beauty therapies include Silkdermic Treatment, which uses microdermabrasion to refine the face or body. Medical beauty treatments include Biostimulation, in which an aesthetic surgeon will inject vitamins into your face to help regenerate the skin's collagen.

You can take home face and body products from Germaine de Capuccini at the spa boutique as well as Italian jewellery—gems to remind you of the importance of maintaining harmony in your life.

Spa Statistics

TYPE OF SPA
Hotel spa

SPA AREA
1,500 sq m (16,150 sq ft)

FACILITIES
9 single indoor rooms; 3 consultation rooms; 1 relaxation lounge; 2 cold plunge pools, 1 jacuzzi, 2 saunas, 2 steam rooms; 1 solarium, 1 sunbed; 1 make-up room, 1 nail salon; 1 cardio studio, 1 gymnasium; 1 indoor swimming pool, 1 outdoor swimming pool; 1 golf course (5 min from the hotel); 2 tennis courts; 1 spa boutique

SIGNATURE TREATMENTS
Aromatherapy Massage, Ayurvedic Massage, Shiatsu Massage, Shirodhara, Stone Therapy, Thalassotherapy, Mud Therapy

TREATMENTS & THERAPIES
Anti-ageing treatments, anti-cellulite treatments, aromatherapy, Ayurvedic treatments, body scrubs, body wraps, bust treatments, electrotherapy, eye treatments, facials, firming and slimming treatments, hand and foot treatments, hot stone therapies, lymphatic drainage, make-up services, manicures and pedicures, massages, purifying back treatments, reflexology, scalp treatments, thalassotherapy, waxing

SPA CUISINE
Savoia Restaurant serves Mediterranean specialities created from fresh, local ingredients. The menu makes provisions for

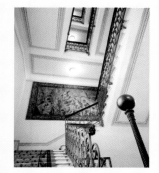

The grand hotel is furnished with valuable art pieces.

various dietary requirements, and the spa's nutritionists work with the chef to help you personalise a dietary plan for the duration of your stay.

ACTIVITIES & PROGRAMMES
Biking, bowls, golf, mini golf, horse riding, tennis, yoga; aqua gym classes

SERVICES
General healthcare, skincare and nutritional consultations; baby-sitting; free transfers to Rome

LANGUAGES SPOKEN BY THERAPISTS
English, Italian

CONTACT
Grand Hotel Palazzo della Fonte
Via dei Villini 7
03015 Fiuggi Fonte (FR)
Italy
T: +39 0775 548 043
F: +39 0775 506 752
E: mbc@palazzodellafonte.com
W: www.palazzodellafonte.com

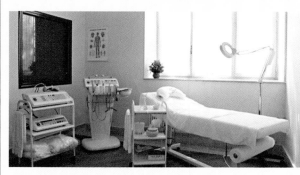

Treatment rooms exude a calm with their simplicity and functionality.

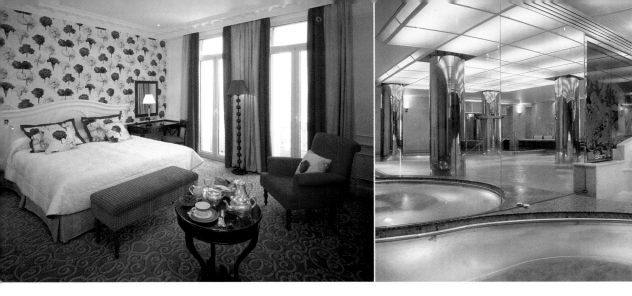

Les Thermes Marins de Monte-Carlo
Monte-Carlo, Monaco

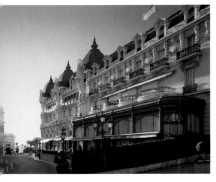

Built by Prince Charles III in 1864, the Hotel de Paris has come to be synonymous with the opulence and fine living standards of Monte-Carlo.

Monte-Carlo: the very name evokes a sense of opulence and refinement and an enduring image of wealth and prestige. The principality of Monaco has long provided the perfect excuse for 19th-century aristocrats and nobility, and today's rich and famous, to escape into the lifestyle that spells out privilege.

Monaco has also been blessed with an idyllic climate. It stands perfectly poised between mountains and the sea, where a special blend of air and sea currents produces the *'belle saison'*—a unique combination of 'being winter and spring'.

Quite fittingly, one of the world's first and most luxurious resorts was founded here in 1863—the Société des Bains de Mer. Today, this association is linked with some of the finest establishments worldwide, including the legendary Hotel de Paris and Les Thermes Marins de Monte-Carlo.

From the turn of the century up to the 1940s, Les Thermes Marins de Monte-Carlo was the European model of modern-day spa baths. In 1995, His Royal Highness, the Sovereign Prince Rainier III, sought a revival of Les Thermes Marins de Monte-Carlo, and thus, Les Thermes Marins de Monte-Carlo was newly and gloriously reborn.

Today, this spa centre—a transparent, light-filled oasis overlooking the Mediterranean Sea—has become the undisputed leader and innovator in seawater therapies, and a place where Monaco and its love affair with water have blossomed in splendour.

The marine therapists at Les Thermes Marins de Monte-Carlo believe in a holistic approach to wellness, so that every spa-goer can attain a perfect harmony between body and mind. The four simultaneous objectives of fitness, health, beauty and relaxation are achieved through the dedicated application of an overall care methodology.

Try a Seaweed Bath to experience the re-charging effect of trace elements reinforced by the use of ground seaweed. Or have two therapists work on you simultaneously with the Under Affusion Massage, rounding off with

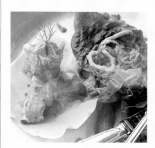

OPPOSITE, LEFT: *The Hotel Hermitage is a charming, timeless establishment with balconies looking over the sea. Guests staying here and at the Hotel de Paris have direct access to the spa.*

OPPOSITE, RIGHT: *The spa's indoor pool opens up to a spectacular solarium with a view. The spa's aqua-fitness centre is widely touted as one of the best in the world.*

LEFT: *The spa is located just behind the Monte-Carlo Casino and commands an outstanding view of the Monte-Carlo port.*

a fine shower of warm seawater combined with an essential oil massage.

You may also wish to awaken your body with one of the shower treatments. The Jet Shower, for example, provides a stimulating jet of seawater to give you a deep massage and firming treatment targeted at decongesting areas of fat and cellulite. This is the perfect remedy for your guilt after having satiated your taste buds at one of Monte-Carlo's many fine gourmet establishments.

To round off your day of self-pampering, book a session for yourself at the Beauty Salon, also managed by Les Thermes Marins de Monte-Carlo. This beauty institute has earned an international reputation with its special therapies such as Sea Peel and Facial Treatment With Ceramides. The therapists will make sure you feel right at home with the rich and the beautiful in Monte-Carlo.

The sun shines in Monte-Carlo for 310 days a year. In this sunshine land, there is only one thing for you to do—indulge your senses and pamper yourself through and through.

Spa Statistics

The chef at l'Hirondelle, the spa restaurant, works together with the spa's micro-nutritionist and dietician to create a menu that is light but packed with flavour.

TYPE OF SPA
Resort spa

SPA AREA
6,600 sq m (71,040 sq ft)

FACILITIES
47 single treatment rooms; 1 flotation chamber; 1 meditation room; 1 relaxation room; 2 consultation rooms; 1 cold plunge pool; 1 reflexology pool; 2 saunas; 1 steam room; 1 solarium; 1 sunbed; 2 labyrinths (connecting the spa to the Hotel de Paris and the Hotel Hermitage); 1 beauty salon; 1 gymnasium; 1 cardio studio; 1 aerobics studio; 2 indoor swimming pools; 1 golf course; 1 tennis court; 1 squash court; 1 spa boutique

SIGNATURE TREATMENTS
Combine Monte-Carlo, Jet Shower, Marine Aerosol, Massage Monte-Carlo, Maxi-Mineral Treatment, Seaweed Bath, Slim Tonic Treatment, Under Affusion Massage

TREATMENTS & THERAPIES
Anti-ageing treatments, anti-cellulite treatments, aqua therapy, aromatherapy, Ayurveda, baths, body bronzing, body scrubs, body wraps, bust treatments, Chinese treatments, electrotherapy, facials, firming and slimming treatments, flotation, hair treatments, hand and foot treatments, heat treatments, holistic treatments, hot stone therapies, hydrotherapy, Indonesian therapies, inhalation therapies, jet lag treatments, lymphatic drainage, make-up services, manicure and pedicure, massages, movement therapies, pre- and post-natal treatments, purifying back treatments, reflexology, salon services, scalp treatments, Thai therapies, thalassotherapy, waxing

SPA CUISINE
Les Thermes Marins de Monte-Carlo's low-calorie restaurant, the l'Hirondelle, offers a '*menu du marche*'. It is considered one of the best representatives of low-calorie cuisine in Europe.

ACTIVITIES & PROGRAMMES
Aerobics, aquaerobics, golf, *tai chi*, tennis, yoga, dance, make-up services, meditation

SERVICES
Consultation for body composition analysis, general healthcare, skincare, nutrition; endermology medical test, weight loss strategy test, neurotransmitter test, saliva hormone test, homocysteine assay, oxidised anti-LDL antibody assay, vitamin E assay E, micro-nutritional profile, stress test; personal training; gift certificates

LANGUAGES SPOKEN BY THERAPISTS
English, French, Italian

ADMISSION
Membership is available but not required for admission.

CONTACT
Les Thermes Marins de Monte-Carlo
2, Avenue de Monte-Carlo
MC 98000
Monaco
T: +377 9216 4946
F: +377 9216 4949
E: thermes@sbm.mc
W: www.montecarlospa.com

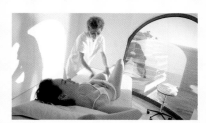

The spa offers a variety of packages such as a six-day Azur Tonic Program, six-day Stress Control Program, and a two-day Mini Wellbeing And Beauty Program, each with a minimum of four treatments a day.

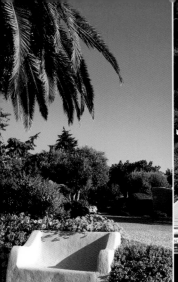
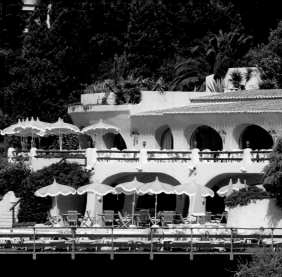
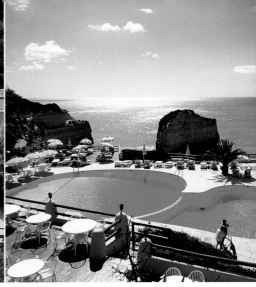

Vilalara at Sofitel Thalassa Vilalara
Lagoa, Portugal

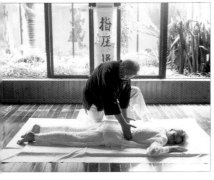

ABOVE: *Eastern healing modalities such as* reiki *and shiatsu (pictured) complement the centre's thalasso cures, and introduce a touch of the exotic.*

OPPOSITE, BOTTOM: *In the thalasso centre's dynamic pool, aquatic exercises are performed as part of the Vilalara Thalassotherapy Programme.*

A colourful and fragrant 10.5-hectare (25-acre) botanical paradise perched above the sandstone cliffs of Portugal's southern coast is peppered with the sinuously curved low-rise buildings that make up the five-star Sofitel Thalassa Vilalara. Guests attracted to water have many ways to enjoy this element, along with the warmth of over 300 days of sunshine per year. There are five outdoor swimming pools, including a separately located one for families and a main seawater pool overlooking the beach. The other three pools are located adjacent to the thalassotherapy centre.

The resort opened in 1967, and two decades later in 1989, Vilalara—the thalassotherapy centre—opened to treat its first guest. The centre's interior is a cavern of mosaics depicting shells and other motifs related to the sea, reflecting the centre's thalasso programmes that focus on the systematic use of seawater and marine-derived ingredients, expertly and precisely administered to ensure an effective cure.

A Thalassotherapy Programme includes a compulsory consultation with the centre's physician who will prescribe a course of four to five treatments a day for six days, based on your needs and goals: these may focus on wellness, smoking-cessation, body shaping or cellulite-reduction. Your sessions, spread over alternating mornings and afternoons, comprise individualised treatment sessions in seaweed application chambers, baths, steam baths, footbaths and shower jets. Group sessions under the supervision of a physiotherapist are held in the centre's two large indoor swimming pools: the jet stream pool (a pool of water jets that you direct to the upper and lower parts of your body), and the dynamic pool where aqua exercises are performed.

The thalasso centre also includes a gym for guests wanting a workout. Guests seeking something different can rebalance their bodies and minds with a range of complementary therapies such as *reiki* and shiatsu from Japan, and beauty services. These are available on an à la carte basis.

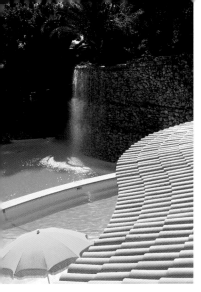

OPPOSITE, LEFT: *The low-rise buildings are nestled in colourful gardens.*

OPPOSITE, CENTRE AND RIGHT: *The restaurants overlook the pool and beyond, a sandy cove of ochre sandstone formations that typify the beauty of Portugal's Algarve region.*

LEFT: *The trio of pools fronting the thalasso centre includes a freshwater grotto, a comfortably heated seawater pool that can be used all year round, and a waterfall pool where you can keep cool during the summer months.*

Spa Statistics

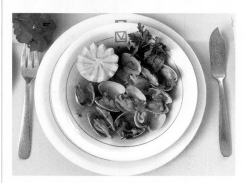

The gastronomic Vilalara Restaurant makes full use of fresh local produce, especially seafood, in its regional specialities such as the 'clam cataplana'. There is also a dietetic restaurant where healthy dishes of 400 calories each are served for guests watching their waistlines.

If your goal is to lose weight, your diet will be limited to 1,000 calories a day, with your lunches and dinners taking place at the 'dietetic restaurant'. A hearty buffet breakfast can be enjoyed in the sunny conservatory-styled breakfast room above the thalasso centre; here a good selection of healthy options is clearly marked out.

To complement its cures for the body, the hotel organises innovative events—such as jazz nights and admiring the starry skies with the help of renowned astronomers—to feed your mind and soul.

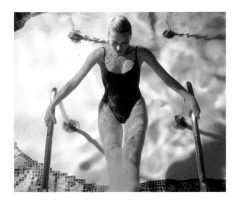

TYPE OF SPA
Thalasso centre

SPA AREA
2,800 sq m (30,140 sq ft)

FACILITIES
20 single treatment rooms for thalassotherapy, 1 pressotherapy room, 1 osteopathy room; 2 consultation rooms; 2 saunas, 1 steam bath; 1 beauty parlour; 1 aerobics studio, 1 gymnasium; 3 indoor dynamic pools (for thalassotherapy); 3 outdoor fresh water pools, 2 outdoor seawater pools (1 heated year-round); 6 tennis courts; 1 spa boutique

SIGNATURE TREATMENTS
18 thalasso treatments

TREATMENTS & THERAPIES
Anti-smoking treatments, anti-cellulite treatments, aqua therapy, baths, body scrubs, body wraps (algae), facials, firming and slimming treatments, hair treatments, hand and foot treatments, holistic treatments, hot stone massage, hydrotherapy, inhalation therapies, lymphatic drainage, manicures and pedicures, massages, reflexology, *reiki*, thalassotherapy. The basic Thalassotherapy Programme, Into Shape, includes 7 nights accommodation, dietetic meals (1,000 calories per day), checkup with spa physician, 24 thalasso treatments, mineral water, a gift and free use of several facilities.

SPA CUISINE
A calorie-controlled diet is available at the Dietetique Restaurant. A healthy selection in the breakfast buffet is available at the breakfast room and terrace above the thalasso centre. Beverages such as teas and juices are available at the Thalasso Bar in the thalassotherapy centre.

ACTIVITIES & PROGRAMMES
Aerobics, aquaerobics, biking, golf, horse riding, petanque, sailing, scuba diving, snorkelling, *tai qi*, tennis, yoga; sports instruction, stretching classes; jazz festivals under the stars in spring, and musical entertainment that includes Portuguese 'Fado' from April to October

SERVICES
Baby-sitting, childcare (from April to October for 5 to 12 year olds); complimentary mineral water during meals and a daily bottle in the room

LANGUAGES SPOKEN BY THERAPISTS
English, French, German, Portuguese, Russian, Spanish

ADMISSION
Priority is given to hotel residents. The thalasso centre is closed on Sundays.

CONTACT
Sofitel Thalassa Vilalara
Praia das Gaivotas
Alporchinhos-Porches
8400-450 Lagoa
Algarve
Portugal
T: +351 282 320 000
F: +351 282 320 077
E: h2987@accor-hotels.com
W: www.thalassa.com or
www.sofitelvilalara.com

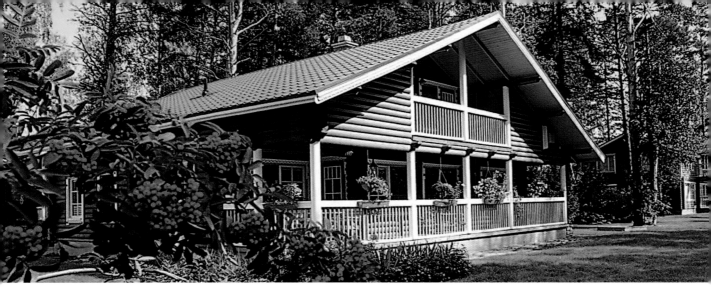

Guerlain Beauty Studio & Spa
at Le Meridien Moscow Country Club
Moscow, Russia

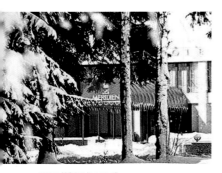

ABOVE: *Winter is one of the most beautiful seasons to visit.*

OPPOSITE, BOTTOM: *The hotel also offers a range of modern conference facilities; the most intimate being the rustically decorated Club House that is set within a log cabin complete with a fireplace.*

Artistes such as tenor Nickolay Baskov and actress Larissa Udovichenko are among prominent Russians who have recently checked into the five-star Le Meridien Moscow Country Club. Just 45 minutes, but a world away from the Red Square and the Kremlin, the property is set within a 120-hectare (297-acre) birch forest.

In the summer months, you can occupy your hours with a battle on the paintball range, scale a climbing wall, or enjoy the sun and surrounding beauty on the lakeside beach while watching pleasure-seekers rowing boats or attempting to fish for their own supper. You may also spot Russian politicians teeing off on the 18-hole golf course designed by Robert Trent Jones Jr. In winter, golf clubs and balls are replaced by snowmobiles, dog sleigh races and cross-country skiing.

To reward yourself after a session of activity, or to pamper yourself, visit the Guerlain Beauty Studio & Spa, a pastel-hued space fragranced by delicate floral scents, and graced with relaxing Oriental instrumental music.

To re-energise your body after sports, opt for an After Sporting Activity (to help eliminate toxins and re-energise you) or a Special Sporting Activity such as Leg Lightness (to bring relief to heavy or swollen legs), which combines massages and hydrotherapy. For a pampering treat, opt for the popular one-hour Facial Guerlain that includes a massage to aid the deep cleansing of the skin.

Besides facials, massages and self-tanning treatments that revolve around the French luxury brand Guerlain, the spa menu includes treatments based on Biosel products, which combine the Asian concept of energy with the traditional European use of ingredients from the sea. To ease tension, book the Comfort Anti-Stress Body Treatment With Oligo-Elements, which includes a rejuvenating massage and hydrotherapy session. To refine your skin and figure, go for the Special

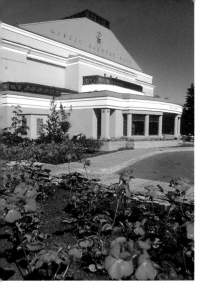

OPPOSITE: *In addition to the hotel's 131 rooms and suites (some with private jacuzzis and saunas), the property is peppered with charming red-roofed timber dachas or vacation cottages (pictured).*

LEFT: *The spa and health facilities are housed in the sports centre (pictured), a hub of social activity where you can have a game of indoor tennis, work out in the gymnasium, or relax after training at the Sports Bar & Café.*

Light Cellulitis Body Care, which involves massage and hydrotherapy. You can then adjourn to the Happy Bar to quench your thirst with freshly squeezed fruit juices.

However, you cannot claim to have been to Russia until you have relaxed your body in the heat of the *bania* and been whipped with a *vennik* by the bathhouse attendant. The attendant has a regular following of clients, and has become as much a feature of the spa as the *bania* is a feature in Russian life.

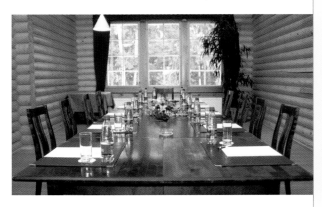

Spa Statistics

TYPE OF SPA
Hotel spa

SPA AREA
300 sq m (3,230 sq ft)

FACILITIES
6 single treatment rooms (1 with bathtub); 1 relaxation lounge; 1 Guerlain facial room; 1 jacuzzi; 2 saunas, 1 steam room; 1 solarium; 1 hair salon, 1 nail salon, 1 Guerlain make-up stand; 1 aerobics studio, 1 cardio studio, 1 gymnasium; 1 children's pool, 1 indoor swimming pool with hydro-massage waterfall; 1 mini football field; 1 outdoor swimming pool; 1 golf course; 1 jogging route (4 km/2.5 miles); 2 indoor tennis courts, 3 outdoor tennis courts, 1 squash court; 1 universal hall for mini football, basketball or volleyball; 1 bar; 1 Guerlain bijoux boutique, 1 spa boutique

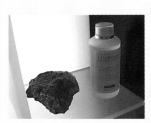

Treatments revolve around face and body products and methods from France's Guerlain and Italy's Biosel. The latter harness natural products from the sea with energetic techniques to enhance balance and wellbeing.

SIGNATURE TREATMENTS
Comfort Anti-Stress Body Treatment With Oligo-Elements, Facial Guerlain, Special Light Cellulitis Body Care

TREATMENTS & THERAPIES
Anti-ageing treatments, anti-cellulite treatments, aqua therapy, aromatherapy, baths, body scrubs, body wraps, bust treatments, facials, firming and slimming treatments, hair treatments, hand and foot treatments, hydrotherapy, jet lag treatments, lymphatic drainage, make-up services, massages, manicures and pedicures, purifying back treatments, waxing; half- or full-day spa programmes

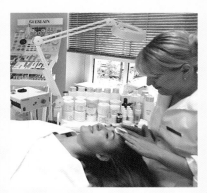

Rejuvenate your skin and relax your body under the pampering hands of the therapists.

PROVISIONS FOR COUPLES
Le Meridien Spa Breaks (packages for two that include accommodation, and body and face treatments)

SPA CUISINE
Freshly squeezed juices, teas and coffees are available at the Happy Bar in the spa. Healthy and light snacks, salads and fruit are available at the Sports Bar & Café. Vegetarian options are available on the menu.

ACTIVITIES & PROGRAMMES
Aerobics, basketball, biking, fencing (on request), golf, horse riding (15 minutes from the resort), mini football, tennis, squash, volleyball; cooking and dance lessons (on request), massage, nailcare and stretching classes; sports instruction

SERVICES
Skincare consultation; private spa parties; baby-sitting; corporate programmes, gift certificates; day-use rooms, free transfers to nearby towns and to the airport

LANGUAGES SPOKEN BY THERAPISTS
English, Russian

CONTACT
Le Meridien Moscow Country Club
Nakhabino, Krasnogorsky District
Moscow Region 143430
Russia
T: +7 095 926 5911
F: +7 095 926 5921
E: le.meridien@mcc.co.ru
W: www.lemeridien-mcc.com

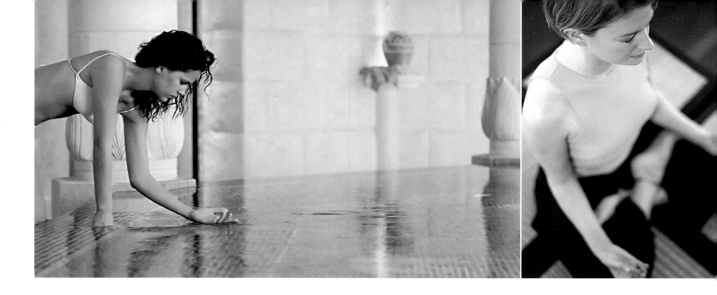

Altira Spa at Mardavall Hotel & Spa
Mallorca, Spain

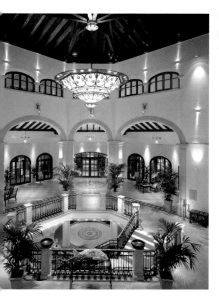

ABOVE: *The hotel is built in a style that typifies the region. The fountain, located by the hotel's main entrance, hints at the tranquillity within.*

OPPOSITE, BOTTOM: *The indoor pool, heated to a comfortable 28 degrees Celsius (82 degrees Fahrenheit), provides ample space for exercise and lounging around.*

Lovers of the sea gravitate to the Mardavall Hotel & Spa, which looks out to the Mediterranean Sea. The hotel, just a few minutes walk from the marina of Puerto Portals, is also a virtual art gallery, with corridors and guest rooms adorned by works of art by contemporary artists who have been inspired by the beauty of the region.

Spa-goers in their quest for health, beauty and serenity can find them all here in the hotel's luxurious Altira Spa: a jewel in the Starwood Spa Collection, which is named after the ancient Greek goddesses of healing (Althea) and beauty (Saphira).

Treatments and therapies designed to soothe and heal are inspired by natural healing methods from around the globe. There is a strong emphasis here on therapies based on Chinese medicine. Treatments such as Acupuncture, Moxibustion or Auriculotherapy are all preceded by personal consultation and supervised by experienced international practitioners. Herbal secrets dating back thousands of years are made relevant to your lifestyle via Oriental Phytotherapy, during which a Chinese physician will prescribe a traditional Chinese herbal recipe or a customised infusion to suit your needs.

In the summer and autumn months, you can enjoy treatments such as Acupuncture and certain massages in the outdoor treatment pavilion in a lovely Mediterranean garden setting. The area contains outdoor pools, and a relaxation room with eight waterbeds. Activities such as Pilates, *tai ji*, yoga and water workouts also take place in this area.

The spa also offers thalasso treatments and packages that harness the healing benefits of ingredients derived from pure marine extracts. One of the most popular, the Thalasso Seaweed Freshness For Legs treatment, relieves heavy, tired legs and is energy-restoring.

Value for money Beauty & Wellness Packages lasting from half a day to five days focus on your goals and interests, such as de-stressing, beauty and body shaping. Three-day programmes that focus on goals

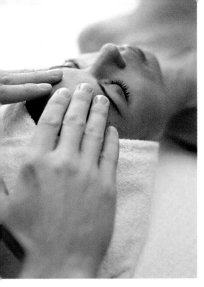

OPPOSITE, LEFT: *Water Balancing, an aquatic massage developed in the USA, takes places in this opulent saltwater pool that combines the mystique of Rome, Egypt and Japan in its décor.*

OPPOSITE, RIGHT: *The spa's wellness mantra, 'the art of doing nothing', borrows from the Chinese phrase 'wei wu wei'. Enjoy a massage, or balance your body and mind with exercises such as tai ji or yoga (pictured).*

LEFT: *If you have only 30 minutes to spare, opt for Stress Recovery Massage (based on Swedish techniques) or Face, Head and Scalp (a pressure point massage).*

Spa Statistics

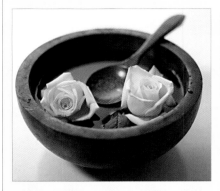

Altira's name, derived from the names of the goddesses of health and beauty, is also symbolic of its mission to heal the body and soothe the soul within beautiful surroundings, using luxurious treatments.

such as relaxation, slimming or enhancing circulation are preceded by a medical examination, and include a daily healthy lunch.

Your treatments may also include Water Balancing—a unique water and sound experience. As your body is buoyed by saltwater, and supported by the nurturing touch of your therapist, the calming underwater music contributes to a relaxing, surreal experience that helps rebalance your entire being.

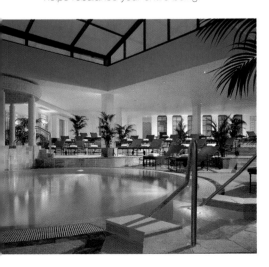

TYPE OF SPA
Hotel spa

SPA AREA
4,700 sq m (50,590 sq ft)

FACILITIES
1 double treatment suite, 1 outdoor treatment pavilion, 3 double treatment rooms, 1 shiatsu room, 7 single treatment rooms; 1 consultation room, 1 relaxation area with 8 waterbeds; 1 jacuzzi; 1 stone sauna, 1 steam room; 2 solariums; 1 hair salon; 1 gymnasium, 1 Pilates studio; 2 indoor swimming pools, 2 outdoor swimming pools; 2 golf courses (10-min drive); 1 spa boutique

SIGNATURE TREATMENTS
Acupuncture Sessions with Consultation, Ayurveda, 'Chinese Medicine' Treatments, thalasso baths and wraps

TREATMENTS & THERAPIES
Acupuncture, anti-cellulite treatments, aqua therapy, aromatherapy, baths, body scrubs, body wraps, bust treatments, Chinese therapies, facials, firming and slimming treatments, hand and foot treatments, hydrotherapy, lymphatic drainage, make-up services, manicures and pedicures, massages, pre- and post-natal treatments, reflexology, scalp treatments, thalassotherapy, waxing. Half-, 1-, 2-, 3-, 5-day spa packages that include treatments and Health Lunch are available.

PROVISIONS FOR COUPLES
1 double treatment suite; 2 double treatment rooms; Couples Massage Of Your Choice

SPA CUISINE
Not available, but provisions for various dietary requirements are available on request.

ACTIVITIES & PROGRAMMES
Aquaerobics, biking, golf, hiking, jogging, Pilates, power walking, *tai ji*, yoga

SERVICES
Personal training; baby-sitting, childcare; corporate programmes; private spa parties; gift certificates; day-use rooms; personal butler service

LANGUAGES SPOKEN BY THERAPISTS
English, German, Spanish

ADMISSION
Membership is available but not required for admission. Non-hotel guests not accompanied by a member pay a day entrance fee to use certain facilities if they are not having a treatment.

CONTACT
Mardavall Hotel & Spa
Passeig Calviá
E-07181 Costa d'en Blanes
Calviá, Palma de Mallorca
Spain
T: +34 (0)971 629 600
F: +34 (0)971 629 602
E: spa@mardavall-hotel.com
W: www.mardavall-hotel.com

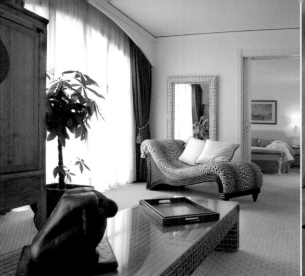
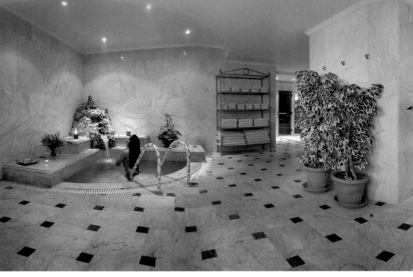

Serenity Spa at Las Dunas Beach Hotel & Spa
Marbella, Spain

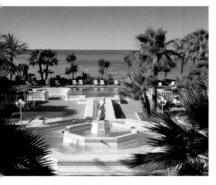

Las Dunas Hotel offers views that span the beaches and the Mediterranean Sea. Day trips can be arranged to the surrounding areas, with their picturesque whitewashed villages and ancient ruins.

Situated right on the stretch of beach between the towns of Marbella and Estepona on Costa del Sol, the Las Dunas Beach Hotel & Spa offers a unique brand of Andalucian hospitality.

Its location represents a special blend of flavours—somewhere between the glitz of Marbella, with its luxury hotels and wealthy tourists, and the more down-to-earth, pueblo charm of Estepona, a former fishing village and farming community that is developing into a quieter holiday resort. Admirably, Las Dunas Beach Hotel & Spa has managed to embrace and capture the uniquely contrasting characters of these two towns.

Andalucians are known for their love of colour, music, socialising, pageants, and partying. This is best reflected in their exuberant local fiestas. The flamingo-coloured Las Dunas Beach Hotel—built in the style of a Spanish hacienda—is a showcase of this exuberance, where guests are treated to magnificently decorated trompe l'oeil murals and where the hotel's Moorish influence is displayed in the landscaped gardens surrounding an ornate traditional Spanish fountain. While it's not quite the Alhambra, Las Dunas does treat its guests to a substantial serving of luxury and style.

The Serenity Spa invites you into an oasis beautifully decorated in honey-coloured marble with black marble detailing. Known for its treatments blending Oriental therapies with Western philosophies, the spa offers a range of innovative face and body treatments, massage therapies and thalassotherapy.

The body treatments, in particular, are a study in exotica. Lime and ginger are used to exfoliate and invigorate the face and body; frangipani oil is concocted into a deliciously comforting body wrap; and a traditional Balinese recipe uses coconut and milk to gently polish and hydrate your skin.

There is even a Strawberry Back Cleanse that promises to leave the skin radiant and glowing—the perfect facial for your back!

Within the spa's range of packages, there is something to suit every itinerary. If you are

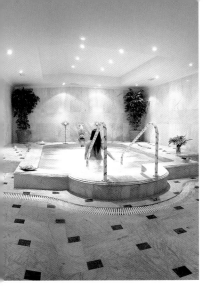

OPPOSITE, LEFT: *The hotel houses 73 rooms and suites. Many of the rooms feature outstanding creations by Belgian artist Marie de Troostembergh.*

LEFT: *The spa has a large jacuzzi, footbaths, a cold plunge pool and a fully equipped gymnasium, and is located next door to the outdoor swimming pool.*

at the hotel for the weekend, for example, you can choose the Oriental package—a favourite treatment of Las Dunas spa-goers, and a truly revitalising experience. You can choose either a Thai or Shiatsu Massage, followed by the Smoothing Body Treatment, a Stress Relieving Body Treatment, a Purifying Facial and a reflexology session.

But if you have three to four days to spend, then by all means take the opportunity of pampering yourself to the fullest, and opt for the Harmony For Body And Soul Package. This includes the Smoothing Body Treatment and Purifying Facial, plus Manual Lymphatic Drainage, Cranial Facial Massage, a stress-relieving Back Massage, a deliciously relaxing and restorative Aromatherapy Massage and a reflexology session.

Whether you are at the Las Dunas Hotel to attend one of the colourful local fiestas or to indulge in its pleasurable spa packages, you will also most certainly be intrigued and touched by the warmth of the Andalucian people and all that the region has to offer.

Spa Statistics

TYPE OF SPA
Hotel spa

SPA AREA
320 sq m (3,440 sq ft)

FACILITIES
5 single indoor treatment rooms; 1 meditation room, 1 relaxation room; 1 cold plunge pool, 1 jacuzzi; 1 sauna; 1 hair salon, 1 nail salon; 1 gymnasium; 1 outdoor swimming pool; 1 golf course; 1 spa boutique selling Elemis and Guinot products

SIGNATURE TREATMENTS
American Body Wrap, Exotic Coconut Rub and Milk Wrap, Exotic Lime And Ginger Scrub, Well Being Massage

TREATMENTS & THERAPIES
Anti-ageing treatments, anti-cellulite treatments, aqua therapy, aromatherapy, baths, body bronzing, body scrubs, body wraps, bust treatments, eye treatments, facials, firming and slimming treatments, hand and foot treatments, heat treatments, hydrotherapy, lymphatic drainage, manicures and pedicures, massages, movement therapies, purifying back treatments, reflexology, salon services, Thai therapies, thalassotherapy, waxing

SPA PACKAGES
Harmony For Body And Soul, Intensive Anti-Cellulite Week, Jet Set Pack (providing for stays of 1 to 7 days), Stress Relief Weekend, Oriental Pack

SPA CUISINE
Available only on request

ACTIVITIES & PROGRAMMES
Golf, hiking, horse riding

SERVICES
Body composition analysis, general healthcare consultation, skin care consultation; baby-sitting, childcare; gift certificates; day-use rooms

LANGUAGES SPOKEN BY THERAPISTS
English, French, German, Italian, Spanish

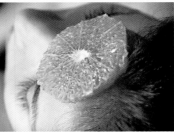

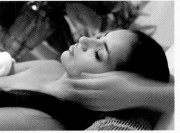

The Serenity Spa offers an à la carte menu featuring eight different facials using top-range Elemis and Guinot products. The most exclusive face treatment is the Elemis Japanese Silk Booster Facial that takes your skin on a journey of total renewal.

ADMISSION
Guests under 16 years of age are not allowed in the spa.

CONTACT
Las Dunas Beach Hotel & Spa
La Boladilla Baja
Crta, Cadiz km 163 500
Estepona 29689
Marbella
Spain
T: +34 (0) 952 794345
F: +34 (0) 952 794825
E: spa@las-dunas.com
W: www.las-dunas.com

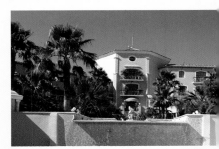

The hotel (pictured) is located near the coastal town of Marbella, a favourite playground of the rich and famous, and renowned for its greens. Guests at the Las Dunas hotel have privileged access to 40 golf courses in the area.

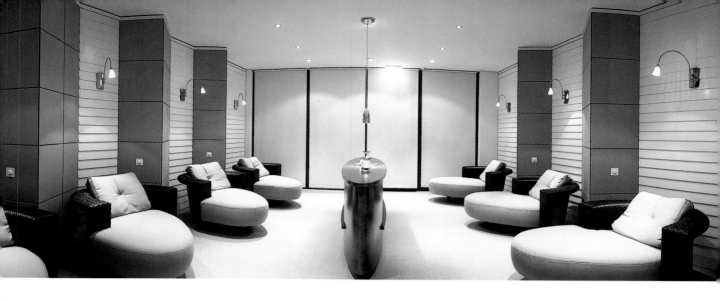

Amrita Wellness at Le Montreux Palace
Montreux, Switzerland

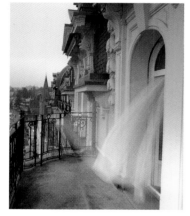

The graceful belle époque style hotel has been immortalised in silver screen classics such as Peter Ustinov's Lady L *starring Sophia Loren and David Niven, and Luc Besson's* Kiss the Dragon *with Jet Li and Bridget Fonda.*

Since 1906, Le Montreux Palace has been a dignified icon in the town that is known around the world for the Montreux Jazz Festival. The region, just an hour's drive from the Geneva airport in the heart of what is dubbed the Swiss Riviera, enjoys relatively mild winters. Illustrious personalities who have signed the guest ledger over the years include German composer Richard Strauss, American jazz great Miles Davis, and former President of the Soviet Union Mikhail Gorbachev.

Below the property's lush gardens is an underground passage that guests in pursuit of an integrated approach to relaxation, health, fitness and nutrition can follow to Amrita Wellness, a purpose-built sanctuary that has a spectacular view of Lac Lehman.

The spa's name comes from the Sanskrit term which means 'elixir of eternal youth'. Its selection of therapies—based on Ayurvedic principles, energy healing, and a blend of Western therapies—and the modern Zen décor harmoniously reflect the wellness centre's East meets West philosophy. The Ayurvedic focus is most evident in its nutritious and delicious spa meals, which are tailored to your *dosha* type.

The signature treatment, the Amrita Ayurvedic Mind & Body Rejuvenation, is a 90-minute session which comprises a gentle body massage, energetic foot stimulation and a *shirodhara* session, in which hot sesame oil is trickled on to your forehead.

Other therapies include classical Eastern massages such as Shiatsu and Tuina, and traditional European spa therapies that include Vichy showers, body scrubs, body wraps, facials, and a range of baths.

Guests who wish to take part in more active pursuits will find these in the centre's fitness area, which features cardio-machines with personal television screens; a training instructor will explain the correct use of equipment before you begin. The fitness area also includes an aerobics room where you can enjoy an energetic aerobics session, or gentler yoga, *qi gong* or *tai ji* classes.

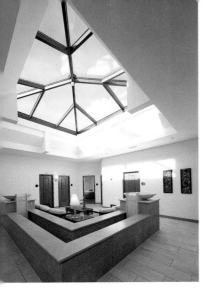

OPPOSITE: *Post-treatment, guests may relax with a healthy beverage at the juice bar, soak in the sun on the outdoor terrace, or luxuriate on designer space-age capsule-like loungers in the roomy relaxation area (pictured).*

LEFT: *The centre's décor revolves around natural elements such as stone, wood, marble, water and light.*

BOTTOM: *The wellness centre's outdoor pool on the lawn is only open during summer, but guests can use the indoor swimming pool (pictured) in all weather.*

Spa Statistics

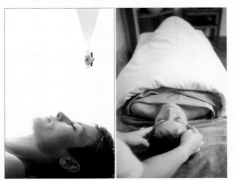

FAR LEFT: *The Amrita Ayurvedic Mind & Body Rejuvenation includes a mentally restorative shirodhara session in which hot oil is dripped and massaged on to your head.*

LEFT: *Treatments revolve around the product ranges from Amrita Private Label and Kerstian Florian. The former offers a blend of essential oils and Ayurvedic influences. The latter reflects the strong kur traditions of European spas, such as the moor mud wrap in the Thermal Contour Treatment (pictured).*

To round up a treatment, you can enjoy a fresh fruit or vegetable cocktail in the juice bar that overlooks the indoor and outdoor pools, and opens to a terrace in the summer.

The centre can tailor treatments to your goals—re-energising your body, calming your mind and spirit, losing weight or stopping smoking—and design customised wellness breaks around your needs and interests. Wellness packages with meals, board and treatments are also available.

TYPE OF SPA
Hotel spa

SPA AREA
1,935 sq m (20,830 sq ft)

FACILITIES
2 double treatment rooms, 1 single treatment rooms; 1 consultation room; 1 relaxation room; 2 cold plunge pools, 3 jacuzzis; 2 saunas, 3 steam rooms; 1 solarium; 1 hair salon; 1 aerobics studio, 1 cardio studio; 1 indoor swimming pool, 1 outdoor swimming pool; 1 golf course (15 km/9 miles from the hotel); 1 spa boutique

SIGNATURE TREATMENTS
Amrita Ayurvedic Mind & Body Rejuvenation, Amrita Elixir Of Youth

TREATMENTS & THERAPIES
Anti-ageing treatments, anti-cellulite treatments, aromatherapy, Ayurvedic treatments, baths, body scrubs, body wraps, Chinese therapies, eye treatments, facials, firming and slimming treatments, hand and foot treatments, hydrotherapy, jet lag treatments, lymphatic drainage, manicures and pedicures, massages, purifying back treatments, reflexology, waxing; 2-night Relaxation Deluxe package, 6-night Ayurveda Experience package, customised wellness breaks

PROVISIONS FOR COUPLES
2 double treatment rooms (including a VIP treatment room with bath and steam shower)

SPA CUISINE
Available at La Brasserie du Palace, and, in summertime, at La Terrasse du Petit Palais. Provisions for dietary requirements available on request. After an Ayurvedic consultation to determine your constitution, a nutrition programme is put in place to help restore balance within your body; information is also given on adapting your diet with the changing seasons.

ACTIVITIES & PROGRAMMES
Aerobics, aquaerobics, *qi gong, tai ji*, yoga

SERVICES
Acupuncture consultation, body composition analysis, medical consultation, naturopathy consultation, nutritional consultation, skincare consultation; personal training, back-training class; gift certificates; day-use rooms

LANGUAGES SPOKEN BY THERAPISTS
English, French, German

ADMISSION
The spa is open to hotel guests and members of the public. Six- or twelve-month memberships are available.

CONTACT
Le Montreux Palace
Grand-Rue 100
CH-1820, Montreux
Switzerland
T: +41 (0) 21 962 1212
F: +41 (0) 21 962 1717
E: amrita@montreux-palace.com
W: www.montreux-palace.com

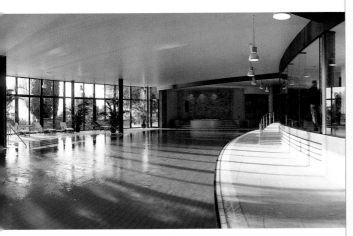

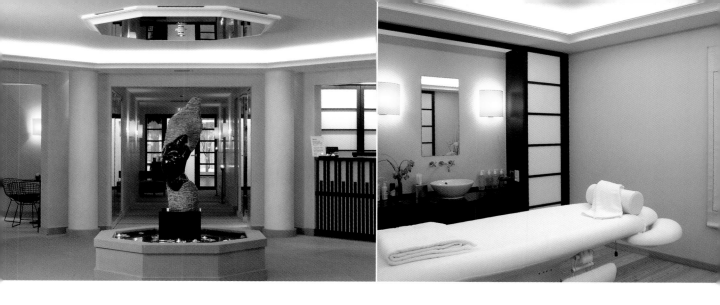

Bellevue Spa at Grand Hotel Bellevue
Saanenland, Switzerland

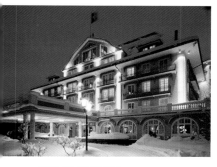

ABOVE: *The Grand Hotel Bellevue stands at the entrance to the village of Gstaad, Saanenland. The area straddles the geographic boundary between the German-speaking and French-speaking parts of Switzerland.*

OPPOSITE, BOTTOM: *The Japanese luxury steam bath can be enjoyed individually or with someone special. Top the session with a drink of Japanese Kombucha, a tea that is fast becoming a trendy beverage for the health-conscious. Legend has it that the Japanese emperor Inkyo took it to cure a severe attack of gastritis. 'Kombu' is the Japanese name of a brown mushroom used to make the tea.*

The setting of the picturesque village of Gstaad is one that seems determinedly cheerful and good-natured. In its surrounding swirl of hills and mountains, one can almost imagine a bevy of happy fairies sunning themselves in the gentle light.

Using light as its central theme, the rooms at the new Grand Hotel Bellevue are designed so as to be bathed in the generous sunlight of Saanenland. The hotel was opened in 2003 and stands in a magnificent parkland replete with mature trees. With just 35 rooms and suites, it excels in personalised service. Guests can choose from rooms or suites with views of a tower, the park or the forest.

The spa attached to the hotel offers a range of treatments that promises the best of East and West. The spa performs its signature Japanese luxury steam bath in a room fit for the most hardened sumo wrestler. The session starts with an aromatherapy steam bath to send you into a state of relaxed bliss. Next, you are ushered to a heated massage table for a special soap-brush massage. This is

followed by a dip in an ergonomically shaped whirlpool. Complete the session with an Asian massage on the Japanese tatami mat.

Another Oriental treat is the Rasul Ritual. A steam bath combines the three elements of water, fire and earth with aromatherapy, and the treatment begins by coating your body with a layer of mud, algae or chalk. Inhale the aromatic fragrances as the temperature is raised slightly. A massage completes the session.

The strong Eastern theme of the spa is balanced by a good selection of European treatments as well. Visit the Salt Inhalation Grotto to cleanse and soothe the respiratory system with a combination of peppermint and eucalyptus essential oils with a marine salt solution; experience the Breuss Massage to release spinal muscular tension; and pamper yourself in a Cleopatra Bath—the ultimate beauty ritual in your quest for smooth, silky skin. If that's not enough, you can round off the treatment with a facial.

The hotel runs an 'Opening Closed Minds Wellness Programme'. This consists of

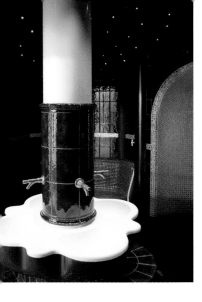

OPPOSITE, LEFT: *Newly opened in the summer of 2003, the Bellevue Spa offers unrivalled comfort and variety. Guests are welcomed in the ornately decorated lobby.*

OPPOSITE, RIGHT: *Enjoy a splendid variety of massages here that will heighten your entire sense of wellbeing.*

LEFT: *Enjoy a steam bath in the traditional Rome-Ottoman tradition. Natural essential oils such as camomile, sage and lavender are added and the combination of steam, health-giving warmth and natural essences will leave you feeling relaxed.*

Spa Statistics

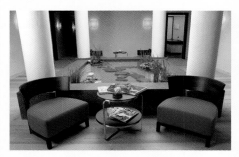

All the facilities at the spa, starting from the waiting room (pictured) where you begin your sojourn of luxurious treatments, are an extension of the light theme in the Bellevue Hotel. The sprawling spa is housed in a transparent chalet built of wood and glass, and lights up like a shining star in the night.

15 special menus that span music, cinema, literature, gastronomy and humidor. Every day, each menu provides two suggestions. These suggestions open up your 'idea bank' to help you combine your hotel stay with, for instance, a Beethoven concert, a ride up the mountains and a relaxing massage at the spa.

The Grand Hotel Bellevue is designed for everyone, from intellectuals to *bons vivants*, and the Bellevue Spa offers an experience that is both intellectual and sensory. A perfect combination, for the perfect stay.

TYPE OF SPA
Hotel spa

SPA AREA
2,500 sq m (26,910 sq ft)

FACILITIES
5 single treatment rooms; 1 meditation room; 2 relaxation rooms; 1 Japanese Luxury Bath; 1 Seraglio Bath Room; 1 soft pack treatment room; 1 cold plunge pool; 1 whirlpool; 3 saunas; 3 steam rooms; 1 solarium; 1 hair salon, 1 nail salon; 1 aerobics studio, 1 cardio studio, 1 gymnasium, 1 Pilates studio; 1 indoor swimming pool; 1 spa boutique; 1 library

SIGNATURE TREATMENTS
Cleopatra Bath; Japanese Luxury Bath; Rasul Ritual

TREATMENTS & THERAPIES
Anti-ageing treatments, anti-cellulite treatments, aqua therapy, aromatherapy, Ayurvedic treatments, body bronzing, body scrubs, body wraps, bust treatments, Chinese therapies, eye treatments, facials, firming and slimming treatments, hair treatments, hand and foot treatments, heat treatments, hot stone therapies, inhalation therapies, lymphatic drainage, make-up services, manicures and pedicures, movement therapies, reflexology, Thai therapies, thalassotherapy, waxing; spa packages combining spa and action, spa and beauty, spa and relax, and spa in Asian style

SPA CUISINE
Not available, but spa-goers can make special requests for vegetarian meals and low-fat diets at the hotel restaurants.

SERVICES
Body composition analysis; personal training; baby-sitting

LANGUAGES SPOKEN BY THERAPISTS
English, French, German, Italian

ADMISSION
Club membership includes rights such as entry into the thermal area; participation in group workouts and personalised training programs. Not all the therapies and treatments are available all year round. Contact spa to check.

CONTACT
Grand Hotel Bellevue
Hauptstrasse
3780 Gstaad
Switzerland
T: +41 (0)337 480 000
F: +41 (0)337 480 001
E: info@bellevue-gstaad.ch
W: www.bellevue-gstaad.ch

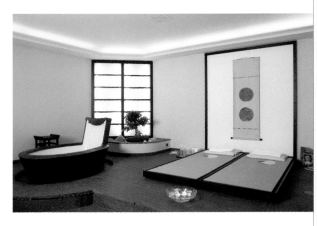

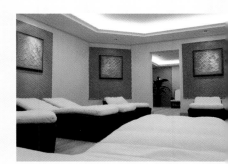

Great attention to detail has gone into every room at the spa, from the meditation room and relaxation room (pictured) to the treatment rooms. Only a small number of select materials are used in the interiors, such as anthracite-coloured stone from China and bleached larch-wood flooring.

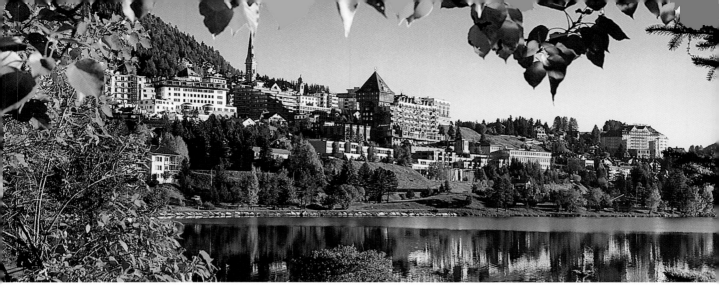

Daniela Steiner Beauty Spa at Badrutt's Palace Hotel
St Moritz, Switzerland

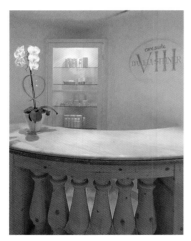

The spa is a space of soothing whites and beiges, and furniture that reflects an alpine atmosphere.

Since 1896, Badrutt's Palace Hotel has been an icon in the glamorous ski resort town of St Moritz, attracting legends such as silver screen star Marilyn Monroe, writer George Bernard Shaw and director Alfred Hitchcock, all of whom have gazed at the Alps and Lake St Moritz through the floor-to-ceiling windows of its Grand Hall.

The hotel traditionally celebrates the start of its winter season—which sees polo matches on frozen lakes, tobogganing, sleigh rides, or skating on the hotel's private ice rinks—on St Nicholas' Day (6 December). As a summer retreat, the Palace is a perfect base for golfing, fishing, mountain biking, rafting, and enjoying open-air concerts.

The Daniela Steiner Beauty Spa is a serene retreat within a retreat. Rituals revolve around the Care Suite Daniela Steiner range of botanical products and treatments which purify and nourish the skin. The focus is on total pampering, so you will rarely be left unattended during a treatment; facials accompany manicures and pedicures; face massages come with body wraps; and facial masks with baths. You can also request for treatments to be personalised to your needs.

As an initiation, opt for 1st Total Cleansing, a two-hour session that includes exfoliation of the scalp, face and body, followed by a relaxing Energy Massage which can be firm or gentle.

Another popular treatment is 2nd Purifying, a stimulating and detoxifying one-hour session that begins with an exfoliation with hot oil and salt, after which you are coddled in a seaweed wrap as you relax on a dry flotation bed.

You may be tempted to lick off the ingredients used in treatments such as Brown Sugar. After your body is exfoliated with hot oil and brown sugar as you lie on a wet table under a shower, your therapist removes the mixture using massaging movements. A lemon herbal mask is applied to your body as you lie on a heated flotation bed.

Crystal Bath is another delicious treatment. It begins with an Energy Massage

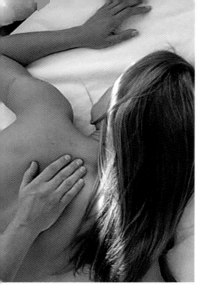

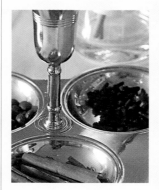

OPPOSITE: *The Palace, as it is affectionately referred to by guests in the know, is often described as a fairy-tale castle in a fairy-tale location overlooking a lake. The 180-room hotel still retains much of its old-world charm after a multi-million dollar facelift completed in 2004, which added discreetly hidden modern features such as Internet access.*

LEFT: *The spa's repertoire includes Classic Body Massage, Shiatsu, Lymph Drainage, Aromamassage and Reflexology. You may also request to have a massage treatment in the privacy of your room.*

using essential oils—typically a blend of angelica, lemongrass, lemon, peppermint and rosemary—applied with rapid movements. This is followed by a soak in a bath scattered with lemon and orange slices; a crystal from the surrounding mountains will have been previously immersed in the water to help enhance your wellbeing.

To share a treat with a partner, book the one-hour Special Skin Care For Two in which you can playfully apply volcanic clay to each other's faces and bodies before basting in a steam room. After showering off the clay, share a Cleopatra Bath of milk, oil and relaxing essences in a large hydrobath.

Grooming treatments that are essential to the immaculate appearance of guests include a range of manicures and pedicures such as Crystal Manicure and Curative Pedicure that work otherwise problem nails into top shape with a natural sheen. Such hand and foot treatments are also popular with guests from neighbouring hotels who come to soak up a part of the Palace's magic in the spa.

Spa Statistics

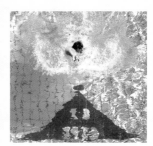

An air of refinement pervades the Palace.

TYPE OF SPA
Hotel spa

SPA AREA
250 sq m (2,690 sq ft)

FACILITIES
10 single treatment rooms; 1 steam room; 1 hair salon; 3 tennis courts; 1 indoor swimming pool, 1 outdoor swimming pool; 1 spa boutique

SIGNATURE TREATMENTS
Brown Sugar, 1st Total Cleansing, 2nd Purifying

TREATMENTS & THERAPIES
Anti-ageing treatments, anti-cellulite treatments, aromatherapy, baths, body wraps, facials, firming and slimming treatments, hand and foot treatments, manicures and pedicures, massages, waxing; spa packages

PROVISIONS FOR COUPLES
Special Skin Care For Two

SPA CUISINE
Not available, but provisions for special dietary needs are available on request.

ACTIVITIES & PROGRAMMES
Tennis

SERVICES
Personal training; baby-sitting, childcare (both at additional cost); gift certificates

LANGUAGES SPOKEN BY THERAPISTS
English, German, Italian, Spanish

The outdoor pool is open during the summer season.

CONTACT
Badrutt's Palace Hotel
Via Serlas 27
CH-7500 St Moritz
Switzerland
T: +41 (0)81 837 2851
F: +41 (0)81 837 2851
E: info@steinercosmetics.com
W: www.badruttspalace.com

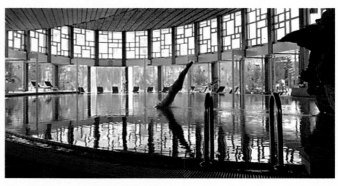

The spa is situated next to this reflective indoor swimming pool. Floor-to-ceiling windows bathe it in plenty of sunshine all year round.

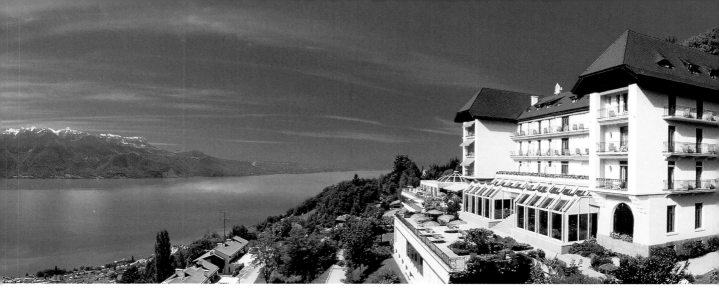

Le Mirador Givenchy Spa
at Le Mirador Kempinski Lake Geneva
Montreux/Vevey, Switzerland

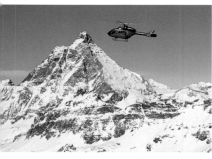

ABOVE: *Travel or sightsee in style by arranging to have a helicopter, yacht or limousine at your disposal.*

OPPOSITE, BOTTOM: *The largest suite, the Duplex Suite, occupies the penthouse level of the hotel. Strikingly modern, its focal point is the open-concept bathroom where you can enjoy a hydro-massage in your bathtub, and a tan from the sunshine streaming through the windows.*

Around Le Mirador Kempinski Lake Geneva, postcard-perfect images abound. From its perch 800 metres (2,620 feet) above the towns of Vevey and Montreux, you enjoy a panoramic view of Lake Geneva, the Alps and the Swiss Riviera. As you explore the surrounding meadows, or follow the hiking and jogging paths through the woods and inhale the fresh mountain air, you are surrounded by a symphony of nature—the twitter of birds, the tinkle of cowbells and the chime of church bells. You may want to explore the region's wineries, or savour these wines and others from around the world from the hotel's award-winning wine cellar.

The scenery is also part of the therapy at Le Mirador Givenchy Spa, where most of the treatment rooms come with a view. This serene sanctuary has a distinctly European focus reflected in both the pampering and the high-tech treatments that beautify your face, refine your figure, and help retain your youth.

The speciality of the house is Exclusively Givenchy, a pampering treatment that comprises a body scrub, a bath with essential oils, and a hydrating wrap. The most exotic massage on the menu is The Canyon Love Stone Therapy, a massage using rounded stones, heated and chilled, from rivers of the American West to rebalance your body and ease muscular aches. The most luxurious offering is the Ylang-Ylang Massage With 4 Hands, in which two therapists simultaneously pamper you in a massage so synchronised that you are unable to tell how many hands are working on you at once. Essential oils derived from ylang-ylang blossoms from Mauritius are used; elderly Mauritians believe that these benefit both body and soul.

To achieve a sun-kissed look, you can bronze yourself at the outdoor pool in summer, or take to the solarium that is enhanced with colour therapy. To further your pursuit of wellness, you may visit the Swiss AntiAge Group

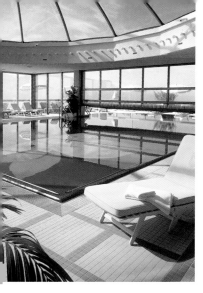

OPPOSITE: *Most of the 81 rooms and suites have balconies from which to admire the view of the lake and the Alps.*

LEFT: *The dramatic glass-domed ceiling over the indoor swimming pool brings the outdoors indoors. In summer, you can enjoy the outdoor pool under the gaily coloured parasols as you watch the clouds drift by. Both outdoor and indoor pool are heated to a comfortable 27 degrees Celsius (81 degrees Fahrenheit), and are linked by a swim-through window.*

where medical experts prescribe technologically advanced treatments to revitalise your cells to combat ageing and rebalance your body. If your goal is to shed some inches, you may want to plan a 9- to 15-day stay at the hotel in conjunction with treatment at the Cambuzat Centre. This programme is based on a psychological behavioural approach to healthy eating and weight loss—based on the principle that the path to wellness lies not just in your body, but also in your mind.

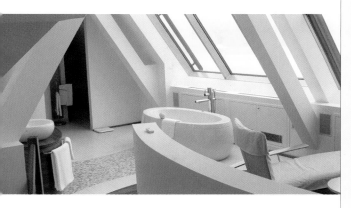

Spa Statistics

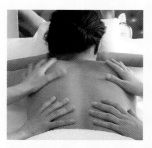

The Ylang-Ylang Massage With 4 Hands seems twice as luxurious with two therapists simultaneously pampering you.

TYPE OF SPA
Hotel spa

SPA AREA
325 sq m (3,500 sq ft)

FACILITIES
9 single treatment rooms; 1 consultation room; 1 relaxation room; 3 jacuzzis; 2 saunas, 2 steam rooms; 1 solarium; 1 hair salon, 1 nail salon; Cambuzat Centre, Swiss AntiAge Group Centre; 1 cardio studio, 1 gymnasium; 1 indoor swimming pool/outdoor swimming pool; 1 golf course (15 min from the hotel), 3 outdoor tennis courts (500 m/1,640 ft from the hotel); 1 spa boutique

SIGNATURE TREATMENTS
Exclusively Givenchy, Special Ylang Ylang Massage With 4 Hands, The Canyon Love Stone Therapy

TREATMENTS & THERAPIES
Aqua therapy, aromatherapy, body bronzing, body scrubs, body wraps, bust treatments, facials, firming and slimming treatments, hair treatments, hand and foot treatments, hot stone therapies, hydrotherapy, massages, purifying back treatments, reflexology, scalp treatments; make-up services, manicures and pedicures, waxing; Spa Day package, Spa À La Carte (with 2 nights accommodation, meals and 1 daily spa treatment), Wellness Experience package (with 6 nights accommodation, meals and 2 spa treatments daily). With the Swiss AntiAge Group

you can have acupuncture, anti-ageing treatments, cellular therapy injections, iridology, laser treatments and lymphatic drainage.

SPA CUISINE
Healthy and light Mediterranean dishes are available at the sunny conservatory-styled Le Patio, or from late spring to early fall, on the restaurant's adjoining terrace. Meals can be adapted to your needs. Cuisine can also be adapted to the needs of clients of the Cambuzat Centre; your mini-bar will be emptied of all temptations if you are undergoing a weight-loss programme.

ACTIVITIES & PROGRAMMES
Aquaerobics, aquagym, biking, golf, hiking, sailing, tennis; cooking classes (on request)

SERVICES
Body composition analysis, general healthcare consultation, nutritional consultation, skincare consultation; personal training; baby-sitting (on request); gift certificates; day spa available

LANGUAGES SPOKEN BY THERAPISTS
Arabic, English, French, German, Italian, Spanish

ADMISSION
Membership is available but not required for admission.

CONTACT
Le Mirador Kempinski
Lake Geneva
1801 Mont-Pélerin
Montreux/Vevey
Switzerland
T: +41 (0)21 925 1770
F: +41 (0)21 925 1112
E: spa@mirador.ch
W: www.mirador.ch

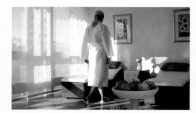

The view through the floor-to-ceiling windows of the relaxation lounge is therapy in itself.

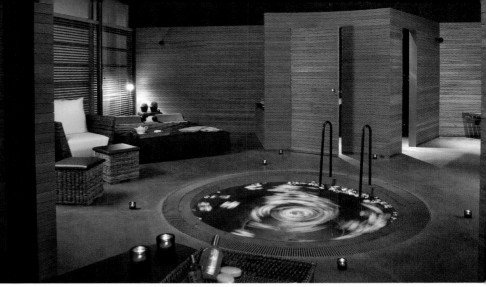

Sparkling Wellness at Park Hotel Weggis
Weggis, Switzerland

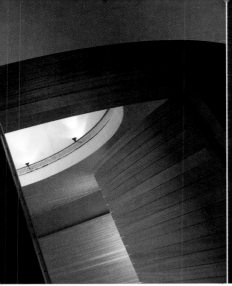

ABOVE: *One way to admire the lake view from the award-winning hotel is from the glass-domed Sunset Bar with a malt whiskey and cigar in hand, accompanied by the tinkling of the ivories. In summer, request for a lakeside spa treatment at a lush secluded spot; on a hot day, try refreshing specials such as the Cooling Full Body Pack With Avocado Oil.*

OPPOSITE, BOTTOM: *The graphic inner courtyard of pebbles and 100-year-old bonsai trees from Japan provides a space for meditative walks. It also gives an inspirational view to those working out in the gym.*

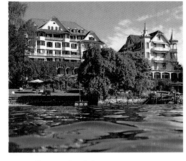

The five-star Park Hotel Weggis' stately Art Nouveau façade belies an interior that is an eclectic blend of Designers Guild fabrics, Murano lighting, Philippe Starck fittings, Molteni furniture and Versace porcelain.

Depending on the package, you will be given a guide to what is known as the 'Sparkling Open Eyes-Path', which features sights to savour and places to quiet yourself among ancient chestnut trees and on walks through nature and rolling parkland overlooking Lake Lucerne and the Alps beyond. To further your path to wellbeing, visit Sparkling Wellness where you can relax and balance both body and mind in an oasis of quietude. Descriptions of treatments on the spa menu are deliberately brief so that you will be pleasantly surprised by the experience.

The spa's modern Asian décor and serene Japanese meditation garden echoes exotic treatments such as the Lomi Lomi Nui and Papaya Peeling. The former massage is performed rhythmically to Hawaiian music

which alternates between gentle and forceful passages, and you may opt to have two therapists massaging two people simultaneously (possible for almost all treatments). Papaya Peeling refreshes your skin, and the fragrance of the fruit transports you to the Caribbean, as do other treatments using Ligne St Barth, a line of products inspired by native Caribbean practices.

Energy healing is emphasised in treatments such as Wellness With Colours (a gentle massage with coloured oils chosen for your needs), Harmony Through Cosmic Light and Spinal Care Integrating Cosmic Light. The latter two involve the therapist gently caressing your body while projecting healing energies to help clear blockages within.

Treatment packages take place in a SPA-Cottage. This gives you the private use of a combination of facilities that may include a sauna/tepidarium or steam bath, hydrotherapy facilities, a solarium and a waterbed. Try Steam-Soap-Enjoy, which begins with a relaxing steam bath, during which your body is

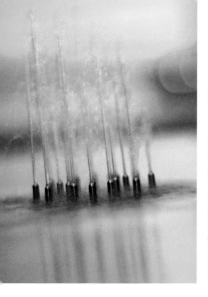

OPPOSITE AND LEFT: *The SPA-Cottage with its mahogany walls, terrazzo floors, and natural materials is both welcoming and relaxing. Within, you may soak your body in a quiet pool, decorated seasonally, enjoy a reflexology session walking around a Kneipp pool lined with smooth pebbles from Malaysia, or relax on a waterbed while sipping tea and listening to meditational or classical music. A SPA-Cottage may be rented by a group of up to four friends for a minimum of two hours, though many guests prefer to rent it for longer periods of time to take advantage of the calm within.*

massaged with fragrant soap suds and rubbed vigorously with a glove. After a cooling shower and a soak in the whirlpool, natural oils are applied to your body.

Sparkling Wellness at Park Hotel Weggis is the first in Switzerland to offer OwnZone training. A trainer will teach you how to optimise your exercise within your heart and health limits. This is accomplished with the help of a heart monitor and a wrist-worn device; this training is included in the Sense of Sport package. After a jog, a walk or cycling, you will be rewarded with a sports massage. For the convenience of exercise enthusiasts, the fitness centre, equipped with the most modern Cybex units, is open 24 hours a day.

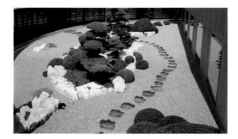

Spa Statistics

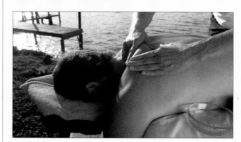

Before your treatment, your therapist may gently enquire about your lifestyle so she can personalise treatments to your needs, and ask if you prefer a treatment that awakens or relaxes. One of the most personalised treatments is the Intuitive Energy Massage, where classic massage techniques are intuitively adapted to enhance your relaxation.

TYPE OF SPA
Hotel spa

SPA AREA
610 sq m (6,570 sq ft)

FACILITIES
6 SPA-Cottages with sauna/tepidarium or steam bath, quiet pool or whirlpool and Kneipp waters, footbath, exhilarating shower, solarium, waterbed, and opportunity to take advantage of treatments, widescreen TV, stereo/CD/DVD player with unique surround sound; 1 beauty salon; 1 gymnasium/cardio studio; 4 golf courses nearby, 1 squash court nearby, 5 tennis courts nearby; 1 meditation garden; 1 spa boutique; 1 audiothek and library (CDs and books can be borrowed and taken into the SPA-Cottages)

SIGNATURE TREATMENTS
Cooling Full Body Pack With Avocado Oil (Summer), Healing Herbal Stamps, Harmony Through Cosmic Light, Lomi Lomi Nui (with 2 or 4 hands), Papaya Peeling, Steam-Soap-Enjoy; Lakeside Treatments

TREATMENTS & THERAPIES
Body scrubs, body wraps, colour therapies, energy therapies, eye treatments, facials, hair treatments (on request), hand and foot treatments, lymphatic drainage, make-up services, manicures and pedicures, massages, purifying back treatments, reflexology, shiatsu, waxing; spa packages, Energyweek and Energy weekend packages include spa treatments, exercises and meals.

PROVISIONS FOR COUPLES
6 SPA-Cottages, which may be decorated romantically; 1 double

outdoor treatment pavilion by the lake; package geared towards romance

SPA CUISINE
Healthy yet delicious gourmet meals are available at the hotel's three restaurants—Restaurant Annex, Restaurant Sparks and Restaurant The Grape—and can also be ordered through room service. The emphasis is not so much on counting calories, but on providing a well-balanced diet that retains the integrity of the ingredients. Vegetarian dishes are available on the menu while provisions for various dietary requirements are available on request.

ACTIVITIES & PROGRAMMES
Biking, golf, kayaking, hiking, horse riding, rock-climbing, sailing, scuba-diving, snorkelling, yoga; cooking, make-up, massage, meditation, nailcare, life-enhancement, lifestyle management, sports and stretching classes; OwnZone training

SERVICES
Colour consultation, nutritional consultation; personal training; childcare; private spa parties; gift certificates; day-use rooms

LANGUAGES SPOKEN BY THERAPISTS
English, French, German, Italian

CONTACT
Park Hotel Weggis
Hertensteinstrasse 34
CH-6353 Weggis
Switzerland
T: +41 (0)41 392 0505
F: +41 (0)41 390 0528
E: wellness@phw.ch
W: www.phw.ch

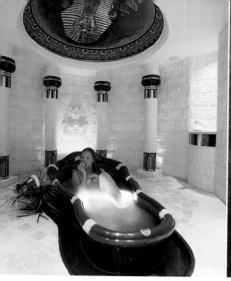
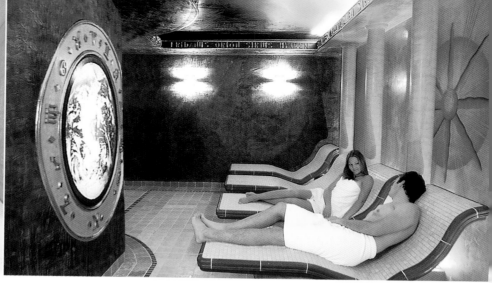

Serenity Spa
at Sheraton Voyager Antalya Hotel, Resort & Spa
Antalya, Turkey

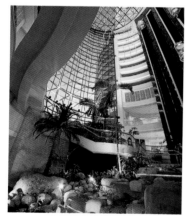

The towering glass atrium is a focal point of the hotel.

At the centrally located Sheraton Voyager Antalya Hotel, Resort & Spa, you are ideally placed to explore the charming old city which dates back to 2 B.C., or to enjoy the refreshing sea air by the harbour and marina. Antalya's sun-kissed beaches along the Mediterranean Sea are a short stroll away through the lush public park that faces the hotel, though you may prefer to opt for a beach shuttle if you are in a hurry. Depending on your preference, opt for a room overlooking the Bey Mountains or the azure sea.

The Serenity Spa on the lower ground floor of the hotel is centrally located, with a corridor that branches off to the fitness centre. This boutique spa, part of the Starwood Spa Collection, offers holistic treatments that aim to rebalance your wellbeing, as well as pamper you with Guinot and Dermalogica facial and body treatments.

Begin your journey into wellbeing by relaxing within the aromatic steam chambers;

refreshing and re-energising yourself under the hot and cold sprays of the Tropical Snail Shower; or cleansing your respiratory tract, boosting your circulation and softening your skin in the steamy atmosphere of the Salt Grotto, an alternative for people who are sensitive to aromatherapy-based steam rooms.

Many of the treatments have a fantasy element woven into them. You may feel like a mermaid during the Oyster Experience in which you are relaxed by a symphony of a multi-jet massage, colour therapy and sedating music as you lie within a giant clam shell.

The Serenity Goddess Massage, during which your body is balanced by two therapists massaging your body in tandem, is heavenly and may make you feel quite like a deity.

In the Japanese Ritual Room—a warm steam room infused with the scent of jasmine—the Japanese Ritual cleanses you in a creamy foaming bath, followed by a relaxing shiatsu massage performed on the floor.

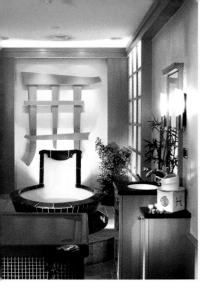

OPPOSITE, LEFT: *You may feel like the legendary Egyptian beauty herself as you sink into the warm waters of the Cleopatra Bath.*

OPPOSITE, RIGHT: *In between treatments, relax in the mild heat of the tepidarium, which fuses decorative elements from the past, present and future.*

LEFT: *The Japanese Ritual Room evokes a sense of the Orient.*

The spa's most popular treatment, especially with celebrity guests, is the Aromatherapy Massage: a superbly pampering experience. This massage restores your body and mind and delights all your senses with oils chosen specially for your needs; 30-, 60- and 90-minute sessions are available.

No trip to Turkey should be without the definitive Turkish experience—the traditional Turkish Bath Massage in which your body is massaged and exfoliated within the traditional Turkish steam room known as the Hamam.

Couples sharing a spa experience benefit not only from the intimacy and privacy, but also from the value for money packages. The Japanese Ritual, for instance, comes at the price of one; and a free Mud Chamber treatment (an exotic treatment in which you can playfully rub healing muds over each others' bodies as you baste in the steamy, aromatic heat) is included when the two of you book the Turkish Bath Massage.

Spa Statistics

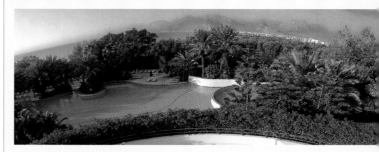

The outdoor swimming pool resembles a lush oasis in the desert.

TYPE OF SPA
Hotel spa

SPA AREA
260 sq m (2,800 sq ft)

FACILITIES
3 single treatment rooms;
1 Japanese Ritual Room;
1 Oyster Experience;
1 Cleopatra Bath; 1 Mud Chamber; 1 jacuzzi; 1 sauna, 1 Hamam, 1 tepidarium;
1 gymnasium, 1 studio;
1 indoor swimming pool,
1 outdoor swimming pool;
4 outdoor tennis courts,
1 squash court; 1 spa boutique

SIGNATURE TREATMENTS
Serenity Goddess Massage, Turkish Bath Massage

TREATMENTS & THERAPIES
Anti-ageing treatments, anti-cellulite treatments, aromatherapy, body scrubs, body wraps, bust treatments, eye treatments, eye enhancements, facials, firming and slimming treatments, holistic treatments, hot stone therapies, hydrotherapy, iridology, lymphatic drainage, massages, purifying back treatments, reflexology, scalp treatments, waxing

PROVISIONS FOR COUPLES
Mud Chamber, Japanese Room, Turkish Bath; Turkish Bath & Mud Chamber. Discounts are given to couples who have certain treatments together.

SPA CUISINE
A Spa Healthy Menu can be enjoyed at the Tropic Terrace, Panoramic Restaurant, Maritime Restaurant, Sundowner Snack

Bar and ordered from Room Service. Provisions for various dietary requirements are available on request.

ACTIVITIES & PROGRAMMES
Aerobics, Pilates; body toning, meditation, *taibo* and stretching classes

SERVICES
Baby-sitting, childcare

LANGUAGES SPOKEN BY THERAPISTS
English, Turkish

ADMISSION
Membership is available but not required for admission.

CONTACT
Sheraton Voyager Antalya Hotel, Resort & Spa
100 Yil Bulvari
Konyaalti Beach
07050 Antalya
Turkey
T: +90 242 238 5555
F: +90 242 238 5570/71
E: reservations.voyager@ sheraton.com
W: www.sheraton.com/voyager

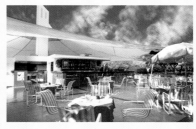

Enjoy the poolside in good weather. Cocktails are served at the Tropic Terrace while Turkish food is available at the Sundowner Snack Bar.

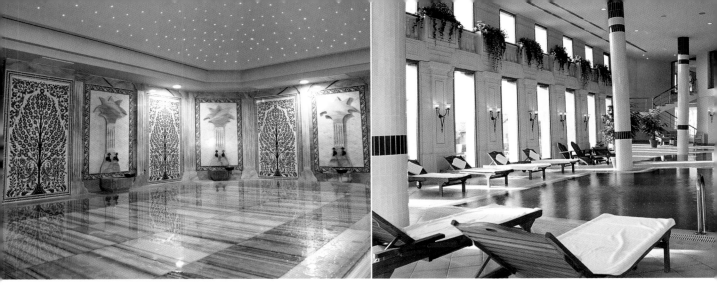

Thermalife Center
at Sheraton Cesme Hotel, Resort & Spa
Cesme, Turkey

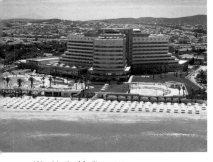

Worship the Mediterranean sun along the beachfront, or at the oasis of a pool fronting this luxurious hotel. Guests staying in the Penthouse Suite have the added privacy of having their own private pool on the rooftop terrace.

Sheraton Cesme Hotel, Resort & Spa, on the western edge of Turkey, close to the Greek island of Chios, is just 8 kilometres (5 miles) away from the picturesque small town of Cesme (meaning 'water spring or fountain'), which is renowned for its charming castle and traditional stone fountains etched with Arabic writing. Its beach is located at a crossroads where hot springs merge with the Aegean Sea.

The fruits of this unique convergence are best enjoyed in the Thermalife Center, a member of the Starwood Spa Collection, which marries the best of thermal and thalasso treatments within the same healing space. Guests of the hotel can easily access this area in pursuit of pleasure and health via the first floor corridor on the western side of the hotel.

In all, the spa offers a variety of 41 single treatments, including 12 different facials. Core treatments revolve around combinations of thermal and thalasso cures which are administered under medical supervision in conjunction with daily aqua gym sessions; the staff also includes nurses, certified masseurs, aestheticians, sports instructors, hydrotherapists and physical therapists.

Thermal and thalasso treatments take the form of balneotherapy, affusion showers, jet showers, and mud and seaweed application. In the Mud Treatment, mud is applied all over your body as a mask—the rich natural minerals it contains help soften and nourish your skin. The treatment is also prescribed for arthritis and rheumatism.

Heat treatments include the Alpha Spa, where you lie on a vibrating massaging bed in a personal capsule of dry heat; this American device offers six anti-stress programmes combined with aromatherapy and seaweed or mud packs to relax your body and enhance your health. Another treatment, the Ionozon Bath, is a steam bath in which a mixture of ozone, oxygen and ionised steam helps

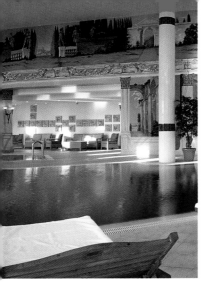

OPPOSITE, LEFT: *In the Sheraton Health Center that adjoins the Thermalife Centre, enjoy a 30-minute Hammam Massage, a quintessential Turkish treatment that takes place in a Turkish bath resplendent with Ottoman architecture and topped with a starlit ceiling.*

LEFT: *The Thermal and Thalasso Pool Hall is a grand bathing area that features pools of water either from the sea or mineral-rich springs.*

increase the oxygen level in your blood, and detoxifies your body through perspiration.

The spa's centrepiece is the Thermal and Thalasso Pool Hall with an 8-metre-high (26-foot) ceiling, tall windows and pillars, paintings, sculptures and huge palm trees. Floor-to-ceiling windows drench the pool area in natural light. It features four therapy pools; a seawater pool, a thermal whirlpool, and a mineral-rich indoor pool that is connected to an outdoor pool by stairs and a water channel. Families or groups of three to five friends can book one of three Luxury Thermal Jacuzzi Family Rooms here.

Besides classical European therapies, the spa also provides treatments such as shiatsu and reflexology which offer an Eastern touch.

Before and after your treatments, you can sip sodas, fresh fruit and vegetable juices or Ayran (a popular Turkish yogurt drink). Regular tea or coffee, espresso or Turkish coffee are available on request.

Spa Statistics

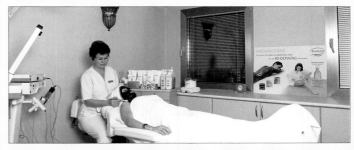

The Thalasso Face Specials ensure that you get the most suitable treatment for your skin's needs: anti-stress, anti-wrinkle and anti-acne. Regenerative and firming masks are also available.

TYPE OF SPA
Mineral springs spa

SPA AREA
3,900 sq m (41,980 sq ft)

FACILITIES
1 double treatment room, 25 single treatment rooms; 1 physiotherapy room; 1 meditation room, 1 relaxation room; 1 Alpha Spa; 1 cold plunge pool, 3 jacuzzis, 1 whirlpool; 2 saunas, 2 steam rooms, 1 Turkish bath (hammam); 2 solariums; 1 hair salon, 1 nail salon, 1 Thalgo Beauty Salon; 1 aerobics studio, 1 gymnasium; 1 indoor swimming pool, 1 outdoor swimming pool; 1 indoor and outdoor thermal pool, 1 indoor thalasso pool; 2 tennis courts; 1 spa boutique

SIGNATURE TREATMENTS
Hammam Massage, Mud Treatment

TREATMENTS & THERAPIES
Anti-cellulite treatments, aqua therapy, aromatherapy, baths, body bronzing, body scrubs, body wraps, bust treatments, Chinese therapies, electrotherapy, eye treatments, facials, firming and slimming treatments, hand and foot treatments, heat treatments, holistic treatments, hydrotherapy, lymphatic drainage, manicures and pedicures, massages, movement therapies, pre- and post-natal treatments, purifying back treatments, reflexology, thalassotherapy, waxing; 3- to 6-day treatment packages are available

PROVISIONS FOR COUPLES
1 double treatment room; The Honeymoon Treatment includes the use of a private whirlpool and an exotic aromatherapy massage

SPA CUISINE
Not available but provisions for various dietary requirements include a diet corner at the breakfast buffet and a salad bar with vegetarian food. The Thermalife Center has a Vitamin Bar serving fresh juices, herbal teas and salads.

ACTIVITIES & PROGRAMMES
Aerobics, aquaerobics (in summer), billiards, boccia, bowling, darts, *tai qi*, tennis, yoga; stretching classes, swimming classes (in summer)

SERVICES
Skincare and nutritional consultations; baby-sitting, childcare; day-use rooms

LANGUAGES SPOKEN BY THERAPISTS
Bulgarian, English, German, Russian, Turkish

ADMISSION
Membership is available but not required for admission. Monthly/seasonal/annual memberships for the Spa and Health Club are available for external guests who reside in Cesme or Izmir.

CONTACT
Sheraton Cesme Hotel, Resort & Spa
Ilica Cad. 35
TR 35940 Cesme, Izmir
Turkey
T: +90 (0)232 723 1240
F: +90 (0)232 723 1856
E: info@sheratoncesme.com
W: www.sheratoncesme.com

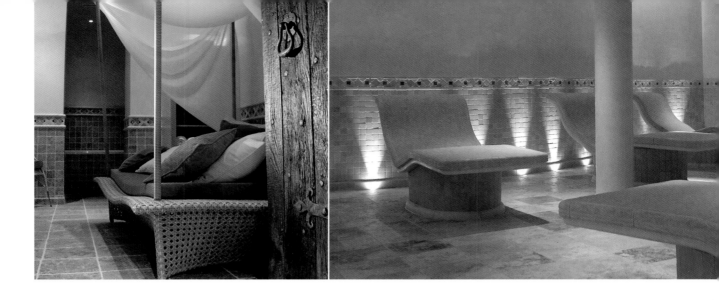

Aquarias at Whatley Manor Hotel
Wiltshire, England, United Kingdom

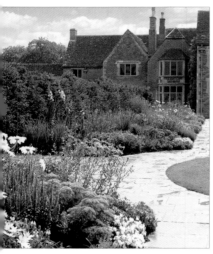

The 900-metre (2,950-foot) driveway leading to the hotel is flanked by lime trees and a wall of 99,000 stones which took two local craftsmen two years to hand-build. The 5-hectare (12-acre) grounds comprising woodlands, meadows and gardens combine the classic elegance of 1920s gardens with contemporary sculptures and sophisticated lighting.

Hosting up to just 46 guests at a time, Whatley Manor in Wiltshire exudes the warmth and privacy of staying in a private home—and a sophisticated and stylish one at that. Instead of your having to check in at the front desk, a manager will attend to all the necessary details in your guestroom, and also see to your comfort throughout your stay. Spoil yourself on classic French cuisine in The Dining Room or enjoy more simple dishes at the informal, chalet-styled Le Mazot. Then be sure to set aside some delightful pampering time for yourself at Aquarias.

Slip on the robe and slippers provided in your room and pad your way to the spa—a sanctuary of relaxation that is open exclusively to hotel residents, members and their guests. The European spa tradition of bathing and taking thermal baths has been reinterpreted here and made luxurious for today's spa-goers. Key features include a figure-eight shaped hydropool and a Thermal Suite comprising a sequence of rooms of differing temperatures; in between, cool down in the Experience Shower where you can enjoy an icy blast infused with mint or a warm tropical rain infused with Maracuja, a tropical flower.

Luxurious treatments using La Prairie products form the core therapies on the spa menu. The house speciality, the Aquarias La Prairie Signature Facial, combines the use of La Prairie Caviar extracts with the alternating use of hot and chilled stones.

The VIP Suite offers a romantic haven where couples can savour five different three-hour treatments within the privacy of the room. These include Total Seclusion (a body polish, flower bath and massage), Aquarias Heaven (an aromatic salt and oil body polish, flower bath and hot stone therapy), Day Dream Cocoon (a body polish, warm oil wrap and massage), La Prairie Experience (a flower bath, customised facial or body treatment and hand treatment) and Aquarias La Prairie Signature Experience (a body polish, flower bath and four-hands massage). Consider celebrating a special occasion by booking the whole space for an entire day.

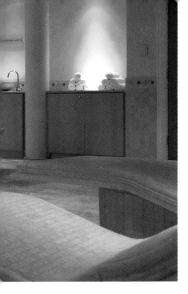

OPPOSITE, LEFT: *Share a sensuous experience with your partner in the VIP Suite by enjoying treatments side by side, sipping champagne while sharing a luxurious flower bath, or daydreaming together on a canopied bed.*

LEFT: *Give yourself at least half an hour before your treatment to enjoy the tepidarium (pictured) and thermal cabins in an ascending sequence of hotness, alternated with cold.*

BOTTOM: *The 8 suites and 15 rooms are dressed with an eclectic selection of antiques from around the world, contemporary furniture, and luxurious bespoke furnishings.*

Spa Statistics

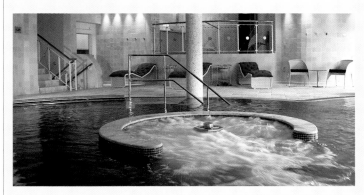

The water element in the figure-eight-shaped hydrotherapy pool is both beautiful and therapeutic. Allow yourself to relax, soothed by a symphony of neck massage fountains and underwater body jets. In the outdoor section which comprises one-third of the pool, recline on an underwater lounger and take in the view beyond the pool's infinite edge to the woodlands and river valley below. The water is heated to a comfortable 34 degrees Celsius (93 degrees Fahrenheit) all year round.

More specialised treatments have to be specifically booked in advance. However, part of the attraction of Aquarias is simply being able to reserve time in advance with a therapist, and letting you get in touch with yourself to decide what form of pampering you wish to take on the day itself.

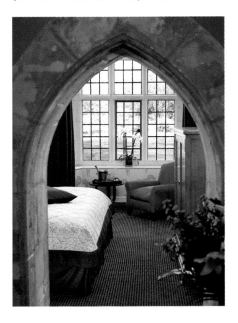

TYPE OF SPA
Hotel spa

SPA AREA
1,500 sq m (16,150 sq ft)

FACILITIES
1 double treatment room, 4 single treatment rooms; 1 relaxation room; 1 Serial Mud Suite, 1 wet room for scrubs; 1 tepidarium; 1 Thermal Suite (comprising 1 Caldarium, 1 Camomile Grotto, 2 Experience Showers, 1 Finnish Sauna, 1 Laconium), 1 sunbed; 1 gymnasium, 1 studio; 1 indoor and outdoor hydropool; 1 café/lounge bar

SIGNATURE TREATMENTS
Aquarias La Prairie Signature Experience, Aquarias La Prairie Signature Facial

TREATMENTS & THERAPIES
Anti-ageing treatments, anti-cellulite treatments, aromatherapy, body scrubs, body wraps, facials, hand and foot treatments, holistic treatments, hot stone therapies, jet lag treatments, massages, pre- and post-natal treatments, reflexology

PROVISIONS FOR COUPLES
1 double treatment room; Aquarias Heaven, Aquarias La Prairie Signature Experience, Day Dream Cocoon, La Prairie Express, Total Seclusion

SPA CUISINE
Light, simple but nutritious and innovative dishes are available for lunch at the spa café/lounge bar, as are fruit juices and teas. Fresh fruit and drinks are available at the poolside, VIP Suite and gymnasium. Provisions for various dietary requirements are catered to on request.

ACTIVITIES & PROGRAMMES
Pilates, *tai chi*, yoga

SERVICES
Body composition analysis, fitness assessment, personal training, skincare consultation

LANGUAGES SPOKEN BY THERAPISTS
Chinese, English, French, German

ADMISSION
The spa is exclusively for members and their guests, and residents of the hotel. Members must be at least 18 years of age, and no guests under 16.

CONTACT
Whatley Manor Hotel
Easton Grey, Malmesbury
Wiltshire SN16 0RP
England
United Kingdom
T: +44 (0)1666 822 888
F: +44 (0)1666 826 120
E: aquarias@whatleymanor.com
W: www.whatleymanor.com

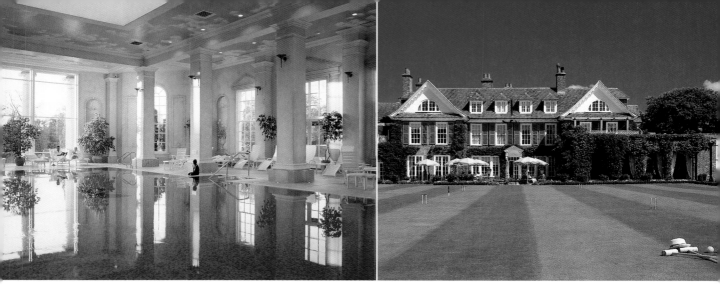

Chewton Glen Spa
at Chewton Glen Hotel, Spa & Country Club
Hampshire, England, United Kingdom

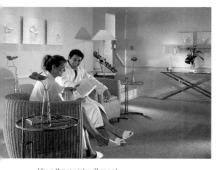

Your therapist will meet you at this waiting room and lead you to your treatment room. Some rooms have a sky light allowing natural light to stream in; this can be closed if your treatment calls for a more cocooning effect.

To step into Chewton Glen is to step into a legend of fabled charm. The tales of Captain Frederick Marryat—whose brother owned the house where he penned *The Children of the New Forest* in 1846—are immortalised in the rooms named after his characters or his ships. Chewton Glen's present owners, who acquired the 8-room property in 1966, groomed it into a luxurious 33-room and 19-suite hotel; their team is renowned for making each guest feel like the lord or lady of the manor.

Day visitors may drive 145 kilometres (90 miles) southwest of London to have lunch or dinner at its Michelin-starred Marryat Room Restaurant. The hotel's trophy cabinet creaks under the weight of its numerous awards, which include Best Small Hotel in the World 2003 by *Gallivanter's Guide*, Best Spa Hotel in Europe 2002 by German magazine *Gala*, and Best Hotel Spa in the UK 2001 by *Professional Beauty* magazine.

The neighbouring New Forest may lure many to the region, but the hotel is a destination in itself where you can linger over afternoon tea in the drawing room, play a game of croquet, or tee off on its 9-hole course within its 53 hectares (130 acres) of parkland. Guests looking to relax, refresh and enliven their bodies, minds and spirits can slip on their Frette bathrobes and pad through the corridors to the Chewton Glen Spa.

Within the spa, which is located over three levels, you can get into shape with the gymnasium's air-machine resistance equipment, attend an exercise class, do laps at the indoor swimming pool, or enjoy a water massage at the hydrotherapy pool. If that sounds too strenuous, opt from among 40 beauty and body treatments which take place in treatment rooms fitted with double doors to reduce external noise.

Popular treatments include a range of body wraps and facials from Clarins, Guinot

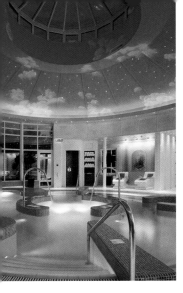

OPPOSITE, LEFT: *The ozone-treated indoor swimming pool resembles a grand Roman bath with its columns and trompe l'oeil frescoes. It overlooks a sundeck and the garden. Adjoining the pool is a steam room for communal bathing.*

OPPOSITE, RIGHT: *The hotel's romantic surrounds and genteel air make it an ideal setting for celebrating a wedding.*

LEFT: *Couples will appreciate the petal-shaped nooks within the hydrotherapy pool. The domed sky light and twinkling lights in the cloud-painted ceiling enhance a beautiful day, but the effect is all the more dramatic on a dark winter's evening. Admire this as you bask on the heated stone loungers.*

and Thalgo, and The Relaxation Spa Day package, which includes a facial, full body massage, Indian Head Massage, and also lunch, refreshments and day use of spa facilities for non-hotel guests. Guests can celebrate the birth of an upcoming child with a Guinot Pregnancy Pampering Treatment.

Exotic therapies from the East that rebalance the mind and body include the gentle Thai Yoga Massage that involves acupressure, stretches and applied yoga to relax the body or banish aches and strains. The Samadhi Synchronized Massage, inspired by yoga, meditation, aromatherapy and holistic healing, offers twice the pampering, for it is performed by two therapists.

Delicious yet healthy options are available at the spa's Pool Lounge, as are desserts and wines. These reflect the spa's philosophy of providing a path to wellness along with a variety of options for guests who may also have the wish to indulge.

Spa Statistics

TYPE OF SPA
Hotel spa

SPA AREA
1,670 sq m (18,000 sq ft)

FACILITIES
10 single treatment rooms; 2 relaxation lounges; 1 indoor hydrotherapy pool, 1 outdoor whirlpool, 1 reflexology pool; 2 saunas, 2 steam rooms; 1 hair salon, 1 nail salon; 1 aerobics studio, 1 gymnasium; 1 indoor swimming pool, 1 outdoor swimming pool; 9-hole golf course, 27-hole sea course (5-min drive), 10 courses (within 30-min drive); 2 indoor tennis courts, 2 outdoor tennis courts; 1 spa boutique

SIGNATURE TREATMENTS
Samadhi Synchronized Massage, Thai Yoga Massage

TREATMENTS & THERAPIES
Acupuncture, anti-ageing treatments, aromatherapy, body bronzing, body masks, body scrubs, body wraps, bust treatments, facials, firming and slimming treatments, hair treatments, hand and foot treatments, holistic treatments, hot stone therapies, hydrotherapy, hypnotherapy, iridology, lymphatic drainage, manicures and pedicures, massages, movement therapies, Neuro Linguistic Programming, pre- and post-natal treatments, purifying back treatments, reflexology, salon services, scalp treatments, Thai therapies, waxing; Spa Days packages

SPA CUISINE
Healthy and light simple choices, fresh fruit juices and smoothies are available at the Pool Bar. Meat and vegetarian options are available. 'Wellness choices' and vegetarian options are available on the menu at the Marryat Room Restaurant that uses fresh local produce and seafood from specialist suppliers. The over-500-long wine list includes organic options. Provisions for various dietary requirements are available on request; advise when booking your stay.

ACTIVITIES & PROGRAMMES
Aerobics, aquaerobics, biking, golf, horse riding (offsite), Pilates, *tai ji*, tennis, yoga; tennis coaching by resident tennis pro.; cooking, make-up services, wardrobe planning, massage, nailcare, life enhancement, lifestyle management and stretching classes; talks by visiting consultants

SERVICES
Body composition analysis, cholesterol screening, general healthcare and nutritional consultation; personal training; child minding (for hotel guests), corporate programmes; gift certificates

LANGUAGES SPOKEN BY THERAPISTS
English, French, German

ADMISSION
Non-hotel guests can enjoy Spa Days, which include treatments, lunch, refreshments, and day use of spa facilities— from Monday to Friday. Country Club memberships are available on an annual basis. Children of 5 and above are welcome, although time and access restrictions apply.

CONTACT
Chewton Glen Hotel,
Spa & Country Club
Christchurch Road, New Milton
Hampshire BH25 6QS
England
United Kingdom
T: +44 (0)1425 275 341
F: +44 (0)1425 272 310
E: spa@chewtonglen.com
W: www.chewtonglen.com

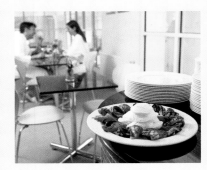

Indulge in a healthy lunch, light snacks or refreshments at the serenely sleek Pool Bar that overlooks the indoor swimming pool.

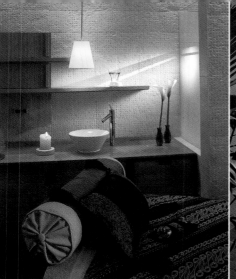
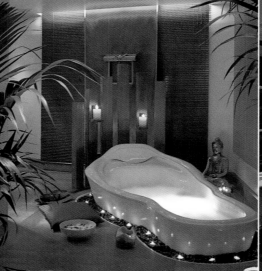
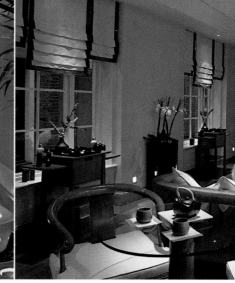

Elemis Day-Spa
London, England, United Kingdom

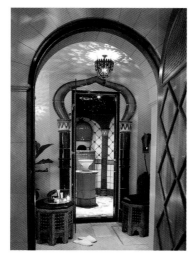

The Arabian Jewel Ritual includes a session in the Rasul, an area that resembles a temple with its exquisite handmade tiles and starry domed roof. This is followed by an Exotic Frangipani Body Nourish Float (inspired by ingredients Polynesian women use to condition their bodies and hair), and a Well-Being Massage (in which warmed oils chosen for your needs are smoothed on to your face and body).

Chic urbanites who do not have enough time to leave the English capital can take a sensory vacation to exotic lands at the Elemis Day-Spa, set within a 1720s townhouse located in a warren of charming cobblestone pedestrian lanes conveniently located just off Bond Street.

It is easy to feel at home here, for the spa's reception lounge resembles a friend's stylish living room where you can browse through a coffee table book and sip a herbal tea or a fruit smoothie as you wait for your 'boarding call' to romantic faraway destinations that may include Bali, Japan, Morocco, Polynesia, Thailand and Tibet.

Your quest for beauty and wellness, restoration and inner peace will lead you to treatment suites gorgeously dressed in hand-made Thai silk drapes of jewelled hues, or into one of three sensory suites.

Sensory Suites are themed to various holistic Day Rituals—each one an all-round experience that recreates the colours, textures, sounds, scents and mood of exotic distant places and ceremonies. Day Rituals may be enjoyed on your own, or as a couple.

In the lavishly appointed Moroccan Moorish Suite on the basement level, for example, you can indulge in The Moorish Ceremony of Dreams. This imaginatively themed treatment promises you the ultimate in pleasurable escapism. It includes an Exotic Frangipani Body Nourish Float (where your body is slathered in a scented oil created from soaked frangipani flowers and coconut, and then cocooned as you float on a waterbed). It also takes you to the Rasul (where you and your partner can apply differently hued *chakra* muds on each others' bodies before basting in the herbal steam).

In the Balinese Suite on the first floor, you can partake of The Balinese Ceremony of Reverence. This includes a Balinese Boreh Hot Spice Therapy: a warming herbal wrap traditionally used by farmers to ease sore muscles after wading through paddy fields.

In the Thai Suite on the penthouse level, you will be supremely pampered with The

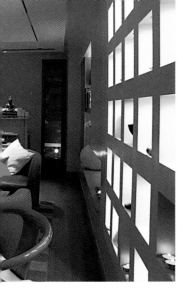

OPPOSITE, LEFT: *The Thai Suite is a sensual heaven topped with a glass atrium lavishly draped in Thai silks. It comprises a relaxation area and two adjoining therapy rooms.*

OPPOSITE, CENTRE: *Luxuriate in a petal-strewn Exotic Jasmine Flower Bath, which combines the play of massage jets, sensual aromas and colour therapy. This bath can be enjoyed as part of the spa's Jasmine Lulur Ritual.*

LEFT: *This haven of calm was designed by The Syntax Group. Your departure to your sensory adventure starts at the reception lounge (pictured).*

Royal Thai Ceremony that includes an Exotic Lime & Ginger Salt Glow, and an Exotic Coconut Rub and Milk Ritual Wrap.

Revolutionary and effective therapies on the spa treatment menu include the Japanese Silk Booster Facial. This special facial uses an advanced formulation of natural silk protein and active plant extracts to refine your skin and maintain its youthful glow.

The Fennel Cleansing Cellulite and Colon Therapy is comprised of a detoxifying body mask and drainage massage to help reduce cellulite, and a non-invasive form of colon cleansing in the form of abdominal massage and reflexology to purify your body.

When the chime of Tibetan cymbals marks the end of your journey and gently brings you back to the present, you will notice yourself breathing more freely. Not only is the air within the spa filled with beneficial aromatic essential oils; your therapist would have also intuitively guided you in your breathing to relax your body in order for you to benefit fully from your journey.

Spa Statistics

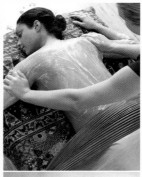

TYPE OF SPA
Day spa

SPA AREA
372 sq m (4,000 sq ft)

FACILITIES
7 single treatment rooms; 1 Balinese Slipper Bath Garden; 1 *rasul* steam chamber; 2 dry flotation beds; 1 sensory relaxation lounge, 1 Thai relaxation lounge (for clients who book The Balinese Ceremony of Reverence, The Moorish Ceremony of Dreams or The Royal Thai Ceremony); 1 spa boutique

SIGNATURE TREATMENTS
Exotic Coconut Rub & Milk Ritual Wrap, Exotic Lime & Ginger Salt Glow, Japanese Silk Booster Facial

TREATMENTS & THERAPIES
Anti-ageing treatments, anti-cellulite treatments, aromatherapy, baths, body bronzing, body scrubs, body wraps, eye treatments, facials, hand and foot treatments, hot stone therapies, jet lag treatments, manicures and pedicures, massages, non-invasive colon therapy, pre- and post-natal treatments, purifying back treatments, scalp treatments; spa packages

PROVISIONS FOR COUPLES
Two-seater *rasul*; Arabian Jewel Ritual, The Balinese Ceremony of Reverence, The Moorish Ceremony of Dreams, The Royal Thai Ceremony

SPA CUISINE
Lunch is provided for guests experiencing The Royal Thai Ceremony. Provisions for various dietary requirements are available on request.

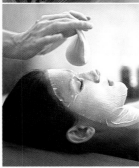

TOP: *In the Exotic Coconut Rub & Milk Ritual Wrap, your skin is polished with coconut, mungbean, spices and lavender, then nourished with oil. Warm milk is poured over your body before you are cocooned in a wrap and left to enjoy a dry float.*

ABOVE: *The Japanese Silk Booster Facial will take the skin on a journey of total renewal. Natural Japanese silk protein, or sulphur compresses, combined with pure plant phytoamine bio-complexes and intelligent algae have been formulated for advanced scientific skincare, producing immediate results.*

SERVICES
Corporate programmes; private spa parties; gift vouchers

LANGUAGE SPOKEN BY THERAPISTS
English

CONTACT
Elemis Day-Spa
2-3 Lancashire Court
Mayfair
London W1S 1EX
England
United Kingdom
T: +44 (0)20 8909 5060
F: +44 (0)20 7499 9558
E: elemisdayspa@elemis.com
W: www.elemis.com

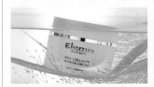

The Pro-Collagen Marine Cream is an anti-ageing cream that increases skin elasticity, suppleness, firmness and hydration levels.

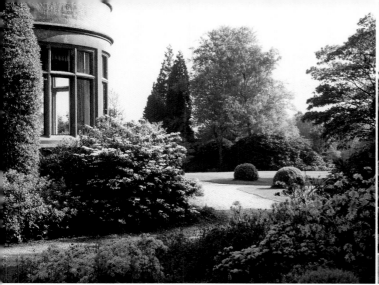

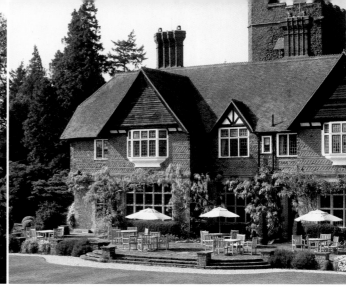

Grayshott Hall Health Fitness Retreat
Surrey, England, United Kingdom

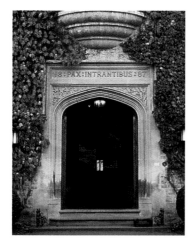

Many guests who return once or twice a year to fine-tune their health, de-stress, lose weight, shake off an unhealthy habit, lift their spirits in winter, or detoxify after a Caribbean holiday of over-indulgence say they feel a calm oozing through the walls as they step through the threshold below the Latin inscription (pictured) 'Pax Intrantibus' (peace as you enter). When you depart, the inscription 'Salus Exuentibus' (health as you leave) is a fitting send-off. The inscriptions date back to 1887.

Grayshott Hall Health Fitness Retreat is just an hour's drive, yet miles away from the stresses of London. The peace and beauty of its 19-hectare (48-acre) gardens is enhanced by the adjoining 283 hectares (700 acres) of land preserved by the National Trust.

The two-level country manor, named by *Spa Management Magazine* as the 1996 Jeffrey Joseph Spa of the Year, is a non-intimidating healing space, with therapists who are professional and reassuring. On arrival, slip into a towelling robe and slippers. The atmosphere is relaxed and casual, even if many prefer to change for dinner.

Five minutes before your treatment, your therapist will meet you and take you to your treatment room. Your first session will be a consultation to devise a treatment programme based on your personal objectives. The à la carte menu contains over 80 treatments—including facials (some designed for men), hydrotherapy, massages (manual and mechanical), body treatments

and, specifically, Natural Therapies—to help you get back on track, physically, mentally or emotionally.

Key Natural Therapies to balance body and mind are Lymphatic Stimulation (skin brushing followed by a massage with aromatherapy oils to detoxify, refresh and energise) and Oriental Wisdom (Chinese *tui na* and Japanese shiatsu massage techniques applied with a blend of essential oils and Chinese herbs to harmonise your meridians and hormonal imbalances, and ease skin problems). Tui-Na Face Massage and Holistic Massage are slow and gentle, but the effects are profound; many people drift into sleep and awaken refreshed, while others find the sessions cathartic. The former has proven so popular, it is now available as a stand-alone treatment that includes a brief tongue analysis and a massage to acupoints on your neck, scalp and head to tone your internal organs. The latter full-body massage is performed so meditatively that it slows down an overactive mind.

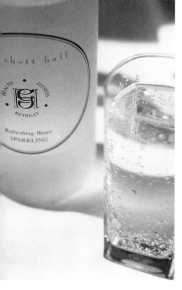

OPPOSITE: *The poetic beauty of the region and the heather-scented air inspired literary greats such as George Bernard Shaw and Arthur Conan Dolye. Grayshott Hall was once a farm where Victorian poet Alfred Tennyson lived for a year.*

LEFT: *Complimentary beverages such as Vivreau (pictured)—spring water bottled on the grounds of Grayshott Hall—are available throughout.*

BOTTOM: *Daily activities and classes, all meals, an exfoliation session with Grayshott Hall's Body Exfoliation Cream, and a treatment consultation are included in the room rate. A complimentary Grayshott Massage (pictured) comes with every night's stay.*

To gain a better perspective of your health, a one-on-one lifestyle consultation may help you manage your stress; a session with a personal trainer may kick-start a workout programme or recommend exercises; and a nutritional consultation and non-invasive BEST (bio-energetic stress test to determine food intolerances) will put you on a path to better eating habits.

Grayshott Hall may be compared to a therapeutic retreat where you can sample a range of therapies, and fitness and relaxation exercises. You will discover those that best suit you, and be inspired to continue on the path of wellness when you return home.

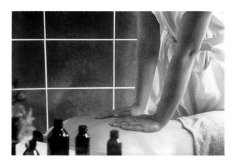

Spa Statistics

TYPE OF SPA
Destination spa

SPA AREA
19 hectares (48 acres)

FACILITIES
75 bedrooms, 35 single treatment rooms; 4 consultation rooms; 2 relaxation rooms; 2 cold plunge pools, 1 whirlpool; 2 saunas, 2 steam rooms; 1 solarium, 1 sunbed; 1 hair salon; 1 aerobics studio, 1 gymnasium, 1 Pilates studio; 1 indoor swimming pool with aqua gym equipment; 1 croquet lawn; 1 golf course (9 hole par 3), 1 putting green; 2 indoor tennis courts, 1 outdoor tennis court; 1 spa boutique

SIGNATURE TREATMENTS
Lymphatic Stimulation, Oriental Wisdom

TREATMENTS & THERAPIES
Acupuncture, Alexander Technique, anti-ageing treatments, anti-cellulite treatments, aromatherapy, Bach Flower Remedies, baths, body bronzing, body scrubs, body wraps, bust treatments, Chinese therapies, chiropody, craniosacral therapy, electrotherapy, eye treatments, facials, firming and slimming treatments, hair treatments, hand and foot treatments, heat treatments, holistic treatments, hot stone therapies, hydrotherapy, hypnotherapy, lymphatic drainage, make-up services, manicures and pedicures, massages, movement therapies, osteopathy, physiotherapy, pre- and post-natal treatments, purifying back treatments, reflexology, salon services, scalp treatments, thalassotherapy, waxing. Some treatments are only available on certain days, so enquire about availability when booking your stay.

SPA CUISINE
Meals are prepared in line with World Health Organization guidelines. Food served in the Main Dining Room is low in saturated fat and calories; this is further reduced in meals served at the Light Dining Room. Meat, fish and vegetarian options are

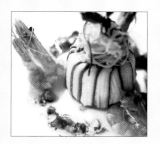

In the past, diet regimes were strictly regimented. These days, meals are attractive to the eye and palette even if they are calorie counted and low in saturated fat.

available at all meals. Provisions for various dietary requirements are available on request—please advise in advance. No alcohol is served.

ACTIVITIES & PROGRAMMES
Aerobics, aquaerobics, badminton (in summer), biking, golf, horse riding, Pilates, *tai chi*, tennis, yoga; cooking and meditation classes, sports instruction; talks on health and alternative health

SERVICES
BEST test (food intolerance and vitamin/mineral deficiency analysis), body composition analysis, fitness assessment; general healthcare consultation, hairstyle consultation (on request), life-coach counselling, nutritional consultation, personal training, skincare consultation; day-use rooms; gift certificates

LANGUAGES SPOKEN BY THERAPISTS
English, French, German, Hebrew, Spanish, Welsh

ADMISSION
There is a minimum of a 2-night stay at Grayshott Hall, but a 4-night stay is recommended.

CONTACT
Grayshott Hall
Headley Road
Grayshott, Near Hindhead
Surrey GU26 6JJ
England
United Kingdom
T: +44 (0)1428 602 020
F: +44 (0)1428 602 001
E: reservations@grayshott-hall.co.uk
W: www.grayshott-hall.co.uk

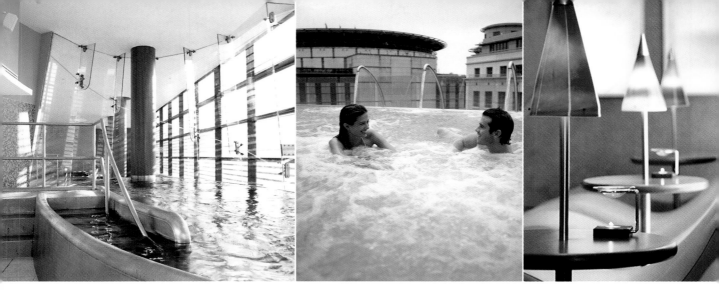

One Spa at Sheraton Grand Hotel & Spa
Edinburgh, Scotland, United Kingdom

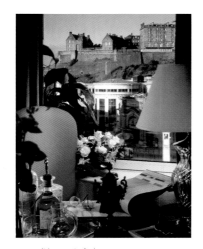

ABOVE: *It is easy to feel at home in the hotel's spacious guest rooms and suites decorated in contemporary Scottish patterns and rich furnishings. A view of Edinburgh Castle from many rooms tops off the experience.*

OPPOSITE, BOTTOM: *A wood and stainless steel bridge over the 19-metre (60-foot) indoor ozone-treated pool leads to a secluded area where the Cleopatra baths are located.*

At the five-star Sheraton Grand Hotel & Spa, you are centrally placed to explore the city's main shopping district of Princes Street, the historic Edinburgh Castle and the distinctive architectural features of the Georgian New Town.

An elevated glass walkway takes you from the hotel building to a stylish six-storey glass structure which resembles a translucent jewelled box: home to One Spa, a gem in the Starwood Spa Collection that was voted in 2003 as 'Favourite UK Hotel Spa of the Year' by *Condé Nast Traveller* and 'Destination/Hotel Spa of the Year' at the British Beauty Awards.

The spa's vibrant colours and organic design help set the scene for renewal and health as you wander through the curved, bone-coloured wood-walled corridors. Relax in the heat of the gold and orange mosaic Laconium, baste in the steam of the rich blue and turquoise Hammam, or buff your body in the stone surrounds of the Wet Plinth Room.

Many holistic treatments on the One Spa menu were drawn from the cultures of China,

Bali and India, adapted to suit modern lifestyles. Many start with a footbath and a salt scrub to soften your skin.

Minds that otherwise find it hard to switch off will let go during the ESPA Optimal Release, which includes a massage using free-flowing movements that release your joints and mental tension. The ESPA Ayurvedic Holistic Body Treatment provides a *marma* massage of vital energy centred on your face and body, as well as a tranquillity inducing *chakra* massage of your head and scalp which is vitality enhancing.

If there is anything twice as good as a massage, it is the ESPA Balinese Synchronised Massage, performed harmoniously by two therapists using stretching and rolling movements and long deep strokes. The oils used are enriched with fragrant spices from Southeast Asia.

Perk up your day with a weekday treat in the form of a 1-hour-25-minute ESPA Life Saving Back Massage (a back cleansing and exfoliation treatment and a tension-releasing

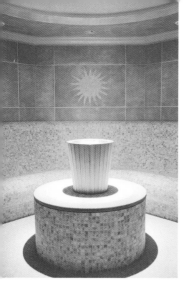

OPPOSITE, LEFT AND CENTRE: *The stainless steel hydropool, located on the roof, five floors above street level, gives you a breathtaking view of the surrounds and a top-of-the-world feeling. This pool can be accessed from an indoor section.*

OPPOSITE, CENTRE: *The relaxation area is a soothing haven.*

LEFT: *Arrive at least 40 minutes before your treatment to relax in the Thermal Suite. Baste in the steamy Hammam, the Aroma Grotto infused with herbal extracts, the Bio Sauna enhanced with coloured lights, the Finnish-styled Rock Sauna and a Laconium (pictured) of dry heat. Then cool off in a Lifestyle Shower with an icy cool mist or warm rainshower.*

aromatherapy massage) or an ESPA Express Facial (with aromatherapy products to refresh and rejuvenate your skin). To rebalance your entire self, try Holistic Pulsing. Gentle rocking techniques, performed as you lie fully clothed on the treatment table, enhance your mobility and release emotional tensions.

Perhaps the best way to enjoy the spa is to book a two-hour session with a therapist; in this way, a treatment can be customised for you according to your interests and needs. This individualised attention is fit for stars such as actor Ralph Fiennes and director Robert Carlisle, who have had their bodies and minds rebalanced in this healing space.

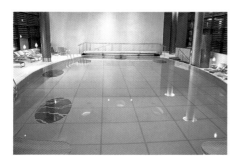

Spa Statistics

TYPE OF SPA
Hotel spa

SPA AREA
3,252 sq m (35,000 sq ft)

FACILITIES
11 single treatment rooms, 1 wet plinth room; 1 consultation room; 1 relaxation room; 1 watsu pool; 2 Cleopatra baths, 1 hydrotherapy bath, 1 outdoor rooftop hydropool; 3 saunas (Rock Sauna, Bio Sauna, Laconium), 2 steam rooms (hammam, aroma grotto), 6 tepidariums; 1 Ice Drench, 2 Lifestyle Showers; 2 nail stations; 1 cardio studio, 1 gymnasium; 1 indoor swimming pool

SIGNATURE TREATMENTS
ESPA Ayurvedic Holistic Body Treatment, ESPA Balinese Synchronised Massage, ESPA Optimal Release

TREATMENTS & THERAPIES
Anti-cellulite treatments, aqua therapy, aromatherapy, Ayurvedic treatments, baths, body scrubs, body wraps, craniosacral therapy, eye treatments, facials, hand and foot treatments, holistic treatments, heat treatments, holistic pulsing, holistic therapies, hot stone therapies, hydrotherapy, jet lag treatments, lymphatic drainage, make-up services, manicures and pedicures, massages, movement therapies, pre- and post-natal treatments, purifying back treatments, reflexology, *reiki*, scalp treatments, Thai therapies, waxing; ESPA Half- and Full-Day Programmes, 1- and 2-day Residential Packages (which include treatments and accommodation)

PROVISIONS FOR COUPLES
Serail Mud Chamber

SPA CUISINE
The spa café, Santini Bis on the 5th floor, serves high-energy light meals. The food is designed to be both tasty and nutritious. You can also enjoy smoothies, isotonic drinks, tea, coffee or herbal infusions throughout the day.

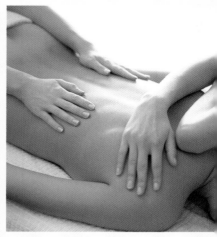

The ESPA Balinese Synchronised Massage performed by two therapists is so seamless it feels like you are being massaged by one therapist with four hands.

SERVICES
Body composition analysis, general healthcare consultation, personal training, skincare consultation; corporate programmes; gift certificates; car parking

LANGUAGES SPOKEN BY THERAPISTS
English, French, Indian (Hindi, Tamil, Malayalam), Russian

ADMISSION
Membership is available but not required for admission. Three types of memberships are available, depending on whether your interests lie in fitness, aqua facilities, or all facilities for a total spa experience. Members receive a personal Lifestyle Assessment and Personalised Programme tailored to their needs, with fitness instructors guiding them to their personal goals.

CONTACT
Sheraton Grand Hotel & Spa
8 Conference Square
Edinburgh
EH3 8AN
Scotland
United Kingdom
T: +44 (0)131 221 7777
F: +44 (0)131 221 7778
E: info@one-spa.com
W: www.one-spa.com

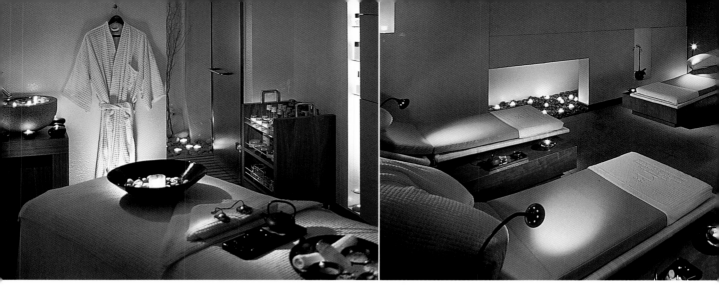

The Spa at Mandarin Oriental, Mandarin Oriental Hyde Park
London, England, United Kingdom

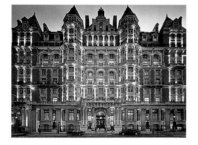

The hotel's Knightsbridge entrance (pictured) became its main entrance in the 19th century as signages were not allowed to face Hyde Park. Queen Victoria allegedly locked the gate to the original Hyde Park entrance during a walk. Even today, the hotel retains the charming tradition of applying for royal permission to open the Hyde Park entrance—otherwise reserved for the royals—to roll out the red carpet for celebrities, foreign dignitaries and guests celebrating special occasions.

Mandarin Oriental Hyde Park straddles the buzz of Knightsbridge, London's prime shopping belt, and the soothing greenery of Hyde Park, where you can enjoy a specially prepared picnic hamper of chilled lobster and champagne during the summer months.

The hotel was conceived in 1889 as a Gentleman's Club: then the tallest building in London. If the hotel's walls could talk, they would tell of summits between heads of states, and royal celebrations where Queen Elizabeth II and the late Princess Margaret learnt to dance.

Like the hotel, The Spa at Mandarin Oriental is a secure haven for those who need to rebalance their bodies, minds and spirits at the nurturing hands of a personal therapist. All spa-goers are pampered like stars; by booking time with a therapist instead of a specific treatment, your session can be personalised to your likes and needs.

Your therapeutic adventure begins as soon as you swap your shoes for spa slippers, slide a crystal bracelet holding your locker key on to your wrist, and descend the granite stairs—decorated with tea lights and single orchids—to the changing areas and the Zen relaxation rooms. In the changing room, each locker is equipped with a personal electronic safe to secure your valuables.

The spa's sleek architectural lines and contemporary Eastern décor hint of holistic treatments that blend Asia's healing cultures with Europe's spa traditions. The resulting luxurious repertoire of facial and body treatments is suited to ladies who lunch; body treatments are also popular with male spa-goers.

A strong Ayurvedic influence is reflected in treatments such as the Ayurvedic Holistic Body Treatment which includes a Marma Massage focusing on the vital energy points on your face and body, and a Chakra Massage focusing on your head and scalp. This revitalising but deeply calming treatment virtually leaves you speechless.

A Thai influence is evident in Optimal Release, a gentle, free-flowing massage that

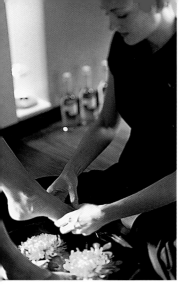

OPPOSITE, LEFT: *Treatment rooms at the spa—named the Best Day Spa 2001 by Health & Beauty Awards and Best UK Hotel Spa 2002 by Condé Nast Traveller (UK)—are a sensual composition of textures: crackled lacquer walls, horsehair panels, granite sinks, wooden floors and a Japanese-inspired bamboo and pebble garden.*

OPPOSITE, RIGHT: *Quiet yourself at the Zen Relaxation Area prior to your treatment. Each lounger—by Japanese designer team, Azumi—can be individually adjusted to suit your preference.*

LEFT: *Your session at the spa begins with a welcoming Foot Ritual—in which your feet are bathed in waters imbued with flowers and essential oils.*

incorporates deep stretches and rocking movements to relieve tension in your muscles and joints, leaving you deeply relaxed.

For an entire day of pampering, opt for packages such as The Ritual. Like other treatments, it begins with a foot ritual and herbal infusion. The Ritual also includes Purifying Herbal Linens (a detoxifying herbal wrap with hot stones); body exfoliation; Detoxifying Sea of Senses (a cleansing algae wrap), Essence Of Earth (a soothing mud wrap) or Oshadi Envelopment (a balancing herbal wrap); and an Ayurvedic Holistic Massage or a Joint Release Massage. However, if you have just under two hours, opt for When Time Is Of The Essence, in which you will be given a facial with eye treatment, and a manicure and pedicure, performed by two therapists.

If you are reluctant to put on your shoes and return to the outside world, linger at leisure in the Zen relaxation room. To continue the spa experience at home, there are ESPA face and body products, Ayurvedic teas, incense, New Age CDs and spa slippers.

Spa Statistics

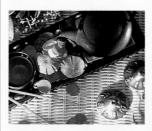

The gentle ching-ching of Tibetan cymbals (pictured) marks the start and end of certain treatments.

TYPE OF SPA
Hotel spa

SPA AREA
50 sq m (538 sq ft)

FACILITIES
8 single treatment rooms; 2 relaxation rooms; 2 sanariums; 2 Vitality Pools (for hydrotherapy); 2 Amethyst Crystal Steam Rooms; 1 gymnasium

SIGNATURE TREATMENTS
Ayurvedic Holistic Body Treatment, Balinese Synchronised Massage, Optimal Release; The Ritual

TREATMENTS & THERAPIES
Anti-cellulite treatments, aromatherapy, Ayurveda, body scrubs, body wraps, eye treatments, facials, hand and foot treatments, holistic treatments, hot stone therapies, Indonesian treatments, jet lag treatments, massages, pre- and post-natal treatments, purifying back treatments, reflexology, scalp treatments; half-day programmes (that include use of the gymnasium), full-day programmes (that include use of gymnasium and lunch in the hotel's The Park restaurant).

SPA CUISINE
Not available, but full-day programmes include a lunch of light Asian specialities at The Park restaurant. Your therapist will be able to advise you on selections that are best suited to your *dosha* type

LANGUAGES SPOKEN BY THERAPISTS
Cantonese, English, French, Hindi, Spanish, Mandarin, Nepali

ADMISSION
Non-hotel guests are required to have a minimum treatment time of 2 hours. Non-hotel guests have access to the gymnasium if they book a half-day or full-day package. The gymnasium is open from 5.30 A.M. to midnight.

CONTACT
Mandarin Oriental Hyde Park
66 Knightsbridge
London SW1X 7LA
England
United Kingdom
T: +44 (0)207 838 9888
F: +44 (0)207 838 9883
E: molonspa@mohg.com
W: www.mandarinoriental.com

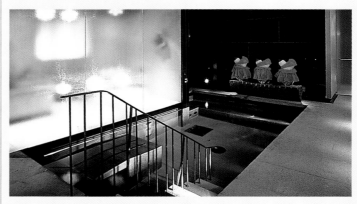

Allow yourself 40 minutes before your treatment to relax yourself in the sanarium (a gentler version of the sauna), the steam room (which features an amethyst to enhance wellbeing) or the Vitality Pool (a sequence of bubbling jets which massage different parts of your body). The 'Three Graces' by British artist Stephen Cox watch over the Vitality Pool in the female heat and water areas (pictured).

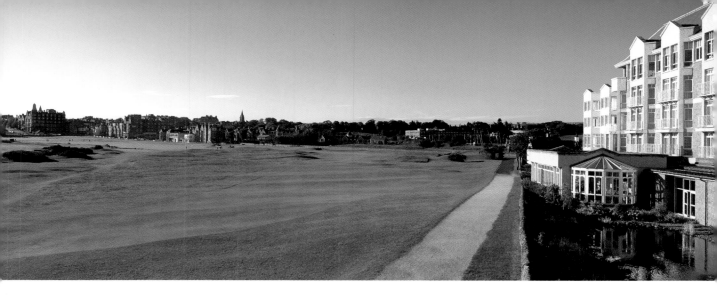

The Spa at Old Course Hotel, Golf Resort & Spa
Kingdom of Fife, Scotland, United Kingdom

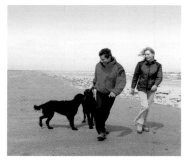

The award-winning Old Course Hotel is situated in St Andrews, which is acknowledged as the home of golf where the game was first played some 500 years ago. In 1995, a golfer playing the infamous Road Hole adjacent to the hotel inadvertently hit a ball into the chimney. The ball bounced on the fire grate and smashed a glass-top table in the Board Room, shocking the meeting in progress!

Built in 1968 to accommodate visitors to the historic university town of St Andrews on Scotland's east coast, the five-star Old Course Hotel, Golf Resort & Spa is situated next to the 17th fairway of the Old Course where its Road Hole is considered the most difficult par 4 in golf. The hotel is also a 2-minute walk from West Sands, the beach immortalised in the movie *Chariots of Fire*.

With nine golf courses in St Andrews, a vicinity that has become synonymous with the sport, the hotel attracts top athletes and golfing celebrities such as actors Michael Douglas and Catherine Zeta-Jones.

The Spa, the centre of wellbeing, is situated in the heart of the hotel on the ground and first floors, and is easily accessible from guest rooms. While one may be tempted to think of it as a sanctuary for golf widows, the property is also a popular romantic destination for couples who are able to enjoy their treatments together in the large treatment rooms, many with stunning views across the Old Course to the sea.

The Spa's signature treatment, the Old Course Golfer's Tonic which reflects the property's sporting heritage, is enticing more men to the spa. Designed to ease aches and pains in the backs and legs of golfers who may feel below par despite a fulfilling game, the treatment begins with a relaxing massage, followed by a luxurious foot treatment, and includes exfoliation, deep massage and a paraffin wax mask on the back and feet.

Hydrotherapy treatments and treatments such as the Cold Marine Facial—which uses marine and plant extracts from Thalgo to refine sensitive skin—are especially fitting, given the Spa's proximity to the sea. Botanical ingredients from Clarins and Pevonia Botanica are used in popular European treatments that include the Paris Method Facial and Kigelia Bust Treatment respectively. Pevonia Botanica's scented candles—designed to activate your smell memory sensor—are especially popular with guests who wish to bring home a memory of the spa experience; these can be purchased from the Spa boutique.

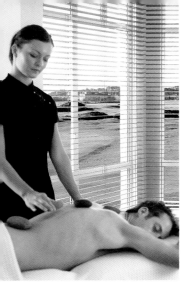

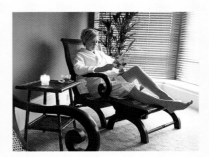

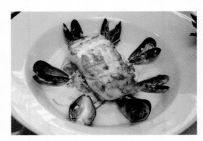

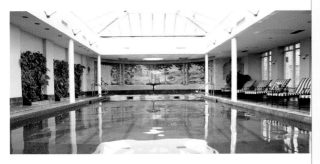

OPPOSITE: *The hotel is just paces from the Road Hole of the Old Course and only a 5-minute stroll from the ancient university town of St Andrews.*

LEFT: *Each therapy suite is unique in décor, and many of them come with a soothing view of the Old Course and the blue sea beyond.*

BOTTOM: *Relax by the sun-loungers or do your laps at the indoor pool, which is bathed in natural light.*

Complementary therapies such as *reiki*, reflexology and kinesiology are also available.

If you are looking to spend a day in the spa while your partner tees off on one of the numerous golf courses, you may want to take advantage of a Spa Day package, which comprises three treatments and a healthy two-course spa lunch. A separate treatment menu is available for men.

Longer packages such as Spa Stays, which include the tellingly named Spa With A Hint Of Golf or Golf With A Touch Of Spa are also available. These include accommodation, meals, spa treatments and golf, giving you the opportunity to enjoy the best of all worlds.

Spa Statistics

TYPE OF SPA
Resort spa

SPA AREA
2,110 sq m (22,680 sq ft)

FACILITIES
12 treatment rooms (all large enough to accommodate couples); 1 relaxation lounge; 1 whirlpool; 1 cardio studio, 1 gymnasium; 1 indoor swimming pool; 1 spa boutique; 1 golf course owned by hotel (and numerous courses in and around the town); 1 fine dining restaurant, 1 seafood bar & restaurant, 2 bars; 1 conservatory; 1 library; gift shops

SIGNATURE TREATMENT
Old Course Golfer's Tonic

TREATMENTS & THERAPIES
Anti-ageing treatments, anti-cellulite treatments, aromatherapy, Ayurvedic treatments, body bronzing, body scrubs, body wraps, bust treatments, Chinese therapies, electrotherapy, eye treatments, facials, firming and slimming treatments, hand and foot treatments, holistic treatments, hot stone therapies, hydrotherapy, lymphatic drainage, manicures and pedicures, massages, pre- and post-natal treatments, purifying back treatments, reflexology, *reiki*, scalp treatments, waxing; packages such as Spa Stays (which include treatments, accommodation, meals and golf), Spa Days (which include treatments and lunch), and seasonable packages such as the Mother & Daughter Mothers' Day Package

PROVISIONS FOR COUPLES
All treatment rooms are large enough to accommodate couples; seasonable packages such as Valentines' Package

SPA CUISINE
Guests may dine at the Sands Seafood Bar & Restaurant or order from the spa menu based on dishes served at the Sands, which are light fusion dishes with an Asian influence. Provisions for various dietary requirements are available on request.

The relaxation room, tastefully decorated with warm walls and plantation furniture, is an inviting space where you can sip a herbal tea.

ACTIVITIES & PROGRAMMES
Pilates, *tai chi*, scenic walks, stretch and flex, yoga

SERVICES
Life-coach counselling; fitness evaluation with related nutritional advice; personal fitness training; baby-sitting, childcare; corporate programmes; gift certificates; spa days

LANGUAGES SPOKEN BY THERAPISTS
Dutch, English, French

ADMISSION
Membership is available, but not required for admission.

CONTACT
Old Course Hotel, Golf Resort & Spa
St Andrews, Kingdom of Fife
KY16 9SP
Scotland
United Kingdom
T: +44 (0)1334 474 371
F: +44 (0)1334 477 668
E: reservations@oldcoursehotel.co.uk
W: www.oldcoursehotel.co.uk

Healthy spa options include a seared fillet of halibut with mussels and vegetable compote (pictured); capriccio of monkfish with pickled vegetables and salsa verde; or home-cured Scottish salmon, pink peppercorns, and lemon and lime cream.

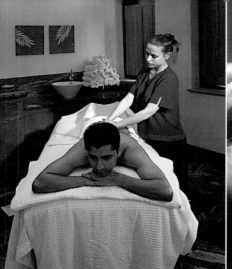
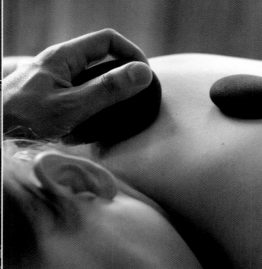
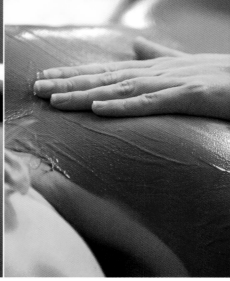

The Spa at Pennyhill Park
Surrey, England, United Kingdom

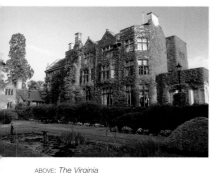

ABOVE: *The Virginia Creeper-clad walls of the hotel appear even more picturesque and romantic when the leaves turn red in autumn.*

OPPOSITE, RIGHT: *As you are lulled by your therapist's intuitive touch, your thoughts may also drift with passing clouds represented by a kaleidoscope of changing colours on the light system above your therapy couch.*

Driving through the gates and up the long driveway towards Pennyhill Park Hotel is almost symbolic of leaving the stresses of the city behind. The 50-hectare (120-acre) property, just under an hour's drive from London, is an idyllic antidote to today's fast-paced hurried lifestyle—a haven of peace surrounded by redwoods and ablaze with rhododendrons.

Pennyhill Park, which has evolved into a 123-room hotel from an English manor built in 1849, still retains the tradition and charm of a genteel country residence. Complementing it is The Spa, which is only open to members and their guests, and hotel residents. This tranquil space is sprawled over three levels in a purpose-built building. You can get fit here by working out in the gymnasium, do a series of laps in the 18-metre (60-feet) outdoor swimming pool, or swim in a ballroom-styled 25-metre (80-feet) indoor pool to the surrealistic accompaniment of underwater music. You may also opt for an aquatic therapy session in an intimate bay within the indoor pool.

An indoor hydropool is connected to the outdoors via a swim-through.

If you are heading to the office after your workout, there are attentive valets in the separate male and female changing areas who will see to it that your office clothes are neatly pressed before you leave.

On entering the spa, you will be given a bathrobe to change into, or if you prefer, a spa suit of wide-legged trousers and a kimono top. Plan to arrive at least 90 minutes before your treatment commences so that you can relax your body in the spa's Thermal Heaven before your treatment. This lavish sequence of heated and chilled rooms includes a fun Schnapps Room infused with essential oils which evoke the scent of the liquor. Cool off in an ice cave which almost resembles an igloo with thick panels of ice, and an icy cool fountain.

On entering the treatment area, you will notice sweet silence instead of piped music. You will, however, be provided with a sound pack with eight different genres of music to listen to in the relaxation area. Music in the

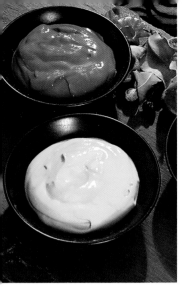

OPPOSITE, LEFT: *Your treatment room is a private sanctuary where you can enjoy a seamless spa session. After a wrap, step straight into the shower, then adjourn back to your therapy couch for a massage.*

OPPOSITE, CENTRE: *Your body is stroked with warm volcanic stones in the Hot Rock Massage which rebalances your energy levels.*

OPPOSITE, RIGHT, AND LEFT: *Your 'Wulima Yulu' (sensory journey) starts with ingredients from the Australian bush. Blends of plants with muds include balancing yellow mud with ylang ylang and mandarin; detoxifying red mud with mint and grapefruit; and warming grey mud with pepperberry.*

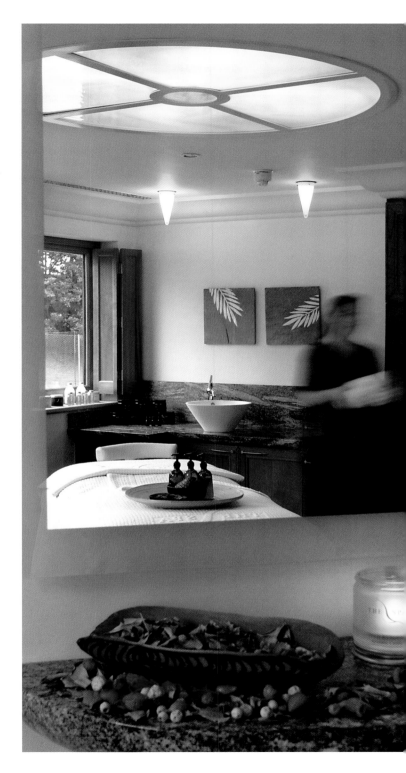

treatment rooms can be individually controlled according to your taste.

If you are visiting the spa with friends or your family, an area comprising two single treatment rooms, a double treatment room, and a lounge area can be closed off for your party when certain packages are booked. This area can also be booked for meetings, and its flat-screen TV for watching DVDs or videos doubles up as a computer screen for business presentations, making it an ideal location for an incentive trip. For brides-to-be, the Bridal Package, which includes pampering treatments and champagne, is a popular option for hen parties.

Spa treatments are designed to help you stay youthful, fit and stress-free. The menu comprises over 50 treatments, with a strong focus on aromatherapy, colour therapy and herbalism, as well as options for men and pregnant women. If you are unsure of what treatments to opt for, book time, and your therapist can advise you on the therapies that best suit your interests when you arrive.

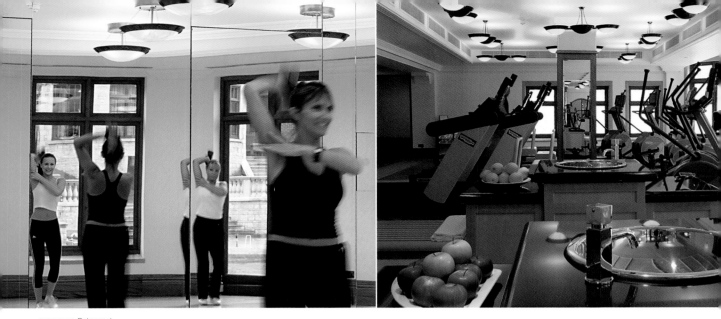

ABOVE LEFT: *Relax and stretch your body with gentle exercises. Classes are designed for small groups of up to 12, but individual sessions can also be arranged.*

ABOVE, CENTRE: *England's rugby team advised on the design of the gymnasium, a veritable fitness playground. While you work out on the latest equipment, you can even surf the Net, check your emails, or play a computer game on a personalised entertainment system. You may also compete with a friend on performance-related computer games. The Bespoke Programme, a personalised workout programme, helps you maximise your workout.*

OPPOSITE, TOP: *Couples may choose to book double treatment rooms.*

BELOW: *The central pedestal in the relaxation room is a delightfully visual steam feature which keeps the air in the room moist.*

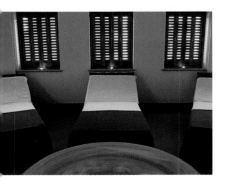

Products used in treatments combine Western technology with Asian and Australian ancient healing secrets. They show a respect for the earth and the human body with their emphasis on purity, efficacy, and social responsibility. Derived from organically grown plants from renewable sources, they contain no artificial colours, fragrances, or animal by-products and are cruelty-free.

Featured prominently on the spa menu are treatments using Li'Tya products inspired by the healing and spiritual techniques of Australian aboriginals, and developed with the wisdom of aboriginal elders. Li'Tya products derived from potent ingredients such as berries, nuts, fruit, clays, muds and desert salts from the Australian bush provide a strong connection to Mother Nature.

Lowanna—which is aboriginal for 'beautiful'—is a 75-minute session that comprises a facial, hand and foot treatment, and head massage. It is a gentle way to initiate first time spa-goers into the spa experience.

The Dreaming is the spa's ultimate treatment that literally pampers you from the roots of your hair to the tips of your toes. Your feet are soaked and massaged in a warm bath enriched with dried flowers native to Australia; your body is exfoliated with your choice of desert salts and aromatherapy oils, then coated with clay. As you are cocooned in a wrap, you will be given a deeply relaxing Paudi Scalp Massage which works the 21 acupressure points on your face and scalp, while your hair is exquisitely conditioned with a Quandong Hair Masque. Your skin will feel velvety smooth after a shower.

The Dreaming continues with a Kodo ('melody') body massage, inspired by aboriginal techniques. As its name implies, the technique—which includes rhythmic movements, spiral motions, and attention to your pressure points—works to improve your energy flow, and enhance your body, mind, balance and wellness. As your complexion is revived and rejuvenated with a facial, your hands are exfoliated and massaged. Your feet are masked and enveloped in Pepperberry and Peat Mud and warm towels, and later massaged, too. When you finally emerge from

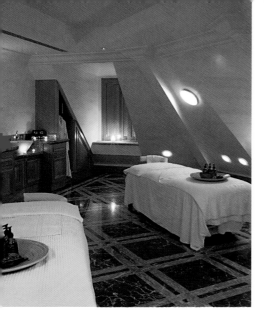

the three-hour session, you may feel like a beautiful butterfly emerging from a cocoon.

Like cuisine served at Café Themis, all spa products used are comprised of organic ingredients. Ingredients used in the spa's private label, simply known as The Spa, smell good enough to eat (and are safe enough if you cannot resist tasting them).

The spa's most decadent hand and foot treatment is the Champagne and Mandarin Manicure or Pedicure—which includes a mask of mandarin and champagne that enhances nail growth, and a protective coat of formaldehyde-free polish. Appropriately, it comes with a serving of delicious chocolates and champagne.

In the Organic Chocolate & Vanilla Body Therapy, your body is exfoliated with a scrub of chocolate, hazelnut and sugar, and massaged with an Organic Vanilla And Citrus Massage Oil. Chocoholics will no doubt find this experience heavenly. To be reminded of this sumptuous experience, bring home The Spa Chocolate And Hazelnut Organic Sugar Scrub from the spa boutique.

Spa Statistics

TYPE OF SPA
Destination spa

SPA AREA
4,180 sq m (45,000 sq ft)

FACILITIES
3 double treatment rooms, 18 single treatment rooms; 1 consultation room; 2 relaxation rooms; 1 cold plunge pool, 1 indoor hydro pool, 1 outdoor hydro pool, 4 reflexology pools (with thrones); 6 Experience Showers; 10 thermal cabins (comprising 1 aromatic steam room, 2 herbal saunas, 1 ice cave, 3 laconiums, 1 Schnapps room, 1 tepidarium, 1 Osmanian Steam); 1 Serial Mud Chamber; 2 grooming areas with vibrating chairs (1 ladies' and 1 men's); 1 exercise studio, 1 gymnasium (incorporating cardiovascular equipment, resistance equipment and free weights); 1 indoor ozonated swimming pool, 1 outdoor ozonated swimming pool; 9-hole golf course, 1 tennis court; 1 spa boutique

SIGNATURE TREATMENTS
Organic Chocolate & Vanilla Body Therapy, The Dreaming

TREATMENTS & THERAPIES
Anti-ageing treatments, anti-cellulite treatments, aqua therapies, aromatherapy, body bronzing, body scrubs, body wraps, eye treatments, facials, firming and slimming treatments, hair treatments, hand and foot treatments, heat treatments, holistic treatments, hot stone therapies, hydrotherapy, jet lag treatments, lymphatic drainage, make-up services, manicures and pedicures, massages, pre- and post-natal treatments, purifying back treatments, reflexology, salon services, scalp treatments, Thai therapies, waxing; spa packages

PROVISIONS FOR COUPLES
3 double treatment rooms. Most treatments can be taken as a couple.

SPA CUISINE
Organic dishes and snacks are served at Café Themis in the spa. The menu comprises a mix and match of 'Healthy' (low in fat and calories) and 'Wicked' (including organic champagne and organic chocolate cakes) options. Vegetarian options are available on the menu, and provisions for various dietary requirements— such as vegetarian, vegan and low-fat—are available on request. The juice bar in the spa serves freshly squeezed organic juices.

ACTIVITIES & PROGRAMMES
Aerobics, archery, golf, Pilates, *tai chi*, tennis, yoga; clay pigeon shooting; Cardio Latino, dance and salsa classes; private make-up lessons; talks by visiting consultants

SERVICES
Body composition analysis, nutritional consultation, personal training, skincare consultation; baby-sitting, childcare; corporate programmes; private spa parties; gift certificates; day-use rooms; personal butler service

LANGUAGES SPOKEN BY THERAPISTS
English, French, German

ADMISSION
The spa is exclusively for members and their guests, and residents of Pennyhill Park Hotel. Annual, 5-year, and lifetime memberships are available. Membership for couples is also available. Members enjoy special prices on treatments and have complimentary use of the Thermal Heaven; residents and guests pay a nominal entrance fee (unless booking a treatment of more than 1 hour). The spa is open only to those aged 16 and above.

CONTACT
Pennyhill Park
London Road, Bagshot
Surrey GU19 5EU
England
United Kingdom
T: +44 (0)1276 486 100
F: +44 (0)1276 486 199
E: enquiries@thespa.uk.com
W: www.thespa.uk.com

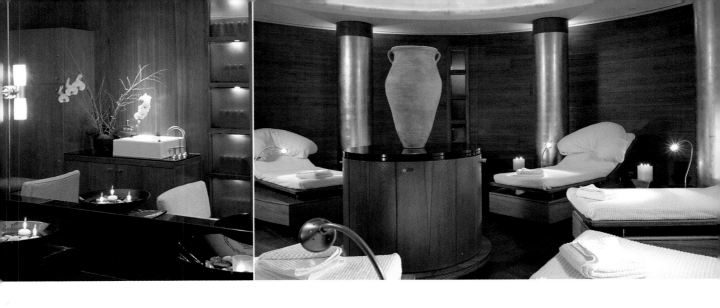

The Spa at Renaissance Chancery Court London
London, England, United Kingdom

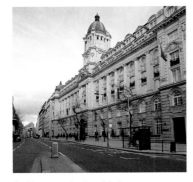

Besides preserving the original building's distinctive features, the hotel's thoughtfulness extends to fitting 7 of its 356 rooms and suites for guests in wheelchairs, and 4 for the hearing-impaired with emergency facilities such as vibrating pillows and flashing beacons.

An imposing bronze-gated carriageway separates the London rush from the hallowed air of the Renaissance London Chancery Court Hotel, just off the cultural and legal pulse of London. This handsome Edwardian landmark, which has starred in period films such as *Howard's End* and *Wilde*, was originally the headquarters of the Pearl Assurance Company from 1914 to 1989.

The hotel is a destination in itself for spa enthusiasts. The Spa at Chancery Court was named 'Day Spa of the Year 2002' at the British Beauty Awards within six months of opening; and spa-goers know they are in good hands, for three of its therapists were nominated for the 'Best Therapist 2003' award by the same body (results were not announced at time of print).

At the spa's reception area, you will exchange your shoes for a pair of jelly reflexology slippers delivered on a wooden tray: a fitting metaphor for leaving behind your worries as you begin your path to rebalance your body, mind and spirit. You will then be led through a labyrinth of slate floors and wooden pathways over a river of pebbles, winding past grey limestone walls and curtains of water. Doors that open to different rooms blend seamlessly with the walls—save for elegant orchids that signify occupied treatment rooms—an effect that is chic yet mysterious.

Allow yourself at least 20 minutes before your treatment to enjoy the heat and wet facilities (located in the segregated changing areas), enhanced with coloured lights. Relax your body in the sauna or steam room (the latter holds an amethyst and is infused with eucalyptus); then cool down at the Lifestyle Shower—a spiral nook of aubergine flecked with gold—with an icy Cool Mist with blue and purple lights, or a warmer Tropical Rainstorm with red and orange lights.

You have a choice of over 40 holistic treatments by ESPA that marry Ayurvedic and Western philosophies; most are designed for both sexes, but others such as the ESPA Flight Reviver (a full body aromatherapy treatment to counter jet lag), and the ESPA Golfer's

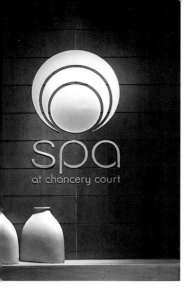

Tonic (a scrub, foot massage with hot stones, head and back massage) are designed for male business travellers. To share a pampering experience with a partner, book the VIP Suite that comes with private amenities such as a shower room and steam bath for two.

The ESPA Holistic Stress Buster With Hot Stone Therapy has become a London ritual like a traditional English afternoon tea at The Lounge in the hotel's lobby, or a lime martini at The Bar. This treatment, which balances the body and mind, begins with a footbath, a full body skin brushing and a scrub. This is followed by an express facial, a scalp massage, and a deep body massage with hot stones— aided by essential oils chosen for your needs—which are placed on vital energy points. Chilled stones may be placed on your face to gently awaken you. If you only have 30 or 40 minutes to spare, opt for a manicure or pedicure which comes with a massage and a healthy lunch bag to go. Whatever your choice, the experience readies you to step back into your shoes to face the world again.

Spa Statistics

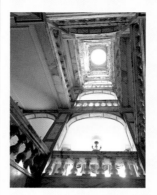

Marble features prominently throughout the hotel. The seven-storey Grand Staircase of rare Pavonazzo marble (pictured) was built to symbolise the stability of the life insurance company which first owned the building.

TYPE OF SPA
Hotel spa

SPA AREA
500 sq m (5,380 sq ft)

FACILITIES
1 double treatment room, 6 single treatment rooms; 1 relaxation lounge; 2 Lifestyle Showers; 2 saunas, 2 Amethyst Crystal Steam Rooms; 1 nail salon; 1 gymnasium; 1 spa boutique

SIGNATURE TREATMENTS
ESPA Holistic Stress Buster With Hot Stone Therapy

TREATMENTS & THERAPIES
Anti-ageing treatments, anti-cellulite treatments, aromatherapy, body scrubs, body wraps, eye treatments, facials, firming and slimming treatments, hair treatments, hand and foot treatments, heat treatments, holistic treatments, hot stone therapies, jet lag treatments, lymphatic drainage, make-up services, manicures and pedicures, massages, pre- and post-natal treatments, reflexology, scalp treatments, waxing; ESPA Full- and Half-Day Programmes; Residential Packages (which include spa treatments, accommodation and breakfast)

PROVISIONS FOR COUPLES
1 VIP couples treatment suite which can be booked for a minimum of 90 minutes;

Spa Full-Day Retreat For Two, Spa Half-Day Retreat For Two (includes treatments, accommodation and English breakfast)

SPA CUISINE
Full-day spa packages include a light lunch in The Lounge. Two-course spa lunches, created by Chef Jun Tanaka, are available at the QC restaurant. Vegetarian options are available on the menu.

SERVICES
Gift certificates

LANGUAGES SPOKEN BY THERAPISTS
English, French, Italian, Spanish

ADMISSION
Hotel guests can enjoy the spa facilities free of charge with a treatment; otherwise, they will be required to pay a nominal fee to use the facilities. Non-residential guests are required to opt for the EPSA Full- or Half-Day Programmes, or a minimum treatment time of 2 hours if selecting from the main treatment list. The gymnasium is exclusively reserved for hotel guests.

CONTACT
Renaissance Chancery Court London
252 High Holborn
London WC1V 7EN
England
United Kingdom
T: +44 (0)20 7829 7058
F: +44 (0)20 7829 7059
E: rhi.loncc.thespa
@renaissancehotels.com
W: www.renaissancehotels.com/loncc

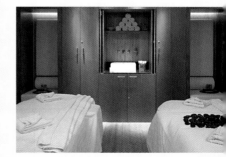

Treatment rooms are elegantly clad in bamboo patterned wood. The VIP treatment suite (pictured), designed for a couple to have a treatment together, reflects Los Angeles glamour, where such rooms are popular with celebrity couples.

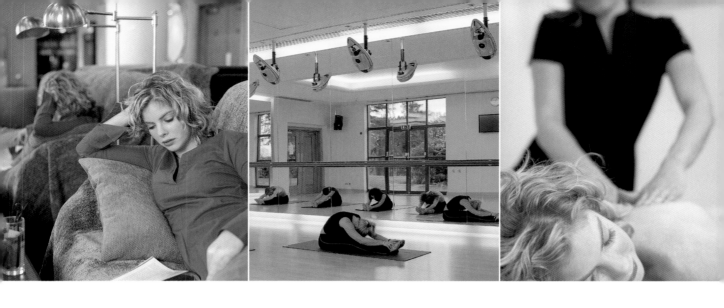

SPA SPC at Stoke Park Club
Buckinghamshire, England, United Kingdom

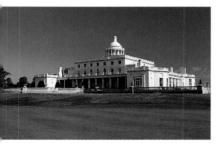

TOP: *SPA SPC won top accolades within months of its opening, including a listing in the 'Ten Best Spas in the UK' by* The Independent *(September 2002), 'Top Spa in UK' by 'W' Magazine and 'Top Ten Spas in the UK' by* Harpers & Queen *(December 2002); and the 'Gold E for Excellence Award' from* Entree Magazine *(October 2002).*

ABOVE: *Two James Bond movies have been filmed here. In one, the most famous game of golf in cinematic history was captured for posterity at the club's golf course.*

OPPOSITE, BOTTOM LEFT: *The indoor swimming pool comes with poolside massage areas and hydro-seat jacuzzis.*

The Stoke Park estate has a recorded history dating back to 1066. Set in a 142-hectare (350-acre) parkland, it is distinctly British. Its line of noble owners from some of England's most powerful families, its royal occupants such as Queen Elizabeth I, and its reputation as having one of the world's finest golf courses combine to make it a club that speaks of eminence and pedigree. In 1908, the estate was turned into Britain's first country club. Today, it is recognised as one of the leading small luxury hotels of the world.

Just a 35-minute drive from Central London, Stoke Park Club underwent a mammoth restoration from 1993 to 2002. The club's largest project to date is the Spa, Health and Racquet Pavilion—where pampering, sports and leisure activities await the guests. SPA SPC is a trend-setting spa concept that offers modern luxury in a refined country setting. Its eclectic treatment menu and packages are highly individualised and utilise the finest product lines from the world's best beauty companies.

Beauty treats take precedence here. The spa's signature SK-II Ultimate Serenity Facial is unique in catering for your own individual needs and skin concerns. The session begins with a consultation, followed by a back and neck massage. The ensuing facial combines pressure point and lymphatic drainage massage with advanced skincare techniques. This procedure promises you refined skin texture and improved elasticity.

But if you are enjoying an extended stay at the hotel, why stop at just one facial? Another signature item on the pampering menu is the Prada Beauty Bio-Firm Facial. By combining the most luxurious range of products with the latest ultrasound technologies, your skin is transformed in a number of indulgent, magical steps. The facial begins with an exfoliation to lift away dead cells and even out skin tone. This is followed by a medley of treatments: soothing eye massage; acupressure to stimulate circulation and draw out toxins; an infusion of strong antioxidants and nutrients; and finally a layer of Tinted Beauty

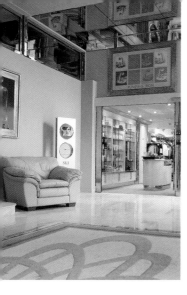

OPPOSITE, CENTRE: *Guests enjoy complimentary use of the Club's facilities such as dance and fitness studios (pictured), a gymnasium and multi-surface tennis courts.*

OPPOSITE, RIGHT: *The treatment menu offers a wide selection ranging from body treatments to holistic therapies.*

LEFT: *The spa offers guests Residential, Half-Day and Day Spa Retreats that include selected treatments, a light lunch and use of the spa facilities. Its modern spa reception area (pictured) makes an interesting contrast to the surrounding estate.*

Finisher for luminosity. This is surely a beauty routine fit for queens and ladies of the manor.

Spa-goers are served herbal teas, organic juices and smoothies at the Spa Bar and the Beach Bar. You can also catch 40 winks in the two deep-relaxation rooms that come complete with Reclining Moon Massage Chairs. All this will ensure you are well-fashioned for that requisite stroll around the historic grounds of the parkland or a fishing expedition at the lake dating back to 1750. At Stoke Park Club, life can finally go back to a time when gentility reigned.

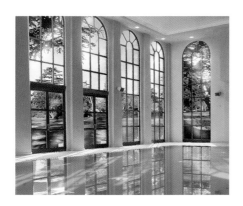

Spa Statistics

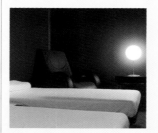

The relaxation rooms also feature custom-made beds with built-in heating and airing systems—perfect for a post-treatment nap.

TYPE OF SPA
Hotel Spa

SPA AREA
5,570 sq m (60,000 sq ft)

FACILITIES
10 indoor treatment rooms; 2 deep-relaxation rooms; 1 hydrotherapy suite; 2 jacuzzis, 2 steam rooms; 1 hair salon, 2 nail stations; 1 cardio studio, 1 fitness studio (offering yoga, Pilates, studio cycling classes), 1 gymnasium; 1 indoor swimming pool; 27-hole championship golf course; 3 indoor tennis courts, 6 grass tennis courts, 4 all-weather tennis courts; 1 carp fishing lake; 1 spa boutique

SIGNATURE TREATMENTS
Prada Beauty Bio-Firm Facial, SK-II Ultimate Serenity Facial

TREATMENTS & THERAPIES
Anti-ageing treatments, anti-cellulite treatments, aroma-therapy, baths, body bronzing, body scrubs, body wraps, eye treatments, facials, firming and slimming treatments, hair treatments, hand and foot treatments, heat treatments, holistic treatments, hot stone therapies, hydrotherapy, Indian head massage, jet lag treatments, life-coach counselling, make-up services, manicures and pedicures, massages, pre- and post-natal treatments, purifying back treatments, reflexology, *reiki*, salon services, scalp treatments, sports massage, waxing

SPA CUISINE
Salads and sandwiches accompanied by herbal teas, fresh juices or smoothies are available at the Beach Bar and the Atrium before and after treatments.

ACTIVITIES & PROGRAMMES
Aerobics, aquaerobics, golf, Pilates, spinning, stretching, tennis, yoga, meditation; life enhancement and lifestyle management classes; sports instruction; talks by visiting consultants

SERVICES
Consultations on body composition analysis, general healthcare, nutrition and skincare; personal training; golf days; tennis, golf and swimming tuition; baby-sitting; corporate programmes; private spa parties; gift certificates; day-use rooms

LANGUAGE SPOKEN BY THERAPISTS
English

ADMISSION
Membership is available but not required for admission. There are several membership categories, such as golf, health, racquet, social and overseas memberships. All members enjoy free access to spa facilities and 10% off treatments.

CONTACT
Stoke Park Club
Park Road, Stoke Poges, Bucks
SL2 4PG
England
United Kingdom
T: +44 (0)1753 717 171
F: +44 (0)1753 717 181
E: info@stokeparkclub.com
W: www.stokeparkclub.com

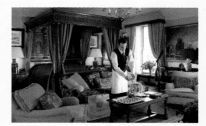

Stoke Park Club boasts 21 bedrooms and suites, each with its own private collection of antique prints, paintings and furniture that its former royal occupants would surely approve of.

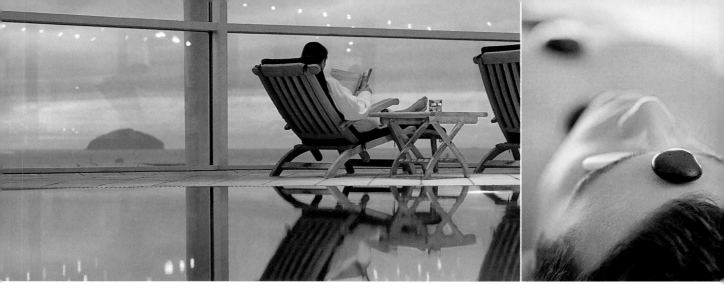

The Spa at The Westin Turnberry Resort
Ayrshire, Scotland, United Kingdom

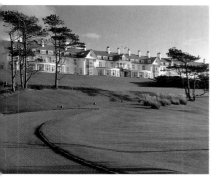

ABOVE: *Rooms and suites are decorated in the style befitting an elegant Edwardian country manor; some rooms have been thoughtfully outfitted for disabled guests.*

OPPOSITE, BOTTOM: *The relaxation room is an inviting space to savour the afterglow of your treatment with a glass of lemon or cucumber water.*

The county of Ayrshire, birthplace of poet Robert Burns, is also home to The Westin Turnberry Resort, which is set between the rolling Scottish countryside and the rugged Atlantic coast. Golfers are among those drawn to the 320-hectare (800-acre) estate which is home to two championship courses and The Colin Montgomerie Links Golf Academy. Enthusiasts of the outdoors can enjoy falconry, clay target shooting, catching their own fish for dinner at the spring-fed loch (ask the chef to cook it for you) or traversing logs and banks in a Jeep Cherokee.

The idyllic surrounds offer the perfect antidote to high-stressed city life, as does The Spa. The Spa, part of the Starwood Spa Collection, reflects the hotel's stately air with dark green hues—traditional to the hotel—and elegant furnishings, with a décor that plays on light and the textures of wood and marble.

The spa menu comprises over 50 holistic ESPA treatments—including a selection specifically for male spa-goers—that are designed to restore the delicate balance between your body, mind and spirit. Treatments marry the best of both worlds: aromatherapy and hydrotherapy from Europe, and Ayurvedic healing philosophies from Asia.

Day Guest programmes, available from Sundays to Thursdays, include treatments and allow non-hotel guests and non-members the use of the spa facilities, swimming pool and gymnasium and a two-course lunch at The Terrace Brasserie. Day Guest programmes include the Pre-Natal Programme For New Beginnings that will coddle and relax pregnant and nursing mothers.

You may feel a deep connection with the earth in your quest to restore your equilibrium. Wraps or 'envelopments' that harness the gifts from Mother Nature include the Oshadi (an Ayurvedic term for plants and herbs used in traditional healing). Envelopment starts with a sea salt and aromatherapy oil exfoliation, followed by a mask of plants and spices which hydrates and warms your skin, helping to ease aching muscles and joints. The use of warm stones has also been incorporated into

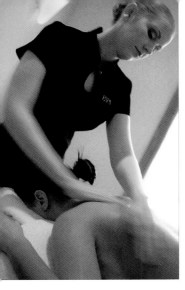

OPPOSITE, LEFT: *The indoor pool is a place for quiet reflection as you admire the view of the Irish Sea through floor-to-ceiling windows.*

OPPOSITE, RIGHT: *Hot Stone Therapy restores equilibrium and revives the body's vital energy.*

OPPOSITE, LEFT: *If you are arriving after a long journey, book the Jet Lag Reviver Massage which helps regulate sleep and energy patterns disrupted by travel. After a day on the links, opt for the Golfers Tonic with a tension-releasing Life Saving Back Massage (pictured).*

Spa Statistics

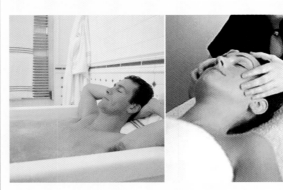

TOP LEFT: *Treatments designed specifically for men include the Marine Hydrotherapy Bath, in which you will be massaged by the multiple jets within the tub.*

TOP RIGHT: *The Blissful Back Face & Scalp targets your centres of stress with a cleansing and exfoliation of your back, a tension-relieving massage and a purifying facial.*

a number of spa treatments, including treatments for the hands and feet.

The spa's signature treatment, the Holistic Total Body Care With Hot Stone Therapy, is an all-encompassing 1-hour-55-minute treatment that begins with a welcoming footbath to relax you. Next comes a full body skin brushing to prepare your skin for the treatment, and then a deep body, face and scalp massage. Hot and cold stones are applied to your vital energy points, lubricated with an individual blend of essential oils. This treatment starts with the 'ching' of cymbals to help clear the room of any unwanted negative energy, and ends on a similar exotic note to rouse you from your reverie.

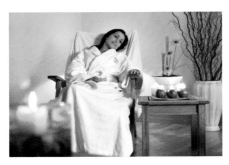

TYPE OF SPA
Resort spa

SPA AREA
1,525 sq m (16,415 sq ft)

FACILITIES
2 hydrotherapy suites, 11 single treatment rooms; 3 relaxation rooms; 1 jacuzzi; 3 saunas, 2 steam rooms; 1 hair salon, 2 nail stations; 1 gymnasium; 1 indoor swimming pool; 2 golf courses in front of main hotel, 2 tennis courts; retail area within spa reception

SIGNATURE TREATMENT
Holistic Total Body Care With Hot Stone Therapy

TREATMENTS & THERAPIES
Anti-ageing treatments, anti-cellulite treatments, aromatherapy, body scrubs, body wraps, eye treatments, facials, hand and foot treatments, heat treatments, holistic treatments, hot stone therapies, hydrotherapy, jet lag treatments, lymphatic drainage, manicures and pedicures, massages, pre- and post-natal treatments, purifying back treatments, reflexology, salon services, waxing; Day Programmes (that include treatments, use of gymnasium, spa facilities, swimming pool and a 2-course nutritious lunch at The Terrace Brasserie).

SPA CUISINE
A lunch menu of light, nutritious contemporary dishes is available at The Terrace Brasserie. The kitchen will do their utmost to ensure the happiness of guests with special dietary requirements or wishes. Salad dishes are available from the in-room dining menu.

ACTIVITIES & PROGRAMMES
Biking, golf, horse riding, Pilates, tennis; talks by visiting consultants

SERVICES
Cholesterol Check, Personal Fitness Evaluation; Gift Voucher

LANGUAGE SPOKEN BY THERAPISTS
English

ADMISSION
Membership is available but not required for admission. 7- or 5-day (Mondays to Fridays) memberships are available. Non-residents and non-members can enjoy individual treatments, but will be required to pay a nominal daily fee if they wish to use the spa's facilities.

CONTACT
The Westin Turnberry Resort
Ayrshire KA26 9LT
Scotland
United Kingdom
T: +44(0) 1655 334 060
F: +44(0) 1655 331 675
E: turnberry@westin.com
W: www.westin.com/turnberry

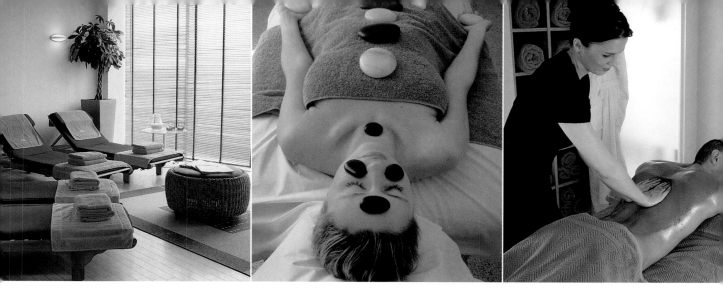

St David's Spa at The St David's Hotel & Spa
Cardiff, Wales, United Kingdom

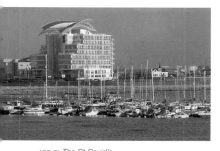

ABOVE: *The St David's Hotel & Spa is surrounded by some of Wales' most important landmark buildings—such as the National Assembly, the Pierhead Building and the Welsh National Opera.*

OPPOSITE, BOTTOM LEFT: *Robbie Williams, Ronan Keating and a list of celebrity sports heroes from the Manchester United and Chelsea football teams and the England Rugby team have helped to make The St David's Hotel & Spa a hip Cardiff address. The hotel has 132 rooms (including 20 suites) with private decked balconies overlooking the bay.*

Cardiff's new Millennium Stadium may have hosted the 1999 Rugby World Cup, but in the past, less athletically inclined tourists may have been prone to giving the capital city a miss. In recent years, however, Cardiff has developed many worthwhile new attractions in addition to its traditional wealth of Welsh cultural relics.

Opened in early 1999, The St David's Hotel & Spa was Wales' first five-star hotel. With its distinctive architecture, the hotel has become a notable landmark in its own right.

The St David's Spa is rapidly gaining renown for its specially tailored spa programmes. Its Residential Spa Experience includes an in-depth consultation session, organic meals, and an attractive variety of spa therapies such as Spa Escape and Spa Detox.

St David's Spa is also one of only five spas worldwide to offer the ESPA Mind & Body treatments. The central philosophy behind these is the Rituals Experience, which enables you to be at one with the heartbeat of nature. Treatments comprise a cultural melting

pot of traditional therapies from China, Bali, India and Europe. In keeping with the ESPA concepts of health and wellbeing, each treatment aims to provide a journey that suits each person's immediate and specific needs.

You have a choice between the one-night and two-night ESPA packages. The Mind & Body one-night programme offers either a rebalancing Ayurvedic Marma Point Massage, or the luxurious Optimal Release Treatment of exfoliation followed by massage. Both of these restorative treatments help to revive exhausted muscles and tired minds via the release of physical and mental tension.

For an overhaul of your lifestyle for even more lasting results, opt for the Spa Experience package. This programme helps you attain your desired goals through a tailor-made personal training session, a Balancing Aromatherapy Massage, Aromatherapy Facial and an Oshadi Envelopment.

The two-night package lets you choose between Oshadi (exfoliation followed by a restorative mask), a soothing Detoxifying

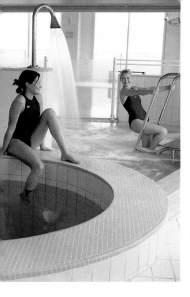

OPPOSITE, LEFT: *The ultra chic spa comes complete with stylishly furnished relaxation areas for more post-treatment bay-watching.*

OPPOSITE, CENTRE: *The spa offers a variety of hot stone therapies, including the Holistic Hand And Nail Treatment Incorporating Hot Stones; Holistic Total Body Care With Hot Stone Therapy; Totally Blissful Back Face And Scalp With Hot Stone Therapy; and a Purifying Herbal Linen Wrap With Hot Stones.*

OPPOSITE, RIGHT: *St David's Spa's special ESPA back massages include exfoliation for cell renewal.*

LEFT: *The many water facilities include the hydro pools, water lounges and swan-neck fountains.*

Algae Wrap, or Restorative Mud Envelopment. The latter combines brushing, exfoliation and warm mud to relieve bodily aches and soothe the skin. It is topped off by a scalp massage.

Whether you are in Wales to tour its castles, visit the National Museum and Gallery, or attend a rugby match at the stadium, The St David's Hotel & Spa offers Cardiff visitors the perfect respite and an ideal opportunity to enhance your personal and physical wellbeing.

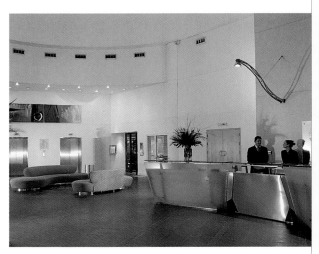

Spa Statistics

TYPE OF SPA
Hotel spa

SPA AREA
20,000 sq m (215,280 sq ft)

FACILITIES
14 single treatment rooms; 2 relaxation rooms; 2 hydro baths, 1 jacuzzi, 1 jet blitz shower, 1 marine hydrotherapy pool, 3 swan-neck fountains; 1 sauna; 1 nail salon; 1 aerobics studio, 1 gymnasium, 1 Pilates studio; 1 indoor swimming pool

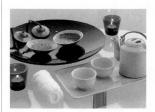

Relax with complimentary servings of herbal tea as you restore your inner equilibrium at the spa.

SIGNATURE TREATMENTS
Ayurvedic Holistic Body Treatment, Balinese Synchronised Massage, Face And Scalp With Hot Stone Therapy, Holistic Total Body Care With Hot Stone Therapy, Optimal Release, Totally Blissful Back

TREATMENTS & THERAPIES
Aromatherapy, Ayurvedic treatments, baths, body bronzing, body scrubs, body wraps, Chinese therapies, eye treatments, facials, hand and foot treatments, holistic treatments, hot stone therapies, hydrotherapy, make-up services, manicures and pedicures, massages, pre- and post-natal treatments, reflexology, scalp treatments, waxing

SPA CUISINE
A buffet style lunch with a different menu every day is served at the spa lounge. Vegan and vegetarian meals are available on request. Guests can also enjoy organic and calorie-controlled spa cuisine at the restaurant and lounge overlooking the bay.

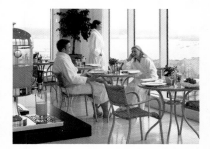

Guests are encouraged to take their lunch at the lounge overlooking the bay.

SPA PACKAGES
The spa offers a good variety of day spa packages and residential packages. Choose from Spa Escape, Spa Experience, Spa Detox, and Mind & Body. ESPA Mind & Body packages are available for 1 or 2 nights.

SERVICES
Aerobics, Pilates, yoga; personal training; skincare and nutrition consultations; corporate programmes; gift certificates; day-use rooms

LANGUAGE SPOKEN BY THERAPISTS
English

ADMISSION
All guests of the hotel automatically receive temporary membership at the spa during their stay. Each of the hotel's floors has a private lift to the spa.

CONTACT
The St David's Hotel & Spa
Havannah Street, Cardiff
CF10 5SD
Wales
United Kingdom
T: +44 (0)2920 454 045
F: +44 (0)2920 313 075
E: spa@thestdavidshotel.com
W: www.roccofortehotels.com

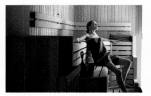

Spa facilities range from the requisite sauna to a specialist Ayurvedic room.

Spa Speak

A glossary of commonly used spa, treatment and fitness terms. Variations may be offered, so it's best to check with the respective spas when you make your booking.

acupoints Points along the meridian channels where the life force accumulates.
acupressure Application of fingertip (and sometimes palm, elbow, knee and foot) pressure on the body's acupoints to improve the flow of *qi* throughout the body, release muscle tension and promote healing.
acupuncture Ancient Chinese healing technique in which fine needles are inserted into acupoints along the body's meridians to maintain health and correct any imbalance.
aerobics Fitness routine that involves a series of rhythmic exercises, usually performed to music. Promotes cardiovascular fitness, improves the body's use of oxygen, burns calories and increases endurance.
aerobics studio Area used for floor exercises.
affusion Hydrotherapy treatment which involves pouring liquid on to a certain part of the body.
affusion shower massage Massage given as you lie under a relaxing, rain-like, warm shower of water or seawater. Increases blood circulation.
after-sun treatment Treatment that soothes skin that has been overexposed to the sun, and cools the over-heated body. May include a cooling bath and a gentle massage with a lotion of soothing ingredients such as cucumber and aloe vera.
aikido Japanese martial art that uses techniques such as locks and throws, and focuses on using the opponent's own energy against himself.
the Alexander Technique Therapy developed by Australian F M Alexander in the 1890s that retrains you to stand and move in an optimally balanced way. Helps reduce physical and psychological problems brought on by bad posture.
algotherapy Use of algae in treatments such as baths, scrubs, body wraps and skin care.
anti-cellulite treatment Treatment that contours the body and reduces cellulite on various parts of the body.
anti-stress massage Typically a 30-minute introductory massage, or one for persons with limited time and who suffer from high levels of stress. Focuses on tension areas such as the back, face, neck and shoulders.
aquaerobics Aerobic exercises performed in a swimming pool where the water provides support and resistance, to increase stamina, and stretch and strengthen muscles.
aqua exercise Gentle exercise in water. May include underwater jets to tone muscles.
aquatic bodywork General term for therapies that take place in warm water, combining the therapist's support with the benefits of water. May include sequences where you are brought underwater. Nurturing and relaxing, encourages feelings of trust and security.
aromatherapy Ancient healing art that dates back to 4,500 B.C.. Refers to the use of essential oils from plants and flowers in treatments such as facials, massages, body wraps, footbaths and hydrobaths.
aromatherapy massage Massage in which essential oils—either pre-blended or specially mixed for your needs—are applied to the body, typically with Swedish massage techniques.
asanas Yoga postures.
aura An electromagnetic field or subtle body of energy believed to surround each living thing. Traditionally thought of as oval in shape, and comprising seven layered bands. Its colour, shape, size and action are believed to reflect your physical, emotional, psychological and spiritual wellbeing.
Aura-Soma Form of colour therapy which has you choose from an array of Equilibrium Bottles or Balance Bottles, each containing two layers of jewel-coloured oils. The therapist will help you relate your choice to your physical, mental, emotional and spiritual wellbeing. Developed in 1984 by Vicky Wall.
Ayurveda Holistic system of healing in India that encompasses diet, massage, exercise and yoga.
Ayurvedic massage Massage that may be performed by more than one therapist directly on the skin to loosen the excess *doshas*. Promotes circulation, increases flexibility, and relieves pain and stiffness. Applied with herbal oil.
baby massage Massage that focuses on the special needs of newborns. Relaxes, improves circulation and relieves common infant ailments. Nurtures and bonds when performed by the infant's parents.
Bach Flower Therapies Thirty-eight flower remedies, each associated with specific negative feelings, developed by Dr Edward Bach in the 1930s. The remedies are derived from solarised flowers that work on a vibrational level to effect emotional change. Flower therapies are also known as **flower essences**.
balneotherapy General term for water treatments that use hot springs, mineral water or seawater to improve circulation, restore and revitalise the body, and relieve pain and stress.
bania Russian version of a sweat bath.
bath Soaking or cleansing the body in water or steam. May employ different temperatures or be infused with salt, flowers, minerals or essential oils.
beauty treatment Treatment to enhance beauty and overall wellbeing. Includes facials, makeovers, manicures, pedicures and waxing.
body bronzing Tanning treatment without the sun. May begin with a scrub to smooth the skin for an even tan.
body composition analysis Evaluation of lean body mass to determine the percentage of body fat to tailor a nutrition and exercise programme.
body mask Regenerating treatment in which the body is slathered with substances such as clay, which may be mixed with essential oil. Detoxifies and hydrates the skin, leaving it radiant.
body scrub Exfoliating body treatment, using products such as salt or herbs, that removes dry, dead skin cells and improves blood circulation. Softens the skin and gives it a healthier glow. Often used for preparing the skin to receive the benefits of massages and wraps. Also known as **body polish**.
body treatment General term that denotes treatments for the body.
bodywork Therapeutic touching or manipulation of the body that uses massage or exercise to relax, ease tension and pain, and treat illnesses. May involve lessons in proper posture or movement. Some modes may treat both the body and mind.
body wrap Treatment in which substances such as seaweed or mud are slathered on the body, which is then wrapped, and sometimes kept under a heated blanket. May be accompanied by a face, head and scalp massage. Detoxifies the system, soothes tired muscles and hydrates the skin.
Bread-Bath Warm room with an oven where you experience heat therapy and aromatic benefits while bread is baked.
brush and tone Use of a loofah, special brush or rough cloth to rapidly brush the body to remove dead skin cells and impurities. Improves circulation. Often used to prepare the body for treatments such as masks and bronzing. Also known as **dry brushing**.
bust treatment Treatment to firm and tone the bust and décolleté.
chair massage Massage performed on you while you remain clothed and seated on a specially designed massage chair. The chair is portable so the massage can be performed almost anywhere. The massage typically concentrates on the back, neck, scalp and shoulders.
chakras According to Indian philosophy, the seven energy centres in the body that are associated with the flow of the body's subtle energy.
champissage Head massage developed by blind Indian manipulative therapist Nehendra Mehta, who popularised his technique in London in the 1980s.
channel To convey energy or thoughts to another person's body or mind.
climatotherapy The therapeutic use of the environment—such as air, climate, atmosphere, temperature, humidity and light—to heal.
cold plunge pool Small pool filled with chilled water to stimulate blood circulation and cool the body quickly, especially after a heat treatment.
colour therapy Use of colour to bring about balance.
complementary therapy Healthcare system not traditionally utilised by conventional Western medical practitioners, and which may complement orthodox treatments. Also known as **alternative therapy**.
compress A hot or cold folded cloth or pad applied to a part of your body.
craniosacral therapy A gentle touch therapy that evaluates and enhances the craniosacral system (comprising the membranes and fluid that surround and protect the brain and spinal cord) to restore balance, ease stress and enhance the body's self-healing process. Developed in the mid-1970s by osteopathic physician John E Upledger.
crystal therapy The use of crystals to balance body and mind. Believed to work on a vibrational level.
cupping Chinese treatment where small glass cups are attached to the skin by a vacuum that is created by placing a lighted match inside each cup to burn up the oxygen. The suction increases the circulation of *qi* and blood.
dance movement therapy Dance as a therapy, with or without music, to help those with emotional problems. The therapist may suggest movements and encourage the participants to innovate their own movements to express themselves.
Dancercise Aerobic exercise derived from modified modern dance steps and movements.
Dead Sea mud treatment Application of mineral-rich mud from the Dead Sea. Detoxifies the skin and body and relieves rheumatic and arthritic pain.
deep tissue massage Firm and deep massage using specific techniques to release tensions, blockages and knots that have built up over time. Believed to release emotional tension. May be adapted to a specific area of tension. Includes sports massage and connective tissue massage. Also known as **deep tissue therapy** or **deep muscle therapy**.
doshas In Ayurveda, the three humours that make up the physical body. According to Ayurvedic philosophy, the five elements of water, fire, air, earth and ether are believed to combine in pairs to form the *doshas*.
dry flotation Tension-relieving treatment in which you 'float' on a platform similar to a waterbed; your body may first be coated in ingredients such as muds, whey, milk or warm oil.
effleurage Long, even massage stroke used to apply lubrication, assess condition of underlying tissues and boost blood and lymph circulation.
energy healing General term to describe a variety of practices aimed at balancing the flow of energy in and around the body. Practitioners generally try to remove blockages, and balance and amplify this energy flow.
enzyme peel Treatment to deep-cleanse skin, usually using ingredients derived from papaya or pineapple.
essential oils Oils extracted from plants and flowers that have specific characteristics which determine their use. They may be sedative or stimulating, and have antibacterial and therapeutic qualities. Usually inhaled or used in treatments such as massages, where they are absorbed by the skin.
exfoliation Removal of dry, dead skin cells and impurities using products such as salt or herbs, or by techniques such as dry brushing. Also known as **scrub**.
eyebrow shaping Grooming of the eyebrows, to suit the facial features.
eye treatment Treatment that focuses on the delicate eye area, generally to combat signs of premature ageing, relieve tired eyes, and reduce puffiness and dryness.
facial Treatment that cleanses and improves the complexion of the face using products that best suit a specific skin type. May include gentle exfoliation, application of a facial mask and moisturiser, and a facial massage. Types of facials include aromatic, oxygenating, whitening and deep-cleansing facials.
facial mask Cleansing facial treatment in which products are applied to the face and left on for a period of time to cleanse pores and slough off dead skin.
facial scrub Exfoliating face treatment that uses products with abrasive ingredients to remove dry, dead skin cells and improve blood circulation. Softens the skin and gives it a healthier glow.
fango Italian for 'mud'.
Farmer's Steam Bath A heat treatment inspired by the old *brechelbath* where flax was prepared for weaving.
fitness facial for men Facial that addresses men's skin types and needs, including shaving burn. May include a face, neck and shoulder massage.
floral bath Bath filled with flowers and essential oils.
flotation therapy Treatment where you float on salt and mineral water at body temperature in an enclosed flotation tank (also known as a **sensory deprivation tank** or an **isolation tank**). The feeling of weightlessness, and the isolation from external sensations and stimuli provide a deep feeling of relaxation and sensory awareness. May be done in complete silence and darkness, or with music and videos.
flower essences Essences derived from solarised flowers that work on a vibrational level to effect emotional change. Based on the work of Dr Edward Bach. Also known as **flower remedies**.
footbath Bath for the feet.
four-handed massage Massage performed by two therapists. Often uses a blend of massage techniques.
fruit acid peel Treatment to renew the skin using mild organic fruit acids.

G5 Deep vibrating massage using a G5 machine that relaxes, stimulates circulation and breaks down fatty deposits.

glycolic facial Facial that uses glycolic acid to break down the bond which holds dry skin on to the face. Exfoliates the top layer, smoothes the skin and softens lines.

gong fu Generic term for martial arts that originated in China.

gymnasium Workout room with weights, and a range of high-tech cardio and variable resistance equipment.

hair services Services for the hair, including cutting, styling, deep conditioning, hair colouring, and washing and blowing dry.

hammam Arabic steam bath.

hay bath Treatment in which the body is surrounded by warm, moist hay. Usually given in conjunction with a dry flotation session.

Healing Dance Aquatic bodywork influenced by watsu's nurturing aspects and WaterDance®'s freedom and range of motions. The therapy also draws on its developer's background in ballet, modern dance, free improvisation and Tragerwork.

herbalism Therapeutic use of herbs and plant-based medicine in treatments and diets to prevent and cure illnesses. Herbal medicine is used by many complementary health disciplines including Ayurveda, homeopathy, naturopathy, and Chinese, Indonesian and Japanese medicines. It may be prepared for internal and external uses through various forms such as pills, teas, oils or compresses. Some healing systems—Traditional Chinese Medicine (TCM), for instance—also use mineral- and animal-based ingredients in herbal medicine. Also known as **herbology**.

herbal steam infusion Steaming with herbs. The heat, moisture and the fragrance of the herbs help to open the pores and promote relaxation.

herbal wrap Treatment where the body is wrapped in hot cloth sheets soaked in a herbal solution for about 20 minutes. Eliminates impurities, softens the skin, and detoxifies and relaxes the body.

high-impact aerobics Aerobics involving jumping, jogging and hopping movements where both feet lose contact with the ground.

holistic approach Integrated approach to health and fitness that takes into account your lifestyle, and mental, physical and spiritual wellbeing.

homeopathy Holistic healthcare practice, based on the concept of 'like cures like', that treats diseases by using minute doses of natural substances that in a healthy person would produce symptoms similar to those already being experienced. Developed by German physician Dr Samuel Hahnemann (1755–1843).

hydrobath Bathtub with water jets that pummel all parts of the body. Seawater may be used, or the water may be infused with essential oils or mineral salts. Relaxes, and stimulates muscle tone and circulation.

hydropool Pool fitted with various high-pressure jets and fountains.

hydrotherapy Therapeutic use of water which includes baths, steam baths, steam inhalation, in-water and underwater massage, soaking in hot springs, and the use of hot, cold or alternating shower sprays.

Indonesian massage Traditional massage of Indonesia that uses deep pressure and specially blended massage oils to ease tension and improve circulation.

inhalation therapy Therapy to aid relaxation and cure breathing problems by inhaling vapours from thermal water or seawater.

iridology Analysis of the marks and changes on the iris, which is divided into areas linked to specific body parts and functions, to diagnose a problem or spot early signs of trouble, in order to recommend appropriate action.

jacuzzi Tub or pool of hot water in which water is swirled about by underwater jets. Two types of massaging effects may be used separately or together: compressed air coming from small holes at the pool's base, and pressure from jets of water at the sides of the pool. Also known as **whirlpool**.

Jahara™ Technique Aquatic bodywork that incorporates footwork patterns and the use of a flotation device known as the Third Arm™.

jamu Indonesian traditional herbal medicine.

Javanese *lulur* Traditional fragrant scrub originating from the royal palaces of Java. A blend of powdered spices, including turmeric and sandalwood, is rubbed on to the body. After the vibrantly coloured paste dries, it is removed with a gentle massage. The skin is then moisturised with yogurt. In Java, the *lulur* is often used to clean and pamper the bride during the week leading up to her wedding.

jet lag treatment Treatment that eases travel-associated aches, pains and stiffness, and helps the body to adjust to a new time zone.

kanpo Japanese traditional herbal medicine. Less commonly used to refer to the Japanese traditional healing system.

kapha In Ayurveda, one of the three *doshas*. *Kapha* types are typically large-sized and stable. *Kapha* is believed to be made up of the elements water and earth.

kinesiology Use of fingertip pressure to locate weakness in specific muscles and diagnose a problem or asymptomatic illnesses. The fingertips are used to massage the appropriate points to disperse toxins and revitalise the flow of energy.

Kneipp baths Herbal or mineral baths of varying temperatures combined with diet and exercise. Kneipp therapy uses hot and cold hydrotherapy treatments to improve circulation.

Kneipp *kur* Treatments combining hydrotherapy, herbology and natural foods for physical and emotional wellbeing, developed in Germany in the mid-1800s by Sebastian Kneipp. Popular in Austria, Switzerland and Germany. The *kur* course of daily treatments uses natural resources, such as algae and thermal mineral water, to remineralise and balance the body.

Kraxen-Stove Herbal heat treatment in which you sit against a hay-filled grating.

kur German for 'cure'. Preventive healthcare system based on the use of natural and spa therapies.

La Stone Therapy® Swedish massage incorporating the use of heated and chilled stones.

labyrinth Ancient meditation tool in which a single winding path leads to a central goal and back out again. Walking a labyrinth is a metaphor for journeying to the centre of understanding and returning with a broadened outlook.

laconium Heat facility of gentle dry heat of about 55 degrees Celsius (131 degrees Fahrenheit).

lap pool Swimming pool with exercise lanes. Standard lap pools are 50 metres (164 feet) in length.

life-coach counselling Counselling sessions that help to solve daily problems, develop harmony with the self and contribute to understanding life's natural philosophy.

light therapy Use of natural or artificial light to heal.

Liquid Sound Sophisticated pools with light and music under and above the water. Aquatic bodywork may be performed in such pools.

lomi lomi Massage originating in Hawaii that uses the forearms and elbows, rhythmical rocking movements, and long and broad strokes.

low-impact aerobics Form of aerobics with side-to-side marching or gliding movements which spares the body from excessive stress and possible injuries.

lymphatic drainage massage Massage that uses a gentle pumping technique to stimulate lymphatic circulation, thus reducing water retention and removing toxins. Lymph drainage can be achieved through manual massage or hydromassage. May be performed on the face and neck, or on the body.

manicure Treatment that beautifies the hands and nails. Hands are soaked and exfoliated with a scrub to remove dead skin cells, cuticles are groomed, and nails are trimmed and shaped. Nails may be buffed to a shine or coated with a polish. May include a hand massage.

manual massage General term for therapist-given massage. Touch helps stimulate endorphin levels, reduce anxiety and pain, and minimise tension. More personal than a mechanical massage.

manuluve Hand and arm treatment comprising a scrub and heated seaweed massage.

marine aerosol treatment Inhalation of ionic seawater mist to cleanse the respiratory system. Alleviates breathing problems caused by asthma or smoking.

marma point massage Ayurvedic massage in which the *marma* points are massaged with the thumb or index fingers in clockwise circles. Focuses on the face, neck, scalp and shoulders.

marma **points** In Ayurveda, the body's vital energy points. It is believed that the dysfunction of any of these points leads to illness.

martial arts Forms of combat and self-defence techniques often practised as sport or fitness regimens.

mask Application of substances such as mud, clay or plants to the face or body in a thick layer. Some may be removed immediately, allowed to dry, or kept moist until they are removed. Some body masks may be combined with a body wrap.

massage Therapy that employs manipulative muscle and soft tissue techniques based generally on concepts of the anatomy, physiology and human function. Relaxes, eases strain and tension, mobilises stiff joints, improves blood circulation, benefits the digestive system, encourages the removal of toxins from the body and creates a sense of wellbeing. Generally delivered by hand, though machines and high-powered water-jets are also used.

masseur Male massage therapist.

masseuse Female massage therapist.

mechanical massage Massage using machines that provide a greater depth than manual massages. Particularly useful for treating muscular male spa-goers. Eases muscle ache and helps break down fatty tissues.

meditation Method of deep breathing, mental concentration and contemplation. During meditation, breathing, brain activity, and heart and pulse rates slow, encouraging the body to relax and achieve a greater sense of inner balance and peace. Relieves stress, removes pain and reduces blood pressure.

meridians Pathways or channels through which vital energy circulates throughout the body. All illnesses are believed to result from an imbalance or blockage of this flow.

meridian stretching Stretching exercises designed to encourage physical and mental flexibility, for the body and mind to perform at their peak. Combines exercise, yoga and Traditional Chinese Medicine (TCM).

microdermabrasion Clinical skin-resurfacing procedure in which a jet of fine crystals is vacuumed across the surface of the face to remove the topmost layer of skin.

mineralise Supply minerals to the body.

moor mud A rich accumulation of waterlogged plant deposits, many of which have medicinal characteristics. Cleanses, detoxifies and helps ease sore muscles.

moxibustion Burning of the dried herb moxa around the acupoints to relieve pain. Applied using cones of moxa directly on the skin, or indirectly with an insulating layer of other herbs.

mud treatment Mineral-rich mud used to detoxify, loosen muscles and stimulate circulation.

multi-jet bath Bath with computerised multiple jets that provide massages to different parts of the body in a precisely timed and rhythmic manner.

myofascial release Use of the fingers, palms, forearms and elbows in long, deliberate, gliding strokes to stretch and mobilise the fascia (connective tissue that surrounds and supports the muscles, organs and bones) to provide long-term relief of pain and promote wellbeing.

nail art Beautification of the nails with patterns, paintings or other decorative motifs.

naturopathy Holistic approach that believes in the body's ability to heal itself. Uses treatments not to alleviate symptoms, but to encourage the body's self-healing mechanisms. Symptoms are viewed not as a part of the illness, but as the body's way of ridding itself of the problem. Also known as **natural medicine**.

neutral bath Bath with water of body temperature. Sedative.

NIA Swahili for 'with purpose'. NIA stands for neuromuscular integrative action, a body-mind fitness activity that encourages personal awareness through graceful dance, martial arts and body-integrative therapies.

nutritional consultation Consultation with a qualified nutritional practitioner to review eating habits and dietary needs. Taking into account your lifestyle, food intolerances, appetite control and weight goals, the nutritionist may compile a nutritionally balanced programme to help you attain optimal health and weight.

onsen Japanese natural hot springs.

organic food Food grown without the use of pesticides or other chemicals.

ovo lacto vegetarian Vegan who consumes milk and egg products.

ovo vegetarian Vegan who consumes egg products.

oxygen breathing therapy Treatment in which oxygen is inhaled through a nasal tube or face mask.

oxygen facial Facial treatment in which a fine mist of oxygen infused with a liquid ampoule is applied to your face.

oxygen therapy Umbrella term describing a wide range of treatments including hyperbaric oxygen therapy, the therapeutic use of ozone and hydrogen peroxide. In spas, it typically describes treatments that supplement your body and skin with oxygen, which are not to be confused with the life-supporting role that oxygen plays in hospitals.

ozone steam bath Individual steam cabinet in which about 99 per cent oxygen and 1 per cent ozone is pumped into the cabinet and mixed with steam.

ozone therapy The use of minute amounts of ozone combined with oxygen. May be mixed with your blood before being reinfused into your body; or injected; or introduced via the rectum, vagina or ear; or administered through the use of an ozone steam bath or by a bag wrapped around your body or limbs.
parafango Combination of fango and mud.
pedicure Treatment that beautifies the feet and toenails. Feet are soaked and exfoliated with a scrub to remove dead skin cells, cuticles are groomed, and nails are trimmed and shaped. Nails may be buffed to a shine or coated with a polish. May include a foot and calf massage.
pediluve Treatment in which feet and legs are dipped in alternate tubs of bubbling jets of warm and cold seawater to improve blood circulation.
pelotherapy Health or beauty treatment using mud packs or mud baths.
personal fitness assessment Programme that assesses your current fitness levels to recommend a suitable exercise programme. May include tests for aerobic capacity, body composition, blood pressure, heart rate, and muscular endurance and strength.
personal training One-on-one personalised workout with a qualified instructor.
physiotherapy Rehabilitative therapy that aids recovery from injury, surgery or disease. Treatments—which include massage, traction, hydrotherapy, corrective exercise and electrical stimulation—help relieve pain, increase strength and improve the range of motion.
phytotherapy Literally, healing through plants. Phytotherapy uses herbs, aromatic essential oils, seaweed and herbal and floral extracts, and may be applied through methods such as massages, wraps, water and steam therapies, inhalation treatments, and the drinking of herbal teas.
Pilates Exercise comprising slow, precise movements with coordinated breathing techniques and special exercise equipment. Its aim is to engage the body and mind, and increase flexibility and strength without building bulk. Developed in Germany by Dr Joseph Pilates in the 1920s.
pitta In Ayurveda, one of the three *doshas*. *Pitta* types are typically medium built and driven. *Pitta* is believed to be made up of the elements water and fire.
pregnancy massage Pre-natal massages dealing with the special needs of a mother-to-be, and ante-natal massages dealing with her needs after she has delivered Some spas have massage tables with a hole in the centre to accommodate a pregnant woman.
pressotherapy Computerised pressure massage that uses a specially designed airbag that compresses and deflates to improve the circulation throughout the feet and legs.
purifying back treatment Deep-cleansing skin treatment for the back, neck and shoulders that removes impurities and excess oils, eases tension, and leaves the skin soft and smooth. Also known as **clarifying back treatment** or **backcial**.
qi 'Vital energy' or 'life force' of the universe and the body. Also known as *ki* (Japanese) and *prana* (Indian).
qi gong Chinese physical exercise of working with or mastering *qi*. Uses breathing and body movement to help develop a powerful *qi*.
rasul Elaborately tiled steam room in which you apply different coloured muds to your body.
reflexology Application of finger-point pressure to reflex zones on the feet—and also hands and ears—to improve circulation, ease pain, relax the body and re-establish the flow of energy through the body. Its underlying theory is that specific areas on the feet, hands and ears correspond with specific body parts, organs and glands, and that the manipulation of those areas can bring about change associated with the corresponding parts.
reiki Healing technique based on ancient Tibetan teachings. The practitioner places his palms over or on various areas of the body for a few moments to energise and balance the body, mind and spirit. Helps treat physical problems and heal emotional stress, and encourages personal transformation.
Rolfing Muscular manipulation and massage therapy that involves deep tissue massage, sometimes painful, to correct musculo-skeletal rigidity, misalignment and chronic pain. Re-educates body movement, improves energy flow and relieves stress. Comprises a series of ten sessions. Developed in the 1900s by Dr Ida Rolf.
Roman bath Historically, a series of rooms and pools of different temperatures that ancient Romans bathed and socialised in. According to ISPA, it is used today to refer to whirlpool bathing areas with benches for more than one person.
salt glow Exfoliating treatment in which the body is rubbed with a mixture of salt and essential oils to remove dry, dead skin cells and stimulate circulation.
sand bath Treatment in which your body is buried under heated sand. Relaxing, and soothes joint aches.
sauna Dry heat in a wood-lined treatment room. The heat causes sweating which helps to cleanse the body of impurities and relax the muscles. Stimulates circulation and refreshes the body. Usually followed by a cold plunge or shower. A Finnish sauna includes the use of *vihtas* (birch twigs) to tap the body to increase circulation and encourage perspiration.
Scotch hose Standing body massage in which a therapist about 3 metres (10 feet) away from you directs a high-pressure shower jet of water at your body. Also known as the **jet blitz**.
shiatsu Massage that uses finger pressure—and also the hands, forearms, elbows, knees and feet—on acupoints. Calms and relaxes.
shirodhara Ayurvedic massage in which warmed medicated oil is dripped steadily on the forehead. Relieves mental tension and calms the mind.
signature treatment Treatment specially created by a spa or spa group, often using indigenous ingredients.
sitz bath Bath in which the bather's hips and feet are immersed in different containers of water, often of contrasting temperatures.
spa Term thought to originate from '*sanitas per aqua*' meaning 'health through water'—or perhaps inspired by the name of a town in Belgium. In Europe, the word was traditionally used to refer to mineral and thermal springs. These days it ideally refers to establishments that provide a professional and integrated approach to health.
spa cuisine Light, healthy meals served at spas. Typically low in calories, fat and salt.
spa menu Selection of treatments and therapies offered by a spa.
spa package Two or more treatments offered together. Often longer in length than individual treatments and good value for money.
sports massage Deep tissue massage directed at muscles used in athletic activities to help the body achieve its maximum physical efficiency. Before physical exertion, it buffers against pain and injury. Afterwards, it helps remove lactic acid and restore muscle tone and range of movement.
steam cabinet Individual steam chamber in which wet heat bathes your body while your head remains in the open air.
steaming Use of hot steam—often infused with essential oils or herbs—to relax the body, soften the skin, and open up the pores to prepare the face or body for treatment. Hair may also be steamed by wrapping it in a hot towel or exposing it to steam.
steam room Tiled room with benches in which steam is generated at high pressure and temperature. The steam opens the pores, eliminates toxins, cleanses the skin and relaxes the body.
step aerobics Aerobic sessions utilising a small platform for stepping up and down.
stone massage The use of warmed and sometimes chilled basalt stones to massage the body using long strokes facilitated by oil. May also be used in facials, manicures, pedicures and reflexology. Also known as **stone therapy**, **hot stone therapy** or **warm stone therapy.**
stress management Techniques to deal with stress and anxiety.
stretching Flexibility workout where various parts of the body are stretched by assuming different positions. Helps increase flexibility and relieve stress and tension.
sweat bath Umbrella term for heat treatment room used for cleansing and relaxation.
Swedish massage Massage in which oils are applied to the body with techniques such as effleurage, petrissage, friction, tapotement and vibration. Relieves stress, tension and muscle pain; improves circulation; increases flexibility; and induces relaxation.
Swiss shower Shower with nine or more hoses spraying water on you from the top and the sides.
tai ji Graceful movement that combines mental concentration with deep, controlled breathing. Regular practice brings about relaxation and good health. Stimulates the energy systems and enhances mental functions.
Thai massage Traditional massage of Thailand that involves a combination of stretching and gentle rocking, and uses a range of motions and acupressure techniques. The massage is oil-free, and performed on a mattress on the floor. Loose pajamas are worn.
thalassotherapy Treatments that harness mineral- and vitamin-rich seawater and seaweed for curative and preventive purposes.
thermal bath Therapeutic use of thermal water rich in salts and minerals.
Traditional Chinese Medicine (TCM) Holistic system of care that sees the body and mind as a whole. Treatments include herbal medicine, physical and mental exercises, and therapies such as acupuncture and moxibustion.
Tragerwork Movement re-education therapy in which the practitioner works on your body using gentle, rhythmic movements, releasing mental and physical stress. Developed in the 1940s by Dr Milton Trager.
treatments for couples Typically treatments that a couple can enjoy together in private with a therapist working on each person. Treatments specially designed for couples usually use an aphrodisiac blend of essential oils.
tui na Chinese system of manual therapy used to treat specific illnesses of an internal nature and musculoskeletal ailments. The hands, arms, elbows and feet may be used.
underwater pressure massage Hydrotherapy treatment in which the therapist directs a pressurised stream of water at your body as you recline in a bath.
vata In Ayurveda, one of the three *doshas*. *Vata* types are typically thin and highly strung. *Vata* is believed to be made up of the elements air and ether.
vegan Person who consumes a vegetable and fruit diet exclusively, and does not eat animal products such as butter, cheese, eggs and milk.
vegetarian Person who consumes mainly vegetables, fruit, nuts, pulses and grains, and who does not eat meat or fish, but eats animal products such as butter, cheese, eggs and milk.
vibrational therapies Therapies such as colour therapy, crystal therapy, homeopathy and flower essences that use substances or treatments that affect your body's natural energy field and filter down to the physical level.
vibratory sauna Personal sauna which bathes your supine body in dry heat as it is relaxed by a vibrating bed, aromatic oils, and perhaps coloured rays of light.
Vichy shower A spray of water from five micro-jets fixed to a horizontal rail which rains down on you as you lie on a table below. May also include a massage. Also known as **affusion shower** or **rain shower**.
vinotherapy The therapeutic use of wine and grapes in beauty and health treatments.
visualisation Technique that involves focusing the mind by consciously creating a mental image of a desired condition to bring about change. May be self-directed or therapist guided. Also known as **imaging.**
Waterbalancing Aquatic bodywork which incorporates elements such as reflexology, *reiki*, Rolfing and Tragerwork.
WaterDance® Aquatic bodywork borrowing elements from Aikido, dance, inversions, massage, rolls, somersaults, and the movements of snakes and dolphins. Also known as **WaTa** or **WasserTanzen**.
water treading Kneipp therapy of walking in calf-deep cold water like a stork. Also known as **water stepping**.
Watsu Aquatic bodywork during which you float in a swimming pool, supported by a therapist who manipulates your body with stretches, rhythmic movements and pressure point massage to bring deep relaxation.
waxing Temporary hair removal method. Warm or cool wax, usually honeycomb wax blended with oils, is applied on to areas of unwanted hair. A cloth is smoothed on to the area and quickly whisked off, pulling the hair off with the wax.
wet area Area in a spa where jacuzzis, saunas, cold tubs, hot tubs, steam baths and pressure showers are located.
yin* and *yang *Yin* is the universal energy force whose characteristics are feminine, cold, dark, quiet, static and wet. *Yang* is masculine, warm, bright, dynamic and dry. In Traditional Chinese Medicine (TCM), true balance and health are achieved when these two opposing forces are in balance.
yoga Ancient Hindu practice comprising focused deep breathing, and stretching and toning the body using various postures. The ultimate goal is to reach your full physical, mental and spiritual potential. Relaxes, and improves circulation, flexibility and strength.

SELECT BIBLIOGRAPHY

Aaland, Mikkel, *Sweat: The Illustrated History and Description of the Finnish Sauna, Russian Bania, Islamic Hammam, Japanese Mushi-Buro, Mexican Temescal and American Indian & Eskimo Sweat Lodge*, Capra Press, 1978

Alexander, Jane, *Mind, Body, Spirit*, Carlton Books, 2001

Ali, Mosarafi and Brar, Jiwan, *Therapeutic Yoga*, Vermilion (an imprint of Ebury Press), 2002

Altman, Nathaniel, *Healing Springs: The Ultimate Guide to Taking the Waters*, Healing Arts Press (a division of Inner Traditions International), 2000

Altman, Nathaniel, *Oxygen Healing Therapies*, Healing Arts Press (a division of Inner Traditions International), 1998

Baggott, Andy, *The Encyclopedia of Energy Healing*, Godsfield Press (a division of David and Charles Ltd.), 1999

Brown, Lulu, *Alternative Medicine*, Hodder & Stoughton, 1999

Chaitow, Leon, *Hydrotherapy: Water Therapy for Health and Beauty*, Vega, 2002

Chiazzari, Suzie, *The Complete Book of Color*, Element Books, 1998

Coghill, Roger, *The Healing Energies of Light*, Gaia Books Ltd., 2000

Cressy, Susan, *The Beauty Therapy Fact File*, Butterworth Heinemann, 1998

Dalgleish, Julia and Dollery, Stuart, *The Health & Fitness Handbook*, Pearson Education Limited, 2001

De La Tour, Shatoiya, *Earth Mother Herbal*, Fair Winds Press, 2002

Eden, Donna, *Energy Medicine*, Jeremy P Tarcher/Putnam, 1999

Endacott, Michael, *The Encyclopedia of Complementary Medicine*, Carlton Books Limited, 1996

Fischer-Rizzi, Susanne, *Complete Aromatherapy Handbook: Essential Oils for Radiant Health*, Sterling Publishing Company, 1990

Gleb, Michael, *Body Learning: An Introduction to the Alexander Technique*, Aurum Press Limited, 1994

Godagama, Shantha, *The Handbook of Ayurveda*, Kyle Cathie Ltd., 2001

Hale, Teresa, *Breathing Free: The 5-Day Breathing Programme that Will Change Your Life*, Hodder & Stoughton, 1999

Kavounas, Alice, *Water: Pure Therapy*, Kyle Cathie Ltd., 2000

Kent, Howard, *Breathe Better Feel Better*, A Quatro Book published by the Apple Press, Quatro Publishing PLC, 1997

Lambert, Mary, *An Introduction to Reiki*, Collins & Brown Limited, 2000

Lark, Liz, *Yoga for Life: Finding and Learning the Right Form of Yoga for Your Lifestyle*, Carlton Books Limited, 2001

Lazarus, Judith, *The Spa Sourcebook*, Lowell House (a division of NTC/ Contemporary Publishing Group, Inc.), 2000

Leavy, Hannelore R and Bergel, Reinhard R, *The Spa Encyclopedia: A Guide to Treatments & Their Benefits for Health & Healing*, Delmar Learning (a division of Thomson Learning Inc.), 2003

Lee, Ginger and Lim, Christine Zita, *Spa Style Asia*, Archipelago Press (an imprint of Editions Didier Millet), 2002

Lipp, Frank J, *Herbalism*, Duncan Baird Publishers Ltd., 2000

Mehta, Mira, *How to Use Yoga*, Lorenz Books (an imprint of Anness Publishing Ltd.), 2001

Mehta, Nerendra, *Indian Head Massage*, Thorsons (an imprint of HarperCollins Publishers), 1999

Mernagh-Ward, Dawn and Cartwright, Jennifer, *Health & Beauty Therapy: A Practical Approach for NVQ Level 3* (2nd Edition), Nelson Thornes, 2001

Mitchell, Emma (General Editor), *Your Body's Energy*, Duncan Baird Publishers, 1998

Neal's Yard Remedies Ltd., *Natural Health & Body Care*, Haldane Manson Ltd., 2000

Norris, Stephanie, *Secrets of Colour Healing*, Dorling Kindersley, 2001

Ody, Pamela, *Practical Chinese Medicine*, Godsfield Press Ltd., 2000

Osborne, Bruce and Weaver, Cora, *17th Century Springs & Spas: In the Footsteps of Celia Fiennes*, Cora Weaver, 1996

Parry, Robert, *Tai Chi*, Headway Life Guides, 1994

Ryrie, Charlie, *The Healing Energies of Water*, Journey Editions (an imprint of Periplus Editions (HK) Ltd.), 1999

Searle, Muriel, *Spas & Watering Places*, Midas Books, 1977

Sedgbeer, Sandra, *The Complete Book of Beauty Treatments*, Thorsons (an imprint of HarperCollins Publishers), 1994

Selby, Anne, H2O: *Healing Water for Mind and Body*, Collins & Brown, 2000

Simmons, John V, *The Beauty Salon and its Equipment* (2nd Edition), Macmillan Press Ltd., 1995

Simon, David, *Vital Energy: The Seven Keys to Invigorate Body, Mind & Soul*, John Wiley & Sons, Inc., 2000

Simpson, Liz, *The Healing Energies of Earth*, Gaia Books Ltd., 2000

Souter, Keith, *Not Just a Room with a Bath*, C W Daniel Company Ltd., 1985

Stillerman, Elaine, *The Encyclopedia of Bodywork: From Acupressure to Zone Therapy*, Facts on File, Inc., 1996

Sullivan, Karen, *Natural Remedies*, Starfire (part of The Foundary Creative Media Company Limited), 2001

Swami Ambikanda Saraswati, *Principle of Breathwork*, Thorsons (an imprint of HarperCollins Publishers), 1999

Ward, John, *Roman Era in Britain*, Methuen & Co. Ltd., 1911; reproduced on website: *http://www.ukans.edu*

Weller, Stella, *The Breath Book: 20 Ways to Breathe Away Stress, Anxiety and Fatigue*, Thorsons (an imprint of HarperCollins Publishers), 1999

Wills, Pauline, *Colour Therapy: An Introductory Guide to the Healing Power of Colour*, Element Books Limited, 2000

Woodham, Anne and Dr Peters, David, *Encyclopedia of Natural Healing: The Definitive Home Reference Guide to Treatments for Mind and Body*, Dorling Kindersley Ltd., 2000

Wright, Janet, *Reflexology and Acupressure*, Hamlyn, 1999

INTERNET RESOURCES

WATER
Aquatic Bodywork
Aqua Wellness, *www.aquawellness.com*
Healing Dance, *aquaticwritings.tripod.com*
Jahara™ Technique Teachers Association, *www.jahara.com*
Liquid Sound, *www.liquid-sound.com*
Network for Aquatic Bodywork, *www.aquanetz.de*
Waterbalancing, *www.waterbalancing.de*
Worldwide Aquatic Bodywork Association, *www.waba.edu*, *www.watsu.com*
Flotation
The Floatation Tank Association, *www.floatationtankassociation.net*
Thalassotherapy
Fédération Internationale de Thalassothérapie, *www.thalassofederation.com*

FIRE
Cyber-Bohemia, *www.cyberbohemia.com/Pages/sweat.htm* (Mikkel Aaland's photographic website with updated information on his book *Sweat*)
Sauna
The Finnish Sauna Society, *www.sauna.fi*

EARTH
Herbalism
College of Phytotherapy, *www.collegeofphytotherapy.com*
National Institute of Medical Herbalists, *www.nimh.org.uk*
Mud
The Dead Sea Research Centre, *www.deadsea-health.org*
Stone Therapy
LaStone Therapy, *www.lastonetherapy.com*

AIR
Climatotherapy
Federation of Climatic Health Resorts of Germany, *www.heilklima.de*
Oxygen and Ozone Therapies
OxygenHealingTherapies.com, *www.oxygenhealingtherapies.com*

HARMONY
Acupuncture
British Acupuncture Council, *www.acupuncture.org.uk*
The British Medical Acupuncture Society, *www.medical-acupuncture.co.uk*
The Alexander Technique
Alexander Technique International, *www.ati-net.com*
Society of Teachers of the Alexander Technique, *www.stat.org.uk*
Colour Therapy
International Association of Colour, *www.iac-colour.co.uk*
Crystal Therapy
Affiliation of Crystal Healing Organizations, *www.crystal-healing.org*
Homeopathy
British Homeopathic Association, *www.trusthomeopathy.org*
The Society of Homeopaths, *www.homeopathy-soh.org*
Labyrinth
The Labyrinth Society, *www.labyrinthsociety.org*
Labyrinthos, *www.labyrinthos.net* (labyrinth resource centre, archive and photo library)
Massage
British Massage Therapy Council, *www.bmtc.co.uk*
The London Centre of Indian Champissage, *www.indianchampissage.com*
Naturopathy
General Council and Register of Naturopaths, *www.naturopathy.org.uk*
Reflexology
Association of Reflexologists, *www.aor.org.uk*
International Institute of Reflexology, *www.reflexology-usa.net*
Reflexology in Europe Network, *www.reflexeurope.org*
Reiki
The Reiki Alliance, *www.reikialliance.org.uk*
Reiki Association, *www.reikiassociation.org.uk*
Shiatsu
The Shiatsu Society (UK), *www.shiatsu.org*
Tai Ji and Qi Gong
Qi: The Journal of Traditional Eastern Health and Medicine, *qi-journal.com*
Taijiquan and Qigong Federation for Europe, *www.tcfe.org*
Yoga
The British Wheel of Yoga, *www.bwy.org.uk*
Yoga Movement, *www.yogamovement.com*
Yoga Research and Education Center, *www.yrec.org*

SPA FEDERATIONS
Day Spa Association, *www.dayspaassociation.com*
European Spa Association, *www.europe-spa.com*
European Spas Association, *www.espa-ehv.com*
International Spa Association (ISPA), *www.experienceispa.com*
The Spa Association, *www.thespaassociation.com*

SPA PUBLICATIONS AND RESOURCES
About Spas, *www.spas.about.com*
Massage Magazine, *www.massagemagazine.com*
Spa Finder Magazine, *www.spafinder.com*
Spa Management Journal, *www.spamanagement.com*
The Spas Research Fellowship, *www.thespas.co.uk*

OTHERS
World Health Organization, *www.who.int*

A listing of the spas featured in Spa Digest, organised in alphabetical order.

Altira Spa at Mardavall Hotel & Spa (Spain) **182**

Amrita Spa at Raffles Hotel Vier Jahreszeiten (Germany) **154**

Amrita Wellness at Le Montreux Palace (Switzerland) **186**

Aquarias at Whatley Manor Hotel (United Kingdom) **200**

Bellevue Spa at Grand Hotel Bellevue (Switzerland) **188**

Better Living Institute at Hotel Royal – Royal Parc Evian (France) **132**

Blue Lagoon Geothermal Spa (Iceland) **166**

Brenner's Spa at Brenner's Park-Hotel & Spa (Germany) **156**

Cala Rossa Spa at Grand Hotel de Cala Rossa (France) **134**

Chewton Glen Spa at Chewton Glen Hotel, Spa & Country Club (United Kingdom) **202**

Daniela Steiner Beauty Spa at Badrutt's Palace Hotel (Switzerland) **190**

Elemis Day-Spa (United Kingdom) **204**

Espace Henri Chenot at Grand Hotel Palace (Italy) **168**

La Ferme de Beauté at Les Fermes de Marie (France) **136**

La Ferme Thermale® Minceur Spa at Les Prés d'Eugénie (France) **138**

GB Spa at Hotel Grande Bretagne (Greece) **162**

Grayshott Hall Health Fitness Retreat (United Kingdom) **206**

Guerlain Beauty Studio & Spa at Le Meridien Moscow Country Club (Russia) **180**

Health & Fitness Centre at Rome Cavalieri Hilton (Italy) **170**

Heubad at Hotel Heubad (Italy) **172**

Liquidrom Therme at the Tempodrom (Germany) **158**

Martinez Givenchy Spa at Hotel Martinez Cannes (France) **140**

Medical Beauty Center at Grand Hotel Palazzo della Fonte (Italy) **174**

Le Mirador Givenchy Spa at Le Mirador Kempinski Lake Geneva (Switzerland) **192**

Naantali Spa at Naantali Spa Hotel & Resort (Finland) **130**

One Spa at Sheraton Grand Hotel & Spa (United Kingdom) **208**

Rogner-Bad Blumau, Hotel & Spa (Austria) **126**

The Saint Gellért Medicinal Bath and Pools at the Danubius Hotel Gellért (Hungary) **164**

Serenity Spa at Las Dunas Beach Hotel & Spa (Spain) **184**

Serenity Spa at Sheraton Voyager Antalya Hotel, Resort & Spa (Turkey) **196**

Spa Cinq Mondes (France) **142**

Le Spa at the Four Seasons Hotel George V (France) **144**

The Spa at the Interalpen-Hotel Tyrol (Austria) **128**

Spa Le Lana at Hotel Le Lana (France) **146**

The Spa at Mandarin Oriental, Mandarin Oriental Hyde Park (United Kingdom) **210**

The Spa at Old Course Hotel, Golf Resort & Spa (United Kingdom) **212**

The Spa at Pennyhill Park (United Kingdom) **214**

The Spa at Renaissance Chancery Court London (United Kingdom) **218**

Sparkling Wellness at Park Hotel Weggis (Switzerland) **194**

SPA SPC at Stoke Park Club (United Kingdom) **220**

Spa Trianon at Trianon Palace Versailles (France) **148**

The Spa at The Westin Turnberry Resort (United Kingdom) **222**

St David's Spa at The St David's Hotel & Spa (United Kingdom) **224**

Thalassa Quiberon at Sofitel Thalassa Quiberon and Sofitel Diététique Quiberon (France) **150**

Thermalife Center at Sheraton Cesme Hotel, Resort & Spa (Turkey) **198**

Les Thermes Marins de Monte-Carlo (Monaco) **176**

Toskana Therme (Germany) **160**

Vilalara at Sofitel Thalassa Vilalara (Portugal) **178**

Villa Marie Spa at Villa Marie Ramatuelle St Tropez (France) **152**

Page numbers in **bold** type refer to entries in
Spa Speak; those in *italic* type refer to an illustration.
Readers should refer to individual spa entries for guid-
ance on treatments and therapies offered by the spas.

acupoints **226**, 86, 96, 100
acupuncture **226**, 100, *100*
　auricular (ear) 100
　auricular points 99
Alexander Technique, the **226**, 89, *89*
alpine warming treatment 50–51
　Kraxen-Stove 40, 50–1, *51*
　Farmer's Steam Bath **226**, 51, *51*
aquatic bodywork **226**, 29–32, *29*
　Healing Dance **227**, 32
　Jahara™ Technique (*see also* Triangular Cervical
　　Support™) **227**, 31, *31*
　Waterbalancing **228**, 30–31, *30*
　WaterDance® (WaTa; WasserTanzen) **228**, 30
　Watsu **228**, 29
aromatherapy **226**, 67, 69–72, *70*
　bath **226**, 72
　massage **226**, 72, *72*
aura **226**, 87, *87*
balneotherapy **226**, 36
basalt stones (*see also* stone therapy) *13*, 67, 81
bath **226**, 11, *11*, 20–22, *20*, *22*, 36
　alternate (contrast hydrotherapy) 21–22
　aromatherapy **226**, 72
　balneotherapy **226**, 36
　Cleopatra Bath *13*
　cold 20–22
　hot **227**, 20, 22
　neutral 21–22
　relaxing bath recipe 21
　seawater 32–33, *32–33*
　seaweed bath recipe 35
　sitz bath **228**, 21
body-mind exercise 101–102
　qi gong **228**, 53, 55, 65, *65*, 101
　tai ji (t'ai chi ch'uan) **228**, 55, 101, *101*
　yoga **228**, 53, 55, 64, *64*, 85, 102, *102*
body wrap **226**
　Dead Sea Mud Wrap **226**, 79
　herbal **227**, 74
　seaweed 35, *35*
　marine muds 80, *81*
breath awareness (breathing) exercise 55, 62–65, *62*
　qi gong (*see under* body-mind exercise)
　meditation **227**, 63, *63*
　visualisation **228**, 63–64
　yoga (*see under* body-mind exercise)
chakras (*see also* colour therapy) **226**, 83, 87, *87*
climatotherapy **226**, 53, 56–57
colour therapy (*see also* chakras) **226**, 91–92, *91*
crystal therapy **226**, 78, *78*
Culpepper, Nicholas 68
dan tian 65, 86
doshas **226**, 14, 85
　kapha **227**, 85
　pitta **227**, 85
　vata **228**, 85
dry heat treatment 45–47
　Bread-bath **226**, 47, *47*
　hot air bath (*laconica*) 11, 42
　sauna **228**, 44–46, *45–47*
　vibratory sauna **228**, 47
elements
　and Chinese philosophy 14–15
　and Greek philosophy 14
　and Indian philosophy 14
enlightenment 102
essential oils **226**, 21, *24*, 26, *26*, 34, 48, 59, 67,
　69–72, *70–72*, 76, 80
facial treatment **226**
　facial steaming recipe 48

facial treatment (cont.)
　oxygen facial **227**, 58–9, *58*
　Avocado and Strawberry Face Mask 76
flotation **226**, 28, *28*
　flotation tank (sensory deprivation tank) **226**, 28
flotation device **226**, 30, *30*
　Styrofoam noodle 31
　Third Arm® *31*
footbath **226**, 26–27, *26*
　alternate 27
　cold 26
　Kneipp water walk 27, *27*
　warm 26
Guérard, Michel 120
healing springs 10–11, 18–19, *18*, 36
　Lourdes, France *18*, 19
　Thermae Bath Spa, England 36
　thermal and mineral water 36–37, *36–37*, 61
　Vichy, France *11*, 36
herbal steam (*see also* alpine warming treatment) **227**,
　50–51
holism 83–86
　Ayurveda **226**, 85, 87
　naturopathy **227**, 84–85
　Traditional Chinese Medicine (TCM) (*see also*
　　phytotherapy) **228**, 86, *86*, 100–101
homeopathy **227**, 88, *88*
hydro-massage 23–25
　affusion shower **226**, 23, *23*
　Scotch hose (jet blitz) **228**, 24
　Swiss shower **228**, 24
　underwater pressure **228**, 24
　jacuzzi (whirlpool) **227**, 25, *25*
hydrotherapy (*see also* bath; footbath; hydro-massage)
　227, 10, 15, 17, 20–32
　Vichy shower (affusion shower; rain shower) **228**, 23
hyperthermia 22
inhalation **227**, 61, *61*, 72
　essential oils **226**, 48, 70–72
　herbal steam **227**, 50–51
　mineral water 61
　oxygen **227**, 58–60, *58–59*
　seawater vapour (marine aerosol) **227**, 61
International Spa Association (ISPA) 10
ions 33, 45, 56–57
Jal Neti nasal douche 61
Kneipp, Sebastian 11, *11*, 15, 20–21, 26, 75
　Kneipp Kurhause 20
labyrinth **227**, 103, *103*
Lentz, Michel 106
massage **227**, 92–97, *93–95*, *97*
　acupressure **226**, 96, *96*
　aromatherapy **226**, 72, *72*
　champissage (head massage) **226**, *94*, 94–95
　deep tissue (deep muscle therapy) **226**, 93–94, *94*
　Hot Stone Massage (Warm Stone Massage) **228**, *13*,
　　15, 81, *81*
　LaStone® Therapy 81, *81*
　lymphatic drainage **227**, 94
　shiatsu **228**, 97, *97*
　shirodhara **228**, 95, *95*
　sports massage **228**, 94, *94*
　Swedish **228**, 93, *93*
　Thai (*nuad bo-ram*) **228**, 97, *97*
　tui na **228**, 96, *96*
medical spa
　balneotherapeutic centre **226**, 11
　climate therapy centre 11
　Kneipp centre 11
　thalassotherapy centre **228**, 11, 32–33, *32–33*,
　　35, 57, 61
　thermal spa 11, 25, 61
Mehta, Nehendra 95
meridians **227**, 86, 96, 100
nadis (*see also* chakras) 87
oxygen bars 59, *59*

oxygen therapy **227**, 58–59
　oxygen breathing therapy **227**, 59
　oxygen facial (*see under* facial treatment)
ozone therapy **227**, 60
　autohaemotherapy 60
　ozone steam bath **227**, 60, *61*
pelotherapy (fangotherapy) **228**, 69, 79–80
　Dead Sea Mud Wrap (*see under* body wrap)
　moor mud bath **227**, 80
　parafango pack **228**, 80
　moor drink 80
　rasul (*see under* wet heat treatment)
phytotherapy **228**, 73–76
　Avocado and Strawberry Face Mask
　　(*see under* facial treatment)
　fruit scrub (*see under* scrub)
　hay bath **227**, 75, *75*
　herbal wrap (*see under* body wrap)
　Papaya and Yogurt Conditioning Mask 76
　Western herbalism **227**, 73
Priessnitz, Vincent 15, 20
reflex points 98, *99*
reflexology **228**, 98–99, *98–99*
reiki **228**, 90, *90*
resort 11, 27
　climate health resort 56–57
scrub
　fruit 76, *76*
　salt (salt glow) **228**, 34, *34*, 43
　Strawberry Herbal Back Cleanse 76
seawater (*see also* thalassotherapy) 32–33, 35, 61
seaweed (*see also* thalassotherapy) 32–33, 35, *35*
sens 97
Seven Pillars of Well-Being 12–13
snow walking 27
spa **228**
　definition of 10
　European experience of 11
spa cuisine programmes **228**
　cuisine minceur 120–123
　La Cuisine Synergique® 106–119
stone therapy **228**, 81, *81*
　Hot Stone Massage (*see under* massage)
　LaStone® Therapy (*see under* massage)
sweat baths **228**, 39–46
　bania **226**, 44
　hammam (Turkish bath) **227**, *40*, 44, *44*
　Roman thermae 11, 42–43
thalassotherapy **228**, 32–35, *32*, 57
　marine aerosol inhalation **227**, 61
　salt scrub (*see under* scrub)
　seawater drink 35
　seaweed body wrap (*see under* body wrap)
　seaweed bath (*see under* bath)
　thalassotherapy centre **228**, 11, 25, 32–33, *32–33*,
　　35, 57, 61
Triangular Cervical Support™ (TCS™) 31
tsubos 97
venniks 44
vihtas (vastas) 45, *46*
vinotherapy **228**, 77
　Caudalie Vinotherapie Spa 77, *77*
vital energy 13, 15, 55, 62, 83, *85*, 86, 101
　ki 83, 90
　prana 55, 83, 87, 102
　qi **228**, 55, 65, 83, 86, 96, 100–101, *101*
water treading (water stepping) **228**, 27
weight loss 47, 74, 106
wet heat treatment 48–49
　facial steaming recipe (*see under* facial treatment)
　rasul **228**, 49, *49*
　steam cabinet **228**, 49
　steam room **228**, 48, *48*
wine (*see also cuisine minceur, under* spa cuisine
　programmes) 77, 120
yin and *yang* **228**, 86

CREDITS

The publisher would like to thank the following for permission to reproduce their material:

Aquarias at Whatley Manor Hotel 7bc (Pete Thorpe), 200tl (Pete Thorpe), 200tr (Pete Thorpe), 200cl (Alistair Hood), 201tr (Pete Thorpe), 201bl (Alistair Hood) **Bar 02 Ltd** 59 **Bath and North East Somerset Council** 43 **Bellevue Spa at Grand Hotel Bellevue** 8–9 **Better Living Institute at Hotel Royal – Royal Parc Evian** 2 (J N Reichel), 6cl (F Subiros), 6bl (J N Reichel), 48 (N Bouchut), 132tl (P Pastor), 132tr (N Bouchut), 132cl (J J Liegeois), 133tl (N Bouchut), 133tr (F Subiros), 133cr (F Subiros), 133bl (J N Reichel) **Blue Lagoon Geothermal Spa** 4–5, 16, 36 **Bridgeman Art Library** 11br *The Baths at Vichy*, from 'Générale Déscription du Bourbonnais' by Nicolas de Nicolay (1517–1583) 1569 (w/c on paper) by French School (16th century) Bibliothèque Mazarine, Paris, France/Archives Charmet; 40 Hammam in Turkey, illustrated plate from *'Moeurs, usages et costumes des Ottomans'* by A Castellan, Paris, c. 1810 (coloured engraving) by French School (19th century), Private Collection/Archives Charmet; 41 *The Tepidarium*, 1853 (oil on canvas) by Théodore Chasseriau (1819–1856) Musée d'Orsay, Paris, France; 55 *Recomposition of Water from Hydrogen and Oxygen: Antoine Laurent de Lavoisier (1743–1794) Experimenting on the Respiration of a Resting Man*, illustration from an educational plate, c. 1860 (colour engraving) (detail of 166602) by French School (19th century), Bibliothèque des Arts Décoratifs, Paris, France/Archives Charmet; 68 Sloane 1975 fol. 44 Representations of Medicinal Plants, illuminated copy of the *Greek Herbal of Pseudo-Apuleius*, c. 1190–1199 (vellum) by English School (12th century) British Library, London, UK; 69 Ms Lat 6966 fol. 154v *Cutting Plants and Preparing Medicine*, from 'L'Antidotaire' by Bernard de Gordon (vellum) by French School, Bibliothèque Nationale, Paris, France/Archives Charmet; 74bl *Dandelion* (colour engraving) by William Kilburn (1745–1818), Private Collection/The Stapleton Collection; 74br *Salviam* from 'A Curious Herbal', 1782 (colour engraving) by Elizabeth Blackwell (fl. 1757–1782), Private Collection/The Stapleton Collection; 84 *The War of the Doctors of the 18th and 19th Centuries*, 1854 (coloured engraving) by French School (19th century), Musée d'Histoire de la Médecine, Paris, France/Archives Charmet; 88br Homeopathic medicine suitcase, 2nd half of 19th century by French School (19th century) Société d'Histoire de la Pharmacie, Paris, France/Archives Charmet **Cala Rossa at Grand Hotel de Cala Rossa** 35cr **Corbis** 19 (Philadelphia Museum of Art), 26, 39 (Images.com), 44 (Hans Georg Roth), 49bl (Bettmann), 58tl, 60 (David Gubernick), 61tr (Hulton-Deutsch Collection), 62 (Robbie Jack), 96tl, 98, 99, 100tl (Rob Lewine) **Daniela Steiner Beauty Spa at Badrutt's Palace Hotel** 80tc **Duncan Baird Publishers, London** 89 (Antonia Deutsch, from *Your Body's Energy*) **Editions Didier Millet** 76tr, 85bc, 96b (Jörg Sundermann), 104–105 (Jörg Sundermann), 106, 120 (Jörg Sundermann) **Elemis Day-Spa** 15tl, 15bl, 72tl, 85tl, 204 (Design Group Syntax) **La Ferme de Beauté at Les Fermes de Marie/Stefano Scata, Erica Lennard, Gilles de Chabaneix, Jean Claude Ligeon, Bertrand Limbour and Philippe Saharoff** 81, 136–137 **La Ferme Thermale® Minceur Spa at Les Prés d'Eugénie** 138tl (Tim Clinch), 138tc (Guy Hervais), 138tr (Tim Clinch), 138cl (Christian Sarramon), 139tl (Tim Clinch), 139br (Christian Sarramon) **Getty Images** 20, 23l (Thomas Barwick), 34 (Thomas Barwick), 37 (Manfred Rutz), 45tr (Ray Massey), 46 (John Pratt), 47br, 52 (Ralf Schultheiss), 53 (Patrick Coughlin), 65 (Chris Cole), 66 (Linnea Lenkus), 67, 70 (Mitch Hrdlicka), 71 (Megumi Miyatake), 72tr (Megumi Miyatake), 73tc (C Squared Studios), 73br (C Squared Studios), 80tr (Chris Sanders), 86 (Kevin Anderson), 90 (Suza Scalora), 94, 100bc **Gunter and Anja Freude** 30 **Haslauer GmbH** 51 **Heubad at Hotel Heubad** 50, 75tr **Hotel Botánico** 25, 72tc **Hutchison Picture Library** 85tr **Images Colour Library** 83 **Irene Vogel/Mario Jahara** 31 **Jeff Saward/Labyrinthos** 103br **Liquidrom Therme at the Tempodrom** 29, 124–125 **Martinez Givenchy Spa at Hotel Martinez Cannes** 1 **Mary Evans Picture Library** 10, 11tl, 11tr, 18tl **Molton Brown Day Spa/Design Group Syntax** 93 **Naantali Spa at Naantali Spa Hotel & Resort** 47tl, 64 **Phototake USA** 54 (Carol Donner), 61tl (Mauritius GmbH) **The Random House Group Limited** 61 (Yoga's Nasal Douche) Extract from *Therapeutic Yoga* by Dr Mosarafi Ali & Jiwan Brar published by Vermilion **Robert Ferre (original drawing)/Vicky Keiser (final graphic)** 103tc **The Robert Harding Picture Library** 78tl, 79, 88tl **Rogner-Bad Blumau, Hotel & Spa** 6tl, 7t, 56, 63, 75br, 95 **The Saint Gellért Medicinal Bath and Pools** 42 **SBBM Ltd** 58tr **Science Photo Library** 87br (Michael Burgess) **Les Sources de Caudalie** 77 **Le Spa at the Four Seasons Hotel George V/David Arraez and Jaime Ardiles-Arce** 144, 145 **The Spa at the Interalpen-Hotel Tyrol** 22, 28, 57 **The Spa at Pennyhill Park** 6tr, 7br, 91, 97tr, 101 **SPA SPC at Stoke Park Club** 24 **Sparkling Wellness at Park Hotel Weggis** 21, 27, 78bl **The Spas Research Fellowship www.thespas.co.uk** 10 **Starwood Spa Collection** 7bl, 12, 13, 14, 15cl, 15br, 17, 32, 38, 45br, 49br, 87tr, 102 **Thalasso Bali at Grand Mirage Resort** 33br, 35cl **Les Thermes Marins de Monte-Carlo** 23tr (Bruno Fabbris), 35br (Jean-Jacques L'Héritier), 80tl (Jean-Jacques L'Héritier), 82 (Gabriel Martinez), 92 (Bruno Fabbris), 97br (Jean-Jacques L'Héritier), 176tl (Joachim Bonnemaison), 176tr (Jean-Jacques L'Héritier), 176cl (Jean-Jacques L'Héritier), 177tl (Ralph Hutchings), 177tr (Antoine Schramm), 177br (Bruno Fabbris) **Vilalara at Sofitel Vilalara Thalassa** 33t **Villa Marie Spa at Villa Marie Ramatuelle St Tropez/Gilles de Chabaneix, Stefano Scata and Serge Alvarez** 152, 153

ACKNOWLEDGMENTS

The publisher would like to thank the following for generously sharing their knowledge, expertise and time:

Alexander Georgeokopoulos, Healing Dance
Prof Angela Schuh, Institute of Medical Balneology and Climatology of University of Munich
Ann Christensen and Sylvie Barbenheim, Amrita Spa at Hotel Vier Jahreszeiten
Beatrice Pinto and Ana Paula Pereira, Vilalara at Sofitel Vilalara Thalassa
David Kompatscher, Hotel Heubad
Deborah Locker, International Spa Association (ISPA)
Emmanuelle Perraud, Fédération Internationale de Thalassothérapie
Izabela Kaczor, Guerlain Beauty Studio & Spa at Le Meridien Moscow Country Club
Jeff Saward, Labyrinthos
Marie Barker, R.G.N., SB Beauty Marketing Ltd and Nora Bode
Mario Jahara, Jahara™ Technique Teacher's Association
Neil Owen and Fiona Humphreys, Thermae Bath Spa
Noella Gabriel and Lucy Toothill, Elemis Day-Spa
Regina Fürmann, Haslauer GmbH
Simon Kelly and Enrida Kelly, Ozone Therapy Equipment UK
Spa Botanica, Sentosa Resort & Spa, Singapore
Tanya Marchese, 02 CLUB Health & Beauty International